Patents eBook Series
"Topics in Anti-Cancer Research"

(Volume 7)

Edited by

Atta-ur-Rahman, *FRS*
Honorary Life Fellow, Kings College, University of Cambridge, Cambridge, UK

&

Khurshid Zaman
Bentham Science Publishers, USA

Topics in Anti-Cancer Research

Volume # 7

Editors: Atta-ur-Rahman, *FRS* and Khurshid Zaman

ISSN (Print): 2468-5860

ISSN (Online): 2213-3585

ISBN (Online): 978-1-68108-627-9

ISBN (Print): 978-1-68108-628-6

©2018, Bentham eBooks imprint.

Published by Bentham Science Publishers – Sharjah, UAE. All Rights Reserved.

General:

1. Any dispute or claim arising out of or in connection with this License Agreement or the Work (including non-contractual disputes or claims) will be governed by and construed in accordance with the laws of the U.A.E. as applied in the Emirate of Dubai. Each party agrees that the courts of the Emirate of Dubai shall have exclusive jurisdiction to settle any dispute or claim arising out of or in connection with this License Agreement or the Work (including non-contractual disputes or claims).

2. Your rights under this License Agreement will automatically terminate without notice and without the need for a court order if at any point you breach any terms of this License Agreement. In no event will any delay or failure by Bentham Science Publishers in enforcing your compliance with this License Agreement constitute a waiver of any of its rights.

3. You acknowledge that you have read this License Agreement, and agree to be bound by its terms and conditions. To the extent that any other terms and conditions presented on any website of Bentham Science Publishers conflict with, or are inconsistent with, the terms and conditions set out in this License Agreement, you acknowledge that the terms and conditions set out in this License Agreement shall prevail.

Bentham Science Publishers Ltd.
Executive Suite Y - 2
PO Box 7917, Saif Zone
Sharjah, U.A.E.
Email: subscriptions@benthamscience.org

**BENTHAM
SCIENCE**

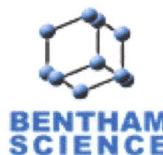

CONTENTS

PREFACE

Topics in Anti-Cancer Research covers important advances in both experimental (pre-clinical) and clinical cancer research in drug development. The book series offers readers an insight into current and future therapeutic approaches for the prevention of different types of cancers, synthesis of new anti-cancer agents, new patented compounds, targets and agents for cancer therapy as well as recent molecular and gene therapy research.

The topics covered in the seventh volume of this series include the role of inflammation in chemotherapy-induced neuromuscular effects, recent advances in nutrigenomics and relevant anti-cancer patents, nanocarriers for on-demand anti-cancer drug release, biochemical mechanisms that control autophagy for treating esophageal cancer, nano-formulations for cancer therapy and nanotaxol.

The comprehensive range of themes covered will be beneficial to clinicians, cancer professionals, immunologists, and R&D experts looking for new anti-cancer targets and patents for the treatment of neoplasms, as well as varied approaches for cancer therapy.

We are obliged to the authors for their contributions and to the reviewers for their comprehensive comments for shaping up the chapters and improving their quality. We extend our thanks to Mr. Mahmood Alam, Mrs. Rafia Rehan and other colleagues for their cooperation in the finalization of this volume.

Atta-ur-Rahman, *FRS*
International Center for Chemical and Biological Sciences
University of Karachi
Karachi 75270
Pakistan

Khurshid Zaman
Honorary Editor
Bentham Science Publishers

INTRODUCTION

Topics in Anti-Cancer Research covers important advances on both experimental (preclinical) and clinical cancer research in drug development. The book series offers readers an insight into current and future therapeutic approaches for the prevention of different types of cancers, synthesizing new anti-cancer agents, new patented compounds, targets and agents for cancer therapy as well as recent molecular and gene therapy research.

The comprehensive range of themes covered in each volume will be beneficial to clinicians, cancer professionals, immunologists, and R&D experts looking for new anti-cancer targets and patents for the treatment of neoplasms, as well as varied approaches for cancer therapy.

The topics covered in the seventh volume of this series include:

- ncRNAs in human cancer
- Taxol to nanotaxol: A journey towards enhanced drug delivery
- Stimuli-responsive nanocarriers for on-demand anti-cancer drug release
- Harnessing biochemical mechanisms that control autophagy for treating esophageal cancer
- Smart nano-formulations for cancer therapy
- The role of inflammation in chemotherapy-induced neuromuscular effects
- Advances in nutrigenomics and relevant anti-cancer patents

List of Contributors

Akyuz, Elvan Yilmaz   Nutrition and Dietetics Department, Health Sciences Faculty, University of Health Sciences, Istanbul, Turkey
Email: elvan.yilmazakyuz@sbu.edu.tr

Ayik, Erdem   Medical School, Department of Pathology, Akdeniz University, Antalya 07070, Turkey
Email: erdemayik@hotmail.com

Aytekin, Ozlem   Nutrition and Dietetics Department, Health Sciences Faculty, University of Health Sciences, Istanbul, Turkey
Email: ozlem.aytekin@sbu.edu.tr

Bayram, Banu   Nutrition and Dietetics Department, Health Sciences Faculty, University of Health Sciences, Istanbul, Turkey
Email: banu.bayram@sbu.edu.tr

Chatterji, Biswa P.   School of Engineering, Ajeenkya DY Patil University, Pune, Maharashtra, 412105, India
Email: biswaprasun@gmail.com

Dash, Aiswarya   School of Engineering, Ajeenkya DY Patil University, Pune, Maharashtra, 412105, India
Email: aiswarya.dash@adypu.edu.in

Elpek, Gulsum O.   Medical School, Department of Pathology, Akdeniz University, Antalya 07070, Turkey
Email: elpek@akdeniz.edu.tr

Feather, Claire E.   Mechanisms of Disease and Translational Research Group, Department of Pathology, School of Medical Sciences, University of New South Wales, Sydney, NSW 2052, Australia
Email: c.feather@unsw.edu.au

Haeri, Azadeh   Department of Pharmaceutics and Nanotechnology, School of Pharmacy, Shahid Beheshti University of Medical Sciences, Tehran, Iran
Email: a_haeri@sbmu.ac.ir

Kaku, Tanvi S.   Department of Biotechnology, St. Xavier's College Autonomous, Mumbai, Maharashtra, 400001, India
Email: tanvikaku@gmail.com

Khan, Maria   Department of Pharmacognosy and Phytochemistry, College of Pharmacy, Taif University, Hawiyah, Taif, Kingdom of Saudi Arabia
Email: 25mariak@gmail.com

Kwok, John B.   Brain & Mind Centre, The University of Sydney, Sydney, NSW 2050, Australia
Email: john.kwok@sydney.edu.au

Lopez-Martinez, Alfonso F.   Centro de Enseñanza Severo Ochoa, Murcia, Spain
Email: alfonsofabio@gmail.com

Mehryab, Fatemeh   Department of Pharmaceutics and Nanotechnology, School of Pharmacy, Shahid Beheshti University of Medical Sciences, Tehran, Iran
Email: f.mehryab@sbmu.ac.ir

Moalem-Taylor, Gila School of Medical Sciences, University of New South Wales, Sydney, NSW 2052, Australia
Email: gila@unsw.edu.au

Moghimi, Hamid R. Department of Pharmaceutics and Nanotechnology, School of Pharmacy, Shahid Beheshti University of Medical Sciences, Tehran, Iran
Email: hrmoghimi@sbmu.ac.ir

Murcia, Laura Department of Genetics and Microbiology, University of Murcia, Murcia, Spain
Email: lauramur@um.es

Navarro-Mendoza, María Isabel Department of Genetics and Microbiology, University of Murcia, Murcia, Spain
Email: mariaisabel.navarro3@um.es

Nicolas, Francisco E. Department of Genetics and Microbiology, University of Murcia, Murcia, Spain
Email: fnicolas@um.es

Pérez-Arques, Carlos Department of Genetics and Microbiology, University of Murcia, Murcia, Turkey
Email: carlos.perez6@um.es

Polly, Patsie Mechanisms of Disease and Translational Research Group, Department of Pathology, School of Medical Sciences, University of New South Wales, Sydney 2052, Australia
Email: patsie.polly@unsw.edu.au

Sultana, Shaheen Department of Pharmaceutics, College of Pharmacy, Taif University, Hawiyah, Taif, Kingdom of Saudi Arabia
Email: shaheen634@yahoo.co.uk

Tutar, Yusuf Nutrition and Dietetics Department, Health Sciences Faculty, University of Health Sciences, Istanbul, Turkey
Email: ytutar@outlook.com

Yusuf, Mohammad Department of Clinical Pharmacy, College of Pharmacy, Taif University, Hawiyah, Taif, Kingdom of Saudi Arabia
Email: yusuf4682@gmail.com

CHAPTER 1

The Role of ncRNAs in Human Cancer and its Related Patents

María I. Navarro-Mendoza[1], Carlos Pérez-Arques[1], Laura Murcia[1], Alfonso F. López-Martínez[2] and Francisco E. Nicolás[1,*]

[1] *Department of Genetics and Microbiology, University of Murcia, Murcia, Spain*

[2] *Centro de Enseñanza Severo Ochoa, Murcia, Spain*

Abstract: The development of the new sequencing technologies has unveiled a new world of regulatory non-coding RNAs (ncRNAs) that is revolutionizing our understanding of the RNA world. New transcripts with non-coding functions are being identified from most of the human genome. Although we have just started to study these ncRNAs, the broad list of regulatory functions assigned to them has assured a prominent role in the regulation of the molecular processes involved in human cancer. This chapter presents a review of the state of the art in the study of ncRNAs and their relationship with human cancer, summarizing the origin, structure and function of the most relevant new classes of ncRNAs. In addition, a selection of recent patents related to ncRNAs and human cancer is included here, analyzing their promising potential in the diagnosis and treatment of human cancer.

Keywords: BARD1, cancer, ceRNAs, HOTAIR, lincRNA, lncRNA, miRNA, ncRNAs, PASR, piRNAs, PROMPT, PTEN, SNORD, sncRNAs, snoRNA, TERRA, tiRNAs, TSS, T-UCR, XIST.

1. INTRODUCTION

The elegant hypothesis of the "RNA world" postulates an ancient first kind of living organisms in which basic functions of life were mostly covered by RNA molecules. Thus, the RNA world hypothesis presents RNA as the most likely compound capable of simultaneously containing genetic information, enzymatic activities and structural properties. It is, therefore, the best compound to imagine a feasible origin of life where the dogma DNA-RNA-Protein is fulfilled entirely by RNA molecules. However, the RNA world hypothesis also confined the ancient

* **Corresponding author Francisco E. Nicolás:** Department of Genetics and Microbiology, University of Murcia, Murcia, Spain; Tel: +34868887136; Fax: 868 88 3963; E-mail: fnicolas@um.es
¶ CPA and MINM contributed equally to this work

Atta-ur-Rahman and Khurshid Zaman (Eds.)

RNA based living organisms as an initial stage of life evolution that shortly was replaced by the current axiom of life-based on the DNA-RNA-Protein scheme, relegating the RNA molecules to a simple intermediate that transfers information from DNA to proteins. This simplistic conception has recently been abandoned since the overwhelming amount of new evidence is positioning RNA as a master regulator controlling most of the molecular processes present in living cells. Hence, the RNA molecules found in living cells are an expanding universe that crossed the limits of protein-coding genes a long time ago. Since the discovery of microRNAs (miRNAs), and powered by the new generation deep sequencing technologies and the ENCODE project, an increasing number of new non-coding RNAs (ncRNAs) are evidencing that our conception of the RNA role in the regulation of cellular processes is not adjusted to the real regulatory capacity of these molecules. Although most of these new ncRNAs have been just discovered and most of their functions are still unknown, their presence in most of the functional genome sequence is manifesting a new RNA world which has assumed predominantly regulatory roles over the majority of molecular processes that confirm a living organism.

The intense structural and functional diversity of ncRNAs define them as a heterogeneous group with a difficult classification. However, among them, there is a subgroup of small RNAs (sRNAs) with constant features that have been deeply studied, these are the sRNAs generated by the RNA interference mechanism (RNAi). RNAi is a negative regulatory mechanism that represses the expression of target RNAs after its activation by the production of double-stranded RNA (dsRNA). It was widely studied in the worm *Caenorhabditis elegans* [1], in plants [2] and fungi [3, 4]. Using mutational studies, the main components of its machinery were identified and characterized [3 - 6]. Thus, an RNA Dependent RNA Polymerase (RDRP) was the first component of the RNAi machinery that was identified [7, 8]. The role of this enzyme is to generate dsRNA from the aberrant RNAs (aRNAs) that are hypothetically produced from the triggering molecules. The crucial role of dsRNA was demonstrated soon after in *C. elegans* in a work that was worthy for the Nobel prize in 2006 [1]. The next gene required in the RNAi pathway codes for a ribonuclease type III known as the Dicer enzyme that slices dsRNA into the small interfering RNAs (siRNAs), a specific type of sRNAs with a fixed size between 19 and 25nt, a 5' phosphate and two nucleotide overhang on the 3' ends [9, 10]. The third enzyme of the RNAi core machinery is the Argonaute protein (Ago) which acts downstream of Dicer, loading siRNAs into the RNA-induced silencing complex (RISC). The RISC uses the guide strand of the siRNA to find complementary mRNA molecules, which are either repressed or directly degraded [3, 11]. This is the canonical RNAi pathway which was firstly described as a host defense mechanism to protect the genome from invasive nucleic acids, such as viruses, transposons and transgenes.

In addition to the canonical pathway and its defensive role, the discovery of other pathways that are endogenously triggered showed that this mechanism is also a regulatory mechanism that controls different cell functions. Hence, the study of the RNAi mechanism has identified an enormous diversity of regulatory functions, such as posttranscriptional regulation of mRNAs, transcriptional regulation and host genome defense [12, 13].

Among all these functions and diversity of RNAi pathways, one of them outstands regarding posttranscriptional gene regulation. It is the microRNA (miRNA) pathway, which has evolved as a fine-tuned regulating mechanism that controls the expression of thousands of different genes in animals. First miRNAs discovered were Lin-4 and Let-7, which are essential regulators for the normal temporal control of diverse postembryonic developmental events in *Caenorhabditis elegans* [14]. This was the starting point that later unveiled thousands of different miRNAs in animals, most of them evolutionarily conserved. Currently, miRNAs are defined as endogenous, single-stranded, short (19-21 nucleotides) RNA molecules that regulate the expression of protein-coding genes [15]. The biogenesis and functional mechanism of miRNAs are similar to other small RNAs, being produced from dsRNA and loaded into a silencing complex in which they act as an RNA guide. Nonetheless, these sRNAs also exhibit many specific features that allow for their own classification. Nowadays, thousands of miRNAs have been identified, and many of them have been experimentally validated. Each miRNA can target hundreds of different mRNAs and each mRNA can be targeted by several different miRNAs. This versatility of miRNAs facilitates the construction of complex regulatory networks that involve an elevated portion of total human genes, becoming key regulators in many complex cellular processes such as development, cell identity, cell cycle and disease [16]. Among these complex processes, human cancer represents a multifactorial disease that is strongly affected by the regulatory potential of miRNAs [17 - 19].

After the revolutionary discovery of miRNAs, the ENCODE project shocked once again our understanding of the RNA world, reporting that 76% of the human genome's noncoding DNA sequences were transcribed and half of the genome might be accessible to transcription factors and other regulatory proteins. Along with this discovery, researchers are reporting the identification of specific ncRNAs from most of the human genome sequences, including intergenic regions, repetitive DNA, introns, promoters and even sense and antisense gene sequences. Unlike the discovery of miRNAs, this current event of firstly identified ncRNA is reporting the characterization of new players with fewer features in common, presenting divergences not only in their biogenesis but also in their structure, size and function. Accordingly, a rising number of new functions associated to these new players are highlighting the functional relevance of ncRNA in the regular development of cellular processes, as well as in the initiation and progress of the human disease. Among all these new RNA regulators, there are ncRNAs that are being identified as significant contributors to the development of human cancer, such as PIWI-interacting RNAs (piRNAs), tRNA derived stress-induced RNAs (tiRNAs), small nucleolar RNAs (snoRNAs), promoter-associated RNAs, large intergenic non-coding RNAs (lincRNAs), Transcribed Ultraconserved Regions (T-UCRs), competing endogenous RNAs (ceRNAs) and other long non-coding RNAs. This chapter focuses on the regulatory functions of ncRNAs and their relationship with human cancer, playing special attention to new developments and associated patents. The most conventional classification of ncRNAs establishes two classes based on sizes that are divided by a threshold of 200 nucleotides (nt): small ncRNAs for those with less than 200nt and long ncRNAs for the remaining ones.

2. SMALL   ncRNAs: miRNAs, piRNAs, tiRNAs, snoRNAs AND paRNAs

2.1. miRNAs

miRNAs were the first regulatory short ncRNAs that were found in animals, and therefore, they have been deeply studied and characterized [14]. They are produced by the RNAi machinery, with special particularities during the early stages of their biogenesis. The main function of these short ncRNAs is the regulation of the target RNAs that share complementary sequence with them by inhibition of translation in animals or direct degradation of targets in plants [7]. Transcription of miRNAs genes generates long, capped and polyadenylated RNAs (pri-miRNAs), which form distinctive hairpin structures [9]. Later, these hairpins are sliced by Drosha (a type of ribonuclease III) in partnership with an RNA-binding protein DGCR8 or Pasha (partner of Drosha), generating 60-70nt stem-loop intermediates (miRNA precursor: pre-miRNA) [15, 20, 21]. These precursors are relocated to the cytoplasm, where they are sliced again by Dicer, another RNase III that generates mature miRNAs (19-24bp). Mature miRNAs are transferred to Argonaute proteins, which are the core of the RISC complex [22]. miRNAs generated by Dicer contains two strands: the functional strand (guide strand) that is transferred to Argonaute proteins and the passenger strand, which was considered not functional, though recent studies suggest that some of them might be also active [23]. Once RISC harbors a functional strand of miRNAs, the complex recognizes complementary sequences in the target mRNAs, usually at the 3′-UTR. The process to represses the expression of the targets can use two different mechanisms: slicing and further degradation of the target mRNA or formation of a stable complex RNA-RISC in which translation is blocked [24, 25]. Nowadays, there are hundreds of human miRNA sequences annotated in the databases [26], with thousands of predicted targets, constructing a regulatory network that encompasses more than 60% of protein-coding genes [27]. Consequently, miRNA can be found regulating most of the essential biological processes of living cells, and therefore, mistakes in their regulatory pathways have been associated with a wide list of diseases [28]. In the case of human cancer, miRNAs have been found deregulated in numerous comparative studies between normal tissues and tumors. Since miRNAs present an enormous regulatory spectrum, they have been found acting both as oncogenes and tumor suppressors. Thus, examples of miRNAs functioning as oncogenes are miR-17-92 cluster, miR-155 and miR-21, which after misregulation provoke a transcriptional activation of their corresponding targets in lung, breast and colon cancers [29]. Inversely, miRNAs miR-15a/16-1, let-7 family and miR-34 family function as tumor suppressors when their targets are repressed [29]. More specific studies have found miR-145 directly involved in the onset and development of colorectal cancer by regulation of MAPK signaling cascade and RNA-RNA crosstalk [30]. Conversely, mir-192 have been found acting as a tumor suppressor thanks to its ability to repress angiogenic pathways in cancer cells by regulation of EGR1 and HOXB9 [31]. Accordingly, with the high number of studies relating miRNAs and cancer, an equivalent of new developments and patents have been published and extensively reviewed [1, 28, 32 - 37]. In this sense, we will review only the most recent advances in the field of miRNAs and their use in cancer therapy (Table **1**). The diagnosis of a specific type of cancer is the field in which most of the miRNA related advances are being developed. Thus, these new developments are mostly based on the identification of a singular profile of miRNAs in a specific type of sample that can be correlated with a particular type of cancer. Among these new advances, different patents presented methodologies to diagnose the most frequent types of malignancies, including breast [38], lung [39, 40], colorectal [41 - 43], gastric [44] and ovarian cancer [45]. In addition, other new advances are presenting methodologies based on the use of miRNAs to treat specific types of cancer. One of them is the work presented by Leedman *et al.*, which proposed a methodology to sensitize cancer cells using miR-7-5pmiRNA. Using this sensitization, and after a DNA alkylating chemotherapeutic agent, the authors claim a significant improvement in the prognosis of melanoma cancers [46]. Another work designed for the treatment of liver cancer presents a combination of miRNA inhibitors (peptide nucleic acid, small interfering RNA, aptamers or antisense RNAs) that act as a repressor of mirRNA-30b, mirRNA-133a and mirRNA-202-5p. This inhibition leads to the repression of cell proliferation through the activation of phosphatase and tensin homolog (PTEN), which were downregulated by hypoxic conditions [47].

2.2. piRNAs

PIWI-interacting RNAs (piRNAs) are small non-coding RNAs produced in the germline cells that inhibit transposons expression in order to maintain genome integrity [48]. They are produced from piRNA precursors that are usually transcribed from intergenic piRNA clusters by a specific mechanism that generates mature piRNAs of 24-30nt in length. The mechanism of action of piRNA-mediated transposon silencing is similar to that of other RNAi pathways in the sense of small RNAs that guide effector complexes to repress target gene transcripts via RNA-RNA base pairing. However, the pathway for the biogenesis of piRNAs presents several differences with the canonical RNAi pathways, such as uniqueness of the specific interaction with PIWI subfamily of Argonaute proteins and Dicer-independence during their generation. Their genomic loci are regions that contain repetitive elements and transcribed transposable elements. Another uniqueness of piRNAs biogenesis is an amplification pathway called "ping-pong", in which the primary piRNAs target their transcripts and induce the recruitment of PIWI proteins to cleave the target transcript and produce secondary piRNAs. The inhibition of transposons and other genetic elements in germline cells during spermatogenesis is accomplished by both epigenetic mechanisms (DNA methylation) and post-transcriptional gene silencing. In consequence of their activity, tumors associated with defects in the normal functioning of piRNAs and piRNA-like transcripts are mainly related to testicular tissues, though have also been linked to other tumor types [49 - 51]. Deregulation of proteins of the piRNAs machinery, such as PIWIL1 and PIWIL2, has been related to several types of tumors and cell cycle arrest [52], anti-apoptotic signaling, and cell proliferation [53]. Due to the limited number of functions associated with these sRNAs, most of the applied advances related to piRNAs are associated with their potential in diagnosing some specific types of cancer (Table 1). A specific application by Zhengdong *et al.* described 197 piRNAs as new biomarkers for diagnosis of bladder carcinoma [54]. However, most applications reporting new uses of piRNAs include these sRNAs in general expression profiles that also describe others ncRNAs as important indicators of cancerous malignancies [55 - 57].

2.3. tiRNAs

Another important class of small ncRNAs is those derived from tRNA, the so-called tRNA-derived stress-induced RNAs (tiRNAs), which are one of the newest members of the ncRNA repertoire. tiRNAs were firstly identified in cells under physiological conditions of stress (human fetus hepatic tissue and human osteosarcoma cells), though they have been found later in other tissues and conditions [16, 58, 59]. These ncRNAs can be generated by a cleavage close to the anticodon position of mature tRNAs, producing two halves (5'-htRNAs and 3'-htRNAs) of 30-40nt length. The enzyme that produces the endonucleolytic cleavage is Angiogenin (ANG), a pancreatic RNase that was previously described for its prominent role in cancer and neurodegenerative disease [60]. Regarding the function of tiRNAs, they have been involved in the inhibition of protein synthesis and the consequent activation of apoptosis [58, 61]. The mechanism of action of tiRNAs during tumor growth and cancer progression is still unknown, though their prominent role in human cancer has been suggested in several studies. For instance, a recent study proposed that tRNA fragments might play important roles in breast and prostate cancer, provoking dissociation of YB-1 from its oncogenic substrates by competitive binding, leading to the destabilization and downregulation of these substrates. Consequently, when these sRNAs are inhibited using anti-sense locked-nucleic acids (LNA)s, *in vitro* cultured cells show an increased cancerous phenotype [16]. Two recent applications propose using tiRNAs for the diagnosis and treatment of human cancer (Table 1). The application presented by Kirino *et al.* proposes a new methodology for the quantification of 5'-htRNAs and 3'-htRNAs in patient samples, which is later used for diagnosis and prognosis [17]. The second application claims to treat and prevent tumors using a pharmaceutical composition based on tiRNAs molecules, which are designed to inhibit protein synthesis and induce apoptosis of cancer cells [18].

2.4. snoRNAs

snoRNA is the only sRNAs found in eukaryotes and in archaea, but not in bacteria (Griffiths-Jones, Nucleic Acids Res, 2005). They are originated from intron sequences of rRNA transcripts, which can generate two groups of snoRNAs based on their secondary structure: C/D-box and H/ACA-box snoRNAs. The C/D-box snoRNAs bind to rRNAs through a typical 10-21bp double helix, and their main function is to promote 2'-O-methylation five bases upstream of the binding site. The H/ACA-box snoRNAs promote base editing (pseudouridylation) after binding to rRNAs sequences (Mattick, Hum Mol Genet, 2005). snoRNAs form complexes with small nucleolar ribonucleoproteins (snoRNPs) and guide them to the target RNAs. These post-transcriptional modifications, methylation and pseudouridylation, facilitate the folding and stability of the target RNAs. Malfunctioning of ribosomes has been previously associated with the transformation of normal cells into tumor cells [62], which correlates with the results of several studies associating defects in the levels of snoRNA to the same alterations provoked by ribosome malfunction [63 - 66]. One of these studies compared 5,473 tumor-normal genome pairs to identify snoRNAs alterations [67], finding that SNORD50A-SNORD50B snoRNA locus was deleted in 10-40% of 12 common types of cancers, and these deletions were associated to reduced survival. Further studies of SNORD50A and SNORD50B RNAs found that they interact with K-Ras, and if this interaction fails, a hyperactivated Ras-ERK1/ERK2 signaling is detected after an overproduction of GTP-bound active K-Ras [67]. In relation to the unbalanced levels of snoRNAs and cancers, most recent patents include snoRNAs in their general methods of cancer diagnosis based on ncRNAs expression profiles (Table **1**) [55, 56, 68] More specifically, Foster and Seedhouse presented an application only devoted to uses of snoRNAs regarding the diagnosis of human cancer. This new development is focused on the snoRNA *HBII-52,* also known as *SNORD115*, which has been found overexpressed in prostate cancer. Thus, the application relates SNORD115 to the diagnosis of prostate cancer, though the disclosure also presents a methodology to identify candidate patients for therapy based on the administration of an effective amount of antagonists against this snoRNA [69].

2.5. Small Promoter Associated RNAs

After the use of new generation technology on massive sequencing for the discovery of new transcripts, one of the first surprises was to find thousands of non-coding RNAs transcribed from promoter regions. These searches revealed the production of several types of RNAs associated with the Transcriptional Start Sites (TSSs) of genes. Some promoter-associated RNAs can be longer than 200nt, however, these long RNAs usually overlap with intergenic regions outside of the promoter, being classified as long intergenic non-coding RNAs (lincRNAs). The different types of promoter-associated RNAs were classified into three groups of ncRNAs: promoter-associated small RNAs (PASRs), TSS-associated RNAs (TSSa-RNAs) and promoter-upstream transcripts (PROMPTs). The main differences between these three classes of promoter-associated RNAs are the position of the promoter where the transcription starts and the size and structure of the mature RNA. PASRs show different sizes, but always present a modified 5'-(capped) end and their transcription starts downstream of TSSs. Their transcription is bidirectional and weak, though they are produced from promoters of highly expressed genes [70, 71]. Similarly, TSSa-RNAs are also weakly produced in both directions from promoters of highly expressed genes. Their unique features are their presence in mouse ES cells and a usual localization between -250 to +50 of TSSs [72]. PROMPTs, however, are produced 0.5 to 2kb upstream of TSSs in a variety of sizes that are never longer than 200bp. They can be easily detected when the RNA exosome is depleted (either naturally or using RNAi) [73]. The transcription origin of promoter-associated RNAs immediately suggests a possible role in the regulation of the same promoter region where they are produced, however, the current lack of evidence is clouding the actual function of these ncRNAs. Nevertheless, their assumed regulatory role and the elevated number of sequences identified in humans (more than 10,000 for TSSa-RNAs and PASRs) indicate a link between diseases and malfunction of these ncRNAs. Accordingly, a recent study found that lack of a HIF-2α promoter PROMPTs downregulates the expression of HIF-2α, affecting the cancerous cell properties associated with colorectal cancer stem cells [74]. Most of the applications associated to the three types of promoters associated RNAs are all restricted to the diagnosis of cancer-based on specific expression profiles of these RNAs in patient samples (Table **1**) [75]. However, due to their regulatory potential, other new developments related to promoter associated ncRNAs described uses for both TSSa-RNAs and PASRs in the regulation of gene expression [76].

2.6. Other Small ncRNAs

Y RNAs are another type of interesting non-conding RNAs (84-113nt) that were found studying autoimmune antibodies against small nuclear RNAs forming ribonucleoprotein in patients with systemic lupus [77]. There are four different Y RNAs (Y1, Y3, Y4 and Y5) transcribed by RNA polymerase III, generating hairpin structures that can interact with Ro60 and La proteins to form Ro-RNP (Ro60 containing ribonucleoprotein complex) [78, 79]. These hairpin structures are similar to pre-miRNAs, and equally can be processed into smaller RNAs (22-36nt), however, their biogenesis does not depend on the silencing machinery [80]. Y RNAs have been mainly involved in DNA replication [81], although misregulation in their production also has been related to cancer [82]. A recent patent based on the detection of circulating Y RNAs proposed them as RNA markers to detect cancerous malignancies [83].

Other interesting small non-coding RNAs are the so-called vault RNAs (vtRNAs), a name assigned to these RNAs since they interact with vault proteins to form vault complexes. These complexes are found associated with nuclear membranes where they may function helping in processes involving transport between cytoplasm and nucleus [84]. Vault RNAs present a size between 86 and 141 nucleotides and are transcribed by polymerase III [85]. The main role of vtRNAs in cancer is a relation with their function helping nucleus-cytoplasm transport since this activity might influence the export of chemotherapeutic drugs out of the nucleus, inducing drug resistance [86]. A recent patent related to vtRNAs found that they can interact with p62, an important factor of cellular autophagy. This invention proposes to modulate the binding of vtRNA to p62 as a novel strategy to influence autophagic flux in cells, which could help in the treatment of diseases associated with reduced autophagy-like cancer [87].

Table 1. Small ncRNAs and Related Patents.

sncRNA	Title	Inventors	Patent Number
miRNAs	Circulating miRNAs as markers for breast cancer	Burwinkel, B., Cuk, K., Zucknick, M., Madhavan, D.C. [38]	US20150197812
	Methods for diagnosing lung cancer using microRNA signatures	Croce, C.M., Calin, G.A., Volina, S.M. [39]	US9051618
	MicroRNA based method for diagnosis of colorectal tumors and of metastasis	Schweiger, M.R., Lehrach, H.M. [41]	US20150247202
	MicroRNA biomarker for the diagnosis of gastric cancer	Too, H., Zhou, L., Zou, R., Yeoh, K.G., So, B.Y., Zhu, F., Yong, W.P.M. [44]	WO2016022076
	MicroRNA biomarkers for ovarian cancer	Lee, A., Shapira, I.M. [45]	WO2015095862
	Cancer therapy using miRNAs	Leedman, P.J., Giles, K.M., Brown, R.A.M.C. [46]	US20150366895
	Pharmaceutical composition comprising microRNA-30B, microRNA-133A, or microRNA-202-5P inhibitor for inhibiting cancer	Lee, Y., Oh, S.Y. [47]	US9295709
	Application of mRNA-6162 as diagnostic marker of lung cancer	Yinghun, H., Yu, W., Pingkun, Z., Teng, M., Qi, W.A. [40]	CN106929599
	Method and system for detecting rectal cancer related microRNA molecular marker by TCGA (the cancer genome atlas) database resources and application of method and system	Rui, C., Na, G., Xiaobo, Li., Qingtao, M., Shenshen, W.M. [42]	CN1066845104
	Compositions and methods used in diagnosing and treating colorectal cancer	Anand, S., Tsikitis, L.C. [43]	WO2018129402
piRNAs	Bladder cancer-related biomarkers and their application piRNA	Zhengdong, Z., Meilin, W., Haiyan, C., Changjun, J., Na, T., Lin, Y.B. [54]	CN103627705
	Gene signatures for cancer prognosis	Stone, S., Gutin, A., Reid, J.G. [55]	WO2015175692
	Gene signatures for renal cancer prognosis	Stone, S., Reid, J., Askeland, E.J., Brown, J.A.G. [56]	WO2015085095
	Compositions and methods of using piRNAs in cancer diagnostics and therapeutics	Zhu, Y.C. [57]	WO2017147594

(Table 1) cont.....

sncRNA	Title	Inventors	Patent Number
tiRNAs	Specific expression of half-tRNA in cancers	Kirino, Y., Honda, S. [17]	WO2015120022
	RNA-induced translational silencing and cellular apoptosis	Anderson, P., Yamasaki, S. [18]	US20110046209
	Gene signatures for cancer prognosis	Stone, S., Gutin, A., Reid, J.G. [55]	WO2015175692
snoRNAs	Gene signatures for renal cancer prognosis	Stone, S., Reid, J., Askeland, E.J., Brown, J.A.G. [56]	WO2015085095
	Methods for diagnosing cancer based on small nucleolar RNA hbii-52	Foster, B., Seedhouse, S.J.M. [69]	US20150354011
	Small RNA molecules and methods of use	Taft, R.J., Simons, C.S. [76]	WO2011120101
	Biomarkers for diagnosis and prognosis of lung cancer	Jiang, F.B. [68]	US20180074059
TSSa-RNAs and PASRs	Small RNA molecules and methods of use	Taft, R.J., Simons, C.S. [76]	WO2011120101
PROMPTs	Cancer diagnostics using non-coding transcripts	Davicioni, E., Erho, N.G., Vergara, C.I.A.C. [75]	WO2013090620
Other snRNAs	Circulating small noncoding RNA markers	Spindler, S., Dhahbi, J.M. [83]	US20160024575
	Modulators of vault RNAs for use in the treatment of diseases	Horos, R., Hentze, M,. Sachse, C. [87]	EP3263704

3. LONG ncRNAs: lincRNAs, T-UCRs, ceRNAs AND OTHER lncRNAs

3.1. lincRNAs

Long intergenic ncRNAs (lincRNAs) are transcript higher than 200nt that are transcribed from the intergenic region, however, beside that premise, they do not share any other feature. LincRNAs are a diverse group of lncRNAs, ranging in sizes from a few hundred to tens of thousands of nucleotides. In humans, more than 3,000 lincRNAs loci have been found thanks to the massive sequencing technologies, though most of them remaining uncharacterized [88]. Some of these lincRNAs present cell-type specific expression and subcellular compartment localization and many of them control the expression of both neighboring genes and distant genomic sequences [89, 90]. The high number of lincRNAs identified and their regulatory functions suggest that they confirm a new regulatory layer which is barely explored and represent a promising field for future discoveries. As expected, the high number of lincRNAs and their regulatory functions shortly led to the discovery of several lincRNAs related to the regulation of genes involved in cancer. For instance, lincRNAs related to the regulation of processes involving the development of cancer are *HOTAIR*, *lincRNA-p21,* and *MALAT-1* [91 - 95]. Chromatin target changes of polycomb proteins have been observed after *HOTAIR* overexpression, which is associated with increased invasiveness and propensity to metastasize in epithelial cancer cells. Oppositely, downregulation of HOTAIR decreases invasiveness, suggesting a strong regulation of cell transformation [91]. Another lincRNA called *LINP1* has also been found overexpressed in cancerous tissues, specifically in human breast cancer. *LINP1* is involved in DNA reparation, serving as a scaffold to link Ku80 and DNA-PKcs in the Nonhomologous End Joining (NHEJ) pathway. Thus, repression of *LINP1* increases the sensitivity of the tumor-cell response to radiotherapy in breast cancer, since target cells are unable to repair the damage associated with the radiation [96]. Overexpression of lincRNAs in tumor cells tissues seems to be a constant in the role of these lncRNAs in cancer. Thus, another lincRNA that has been found overexpressed in tumor cells is *NEAT1*, which helps to the progression of gastric cancers. Similarly to *LIMP1*, repression of *NEAT1* is associated with the suppression of tumorigenic features in gastric cancer cells [97]. Inventions related to lincRNAs proposed treatments based on the downregulation and targeting of known lincRNAs such as *HOTAIR* and *LIVE* (Table **2**). Thus, the potential use of *HOTAIR*-inhibiting small RNAs in the preparation of anti-prostate cancer drugs is exploited using a formula of different siRNAs against the sequence of *HOTAIR*, which is proposed to inhibit cell invasion and migration ability of cancer cells [98]. Regarding LIVE lincRNA, a recent application showed its involvement in the promotion of angiogenesis. This application proposes to arrest tumor growth by inhibition of angiogenesis after silencing of *LIVE* in the affected area [99].

3.2. T-UCRs

Ultraconserved Regions (UCRs) are genomic sequences with 100% identity between orthologous regions of human, mouse, and rat genomes. These sequences are frequently located at fragile sites and other cancer-associated genomic regions. Transcription of UCRs generates noncoding RNAs known as T-UCRs, which can be expressed either ubiquitously or in a tissue-specific pattern [100 - 102]. The misregulation of T-UCRs expression and their role in human cancers depend on two different mechanisms of action: they can serve as direct targets of miRNAs, acting as a decoy for those miRNAs [103] (described in the next section: ceRNAs); or by epigenetic hypermethylation of CpG island promoters [104]. When T-UCRs act as a decoy for miRNAs, they share significant antisense complementarity with the target miRNAs, thus miRNAs form stable complexes with T-UCRs and remain functionally blocked. Hypermethylation of UCR CpG islands has been found in a large number of primary human tumors, revealing that these regions might play a general role regulating different types of cancers, such as hepatocellular carcinoma, prostate cancer, neuroblastoma, colorectal cancer and leukemia [105] (revised in [104]). More specifically, a study focused on bladder cancer found that ultraconserved RNA *uc.8+* was highly expressed in these tissues. When *uc.8+* was downregulated by RNA silencing, cancerous features like cell invasion, migration, and proliferation were reduced. The action mechanism of *uc.8+* is to block the function of miR-596, which results in an increased expression of MMP9 and its consequent improved invasiveness in bladder cancer cells [106]. Similarly, a more recent study found that increased transcription of *uc.339* is upregulated in non-small cancer lung cells results in the repression of *miR-339-3p, -663b-3p,* and *-95-5p.* Consequently, expression of Cyclin E2, a direct target of all these microRNAs is increased, promoting cancer growth and migration [103]. Although T-UCRs are well-known lncRNAs compared to other groups of ncRNAs and despite the numerous links between them and different types of cancer, only a few patents are dedicated to their uses in human cancer. One of these inventions described the uses of thirteen T-UCRs in the diagnosis and treatment of colon cancer [107]. Other general patents include T-UCRs in their claims, though as a part of many other ncRNAs that are used as diagnostic marker of human cancers (Table **2**) [75, 108].

3.3. ceRNAs

Competing endogenous RNAs (ceRNAs) are a heterogeneous group of lncRNAs that act as decoys or molecular sponges with the ability to sequester the active pool of miRNAs, preventing their action on the canonical target mRNAs. The sequence of ceRNAs contains numerous target sequences that are recognized by miRNAs (called miRNA response elements, MRE) in which miRNAs remains blocked. Structurally distant molecules with different biogenesis origins such as circular RNAs (circRNAs), pseudogene transcripts and other lncRNAs are part of the group ceRNAs, sharing all of them the same function: repression of miRNAs. Since miRNAs possess a fundamental role in the development of several types of cancer, ceRNAs also become an important key element regulating the molecular processes involved in this disease. Several studies have dissected the role of specific ceRNAs the regulation of oncogenes and tumor suppressor genes. For instance, the ceRNAs *CNOT6L, VAPA,* and *ZEB2* can act as regulators of *PTEN,* a key tumor suppressor gene that is associated with multiple human cancers, as well as its own non-coding pseudogene *PTENP,* which at the same time also can function as a ceRNAs [109, 110]. Similarly, there are other pseudogenes acting like ceRNAs, such as *BRAFP1* and *KRAS1P,* corresponding to the oncogene BRAF and the proto-oncogene KRAS, respectively [110, 111]. A prominent example of patented applications related to ceRNAs is a recent patent dedicated to a lncRNA called *BARD1 9'L,* which is a ceRNA functioning as a decoy for miRNAs targeting the oncogene *BARD1*. *BARD1 9'L* is transcribed from within an intron of *BARD1* that has its own promoter and possess several MREs in a region similar to the 3′UTR region of *BARD1*. These MREs are targets for microRNAs miR-203 and miR-101, which can repress the expression of *BARD1* and other cancer-associated mRNAs, antagonizing the tumor suppressor effect of these miRNAs. The application proposes *BARD1 9'L* as a new promising treatment target since it has been found abnormally over-expressed in several human cancers [112].

3.4. Other lncRNAs

LincRNAs, T-UCR, and ceRNAs can be classified in specific groups of lncRNAs using criteria such as the origin of transcription, conservation or function, respectively. However, many other single lncRNAs have been found with no common features to be associated with a specific group. One of these lncRNAs is *XIST*, a long RNA of 17kb that is involved in the X chromosome inactivation that occurs in mammals. A high expression level of *XIST* in one the two X chromosomes will determine its silencing by recruitment of the polycomb complex. Conversely, a low expression level of XIST in the other X chromosome-mediated by another lncRNA called *TSIX*, which is the antisense version of *XIST*, will assure the activation of this chromosome [113]. Besides X chromosome inactivation, *XIST* has also been found related to human cancer. Thus, XIST transcript might repress the function of miR-152, helping tumor progression in human glioblastoma [114]. Similarly, overexpression of *XIST* has been associated with BRCA1-like breast cancer, correlating with a poor outcome [115]. Another well-studied lncRNA is the telomeric repeat-containing RNA (*TERRA)*, an RNA transcribed from the ends of the chromosomes, that is involved in the maintenance of the correct length of the telomeric regions by regulating telomerase activity and heterochromatin formation in these regions. In this process, the length of shortened telomeres is increased by homologous recombination with other telomeres, promoted by TERRA DNA-RNA hybrid formed at chromosome ends [116]. Similarly to XIST, alterations in TERRA expression have also been related to cancerous processes. TERRA misregulation might be behind of genome-wide alteration of gene expression in telomere-elongated cancer cells. For instance, up-regulated TERRA and elongated telomeres suppress genes involved in the innate immune system (*STAT1, ISG15, and OAS3*), which counteracts and represses cancer malignancy [117]. Since changes in the expression levels of *XIST* and *TERRA* have been related to human cancers, both of them appear included in patents describing new biomarkers for the diagnosis of different types of cancer (Table **2**) [118, 119]. In addition, recently discovered ncRNAs like SAILOR have been found expressed in aggressive cancer, with an associated application providing methods and compositions for evaluating these new players and their role in the aggressiveness of cancer [120]. Another interesting lncRNA is PANDAR (the promoter of CDKN1A antisense DNA damage-activated RNA), which has been involved in cisplatin resistance in ovarian cancer. Recent studies have found that overexpressed PANDAR correlates with cisplatin resistance, although the exact mechanism for this chemoresistance is still unclear. These studies also found that misregulation of PANDAR might be dependent on p53 and SRFS2 [121].

Table 2. Long ncRNAs and Related Patents.

Long ncRNAs	Title	Inventors	Patent Number
lincRNAs	Applications of targeted HOTAIR-inhibiting small RNA in preparation of anti-prostate cancer drugs	Xiaodong, J., Yi, Z., Rikao, Y., Alin, J., Xiaolin, Y., Jiajie, F.A. [98]	CN201510264863
	Novel lincRNA and interfering nucleic acid molecules, compositions and methods and uses thereof for regulating angiogenesis and related conditions	Marsden, P.A., Das, S., Wang, J.J., Wu, M.Y. [99].	WO2015042720
T-UCRs	Ultraconserved regions encoding ncRNAs	Croce, C.M.U. [107]	EP20130175161
	Thyroid cancer diagnostics	Davicioni, E., Haddad, Z., Wiseman, S.M.T. [108]	WO2014043803
ceRNAs	Novel non-coding RNA, cancer target and compounds for cancer treatment	Irminger-Finger I. [112]	US20160319276
Other lncRNAs	Biomarkers for the identification of chemosensitivity	Birnbaum, D., Charafe-Jauffret, E., Ginestier, C., Salvador, M.B. [118]	US20160040251
	Methods and compositions for identifying undifferentiated stem cells and assessing cell health	Lee, J.T., Zhang, L.M. [119]	US20110008784
	Long non-coding RNA expressed in aggressive cancer	Kohwi-Shigematsu, T., Kohwi, Y., Ordinario, E.C., Balamotis, M.A., Han, H.J. [120]	US20170067125

CURRENT & FUTURE DEVELOPMENTS

The unprecedented number of non-coding RNAs discovered with the new sequencing technologies has revealed that the ancient RNA world present at the beginning of life evolution did not just disappear in benefit of a DNA based living cell. Instead, this ancient RNA world crafted a DNA genome serving as a mold for thousands of RNAs liberated from gene coding duties. Our current understanding of this new RNA world is mostly limited to the observation and detection of these unknown ncRNAs, with a scarce comprehension of both their specific and global functional roles. The variety of sizes, structures and biogenesis mechanisms of these ncRNAs correlates with the broad panel of biological functions in which they might be involved. Consequently, a great effort in the fields of bioinformatics, functional genomics and functional genetics will be required to identify all the functional roles that ncRNAs can play in a living cell. In this sense, the lack of conserved domains or functional motifs will complicate the study of these regulatory molecules. Studies based on the spatial-temporal expression, interaction with other regulatory factors and mutational approaches will be crucial. Regarding the relation between ncRNAs and cancer, their broad regulatory potential involves them in most of the biological functions found in living organisms, which ineluctably connects with the numerous cellular processes that result in cancerous malignancies. The regulatory potential of ncRNAs directly interrelates with the common factor found in all types of cancer: a misregulated genetic pathway that leads to uncontrolled proliferation. In this regard, the key for future developments will depend on the current efforts to identify particular functions of new ncRNAs. The expansion in the knowledge of the ncRNA world will represent a revolution in cancer research, diagnosis and treatment.

CONSENT FOR PUBLICATION

The authors confirm consent for the publication of this chapter.

CONFLICT OF INTEREST

The authors confirm that this chapter content has no conflict of interest.

ACKNOWLEDGEMENTS

This work was supported by "Ministerio de Economía y Competitividad" of Spain government. Department of Science under Contract No. BFU2015-62580-ERC.

DISCLOSURE

"Part of this article has previously been published in Recent Patents on Anti-Cancer Drug Discovery 2017; 12(2): 128-135 as Role of ncRNAs in Development, Diagnosis and Treatment of Human Cancer."

REFERENCES

[1]   Nicolas FE, Lopez-Gomollon S, Lopez-Martinez AF, Dalmay T. Silencing human cancer: identification and uses of microRNAs. Recent Pat Anticancer Drug Discov 2011; 6(1): 94-105.
[http://dx.doi.org/10.2174/157489211793980033] [PMID: 21110826]

[2]   Baulcombe D. RNA silencing in plants. Nature 2004; 431(7006): 356-63.
[http://dx.doi.org/10.1038/nature02874] [PMID: 15372043]

[3]   Fulci V, Macino G. Quelling: Post-transcriptional gene silencing guided by small RNAs in *Neurospora crassa*. Curr Opin Microbiol 2007; 10(2): 199-203.
[http://dx.doi.org/10.1016/j.mib.2007.03.016] [PMID: 17395524]

[4]   Nicolás FE, Ruiz-Vázquez RM. Functional diversity of RNAi-associated sRNAs in fungi. Int J Mol Sci 2013; 14(8): 15348-60.
[http://dx.doi.org/10.3390/ijms140815348] [PMID: 23887655]

[5]   Calo S, Nicolás FE, Lee SC, *et al*. A non-canonical RNA degradation pathway suppresses RNAi-dependent epimutations in the human fungal pathogen *Mucor circinelloides*. PLoS Genet 2017; 13(3): e1006686.
[http://dx.doi.org/10.1371/journal.pgen.1006686] [PMID: 28339467]

[6]   Trieu TA, Calo S, Nicolás FE, *et al*. A non-canonical RNA silencing pathway promotes mRNA degradation in basal fungi. PLoS Genet 2015; 11(4): e1005168.
[http://dx.doi.org/10.1371/journal.pgen.1005168] [PMID: 25875805]

[7]   Bartel DP. MicroRNAs: Genomics, biogenesis, mechanism, and function. Cell 2004; 116(2): 281-97.
[http://dx.doi.org/10.1016/S0092-8674(04)00045-5] [PMID: 14744438]

[8]   Calo S, Nicolás FE, Vila A, Torres-Martínez S, Ruiz-Vázquez RM. Two distinct RNA-dependent RNA polymerases are required for initiation and amplification of RNA silencing in the basal fungus *Mucor circinelloides*. Mol Microbiol 2012; 83(2): 379-94.
[http://dx.doi.org/10.1111/j.1365-2958.2011.07939.x] [PMID: 22141923]

[9]   Basyuk E, Suavet F, Doglio A, Bordonné R, Bertrand E. Human let-7 stem-loop precursors harbor features of RNase III cleavage products. Nucleic Acids Res 2003; 31(22): 6593-7.
[http://dx.doi.org/10.1093/nar/gkg855] [PMID: 14602919]

[10]   de Haro JP, Calo S, Cervantes M, Nicolás FE, Torres-Martínez S, Ruiz-Vázquez RM. A single dicer gene is required for efficient gene silencing associated with two classes of small antisense RNAs in *Mucor circinelloides*. Eukaryot Cell 2009; 8(10): 1486-97.
[http://dx.doi.org/10.1128/EC.00191-09] [PMID: 19666782]

[11]   Cervantes M, Vila A, Nicolás FE, *et al*. A single argonaute gene participates in exogenous and endogenous RNAi and controls cellular functions in the basal fungus *Mucor circinelloides*. PLoS One 2013; 8(7): e69283.
[http://dx.doi.org/10.1371/journal.pone.0069283] [PMID: 23935973]

[12]   Fu Y, Lee H, Collins M, *et al*. Cloning and functional characterization of the *Rhizopus oryzae* high affinity iron permease (rFTR1) gene. FEMS Microbiol Lett 2004; 235(1): 169-76.
[PMID: 15158278]

[13]   Nicolás FE, Vila A, Moxon S, *et al*. The RNAi machinery controls distinct responses to environmental signals in the basal fungus *Mucor circinelloides*. BMC Genomics 2015; 16(1): 237.
[http://dx.doi.org/10.1186/s12864-015-1443-2] [PMID: 25880254]

[14]   Lee RC, Feinbaum RL, Ambros V. The *C. elegans* heterochronic gene lin-4 encodes small RNAs with antisense complementarity to lin-14. Cell 1993; 75(5): 843-54.
[http://dx.doi.org/10.1016/0092-8674(93)90529-Y] [PMID: 8252621]

[15]   Denli AM, Tops BBJ, Plasterk RHA, Ketting RF, Hannon GJ. Processing of primary microRNAs by the microprocessor complex. Nature 2004; 432(7014): 231-5.
[http://dx.doi.org/10.1038/nature03049] [PMID: 15531879]

[16]   Saikia M, Hatzoglou M. The many virtues of tRNA-derived stress-induced RNAs (tiRNAs): Discovering novel mechanisms of stress response and effect on human health. J Biol Chem 2015; 290(50): 29761-8.
[http://dx.doi.org/10.1074/jbc.R115.694661] [PMID: 26463210]

[17]   Kirino Y, Honda S. Specific expression of half-tRNA in cancers. WO2015120022, 2015.

[18]   Anderson P, Yamasaki S. RNA-induced translational silencing and cellular apoptosis. US20110046209, 2011.

[19]   Nicolas FE. Role of ncRNAs in development, diagnosis and treatment of human cancer. Recent Patents Anticancer Drug Discov 2017; 12(2): 128-35.
[http://dx.doi.org/10.2174/1574892812666170105113415] [PMID: 28056753]

[20]   Gregory RI, Yan K-P, Amuthan G, *et al.* The microprocessor complex mediates the genesis of microRNAs. Nature 2004; 432(7014): 235-40.
[http://dx.doi.org/10.1038/nature03120] [PMID: 15531877]

[21]   Lee Y, Ahn C, Han J, *et al.* The nuclear RNase III Drosha initiates microRNA processing. Nature 2003; 425(6956): 415-9.
[http://dx.doi.org/10.1038/nature01957] [PMID: 14508493]

[22]   Zeng Y, Cullen BR. Sequence requirements for micro RNA processing and function in human cells. RNA 2003; 9(1): 112-23.
[http://dx.doi.org/10.1261/rna.2780503] [PMID: 12554881]

[23]   Leuschner PJF, Ameres SL, Kueng S, Martinez J. Cleavage of the siRNA passenger strand during RISC assembly in human cells. EMBO Rep 2006; 7(3): 314-20.
[http://dx.doi.org/10.1038/sj.embor.7400637] [PMID: 16439995]

[24]   Humphreys DT, Westman BJ, Martin DIK, Preiss T. MicroRNAs control translation initiation by inhibiting eukaryotic initiation factor 4E/cap and poly(A) tail function. Proc Natl Acad Sci USA 2005; 102(47): 16961-6.
[http://dx.doi.org/10.1073/pnas.0506482102] [PMID: 16287976]

[25]   Bagga S, Bracht J, Hunter S, *et al.* Regulation by let-7 and lin-4 miRNAs results in target mRNA degradation. Cell 2005; 122(4): 553-63.
[http://dx.doi.org/10.1016/j.cell.2005.07.031] [PMID: 16122423]

[26]   MicroRNA database website. Available at: http://www.mirbase.org/ (Accessed on: December 4 2016).

[27]   Selbach M, Schwanhäusser B, Thierfelder N, Fang Z, Khanin R, Rajewsky N. Widespread changes in protein synthesis induced by microRNAs. Nature 2008; 455(7209): 58-63.
[http://dx.doi.org/10.1038/nature07228] [PMID: 18668040]

[28]   Nicolas FE, Lopez-Martinez AF. MicroRNAs in human diseases. Recent Pat DNA Gene Seq 2010; 4(3): 142-54.
[http://dx.doi.org/10.2174/187221510794751659] [PMID: 21288192]

[29]   Lujambio A, Lowe SW. The microcosmos of cancer. Nature 2012; 482(7385): 347-55.
[http://dx.doi.org/10.1038/nature10888] [PMID: 22337054]

[30]   Mazza T, Mazzoccoli G, Fusilli C, *et al.* Multifaceted enrichment analysis of RNA-RNA crosstalk reveals cooperating micro-societies in human colorectal cancer. Nucleic Acids Res 2016; 44(9): 4025-36.
[http://dx.doi.org/10.1093/nar/gkw245] [PMID: 27067546]

[31]   Wu SY, Rupaimoole R, Shen F, *et al.* A miR-192-EGR1-HOXB9 regulatory network controls the angiogenic switch in cancer. Nat Commun 2016; 7: 11169.
[http://dx.doi.org/10.1038/ncomms11169] [PMID: 27041221]

[32]   Jain CK, Gupta A, Dogra N, Kumar VS, Wadhwa G, Sharma SK. MicroRNA therapeutics: The emerging anticancer strategies. Recent Pat Anticancer Drug Discov 2014; 9(3): 286-96.

[http://dx.doi.org/10.2174/1574892809666140307101519] [PMID: 24605908]

[33] Zhao Q, Li P, Ma J, Yu X. MicroRNAs in lung cancer and lung cancer bone metastases: Biomarkers for early diagnosis and targets for treatment. Recent Pat Anticancer Drug Discov 2015; 10(2): 182-200.
[http://dx.doi.org/10.2174/1574892810666150120163617] [PMID: 25600282]

[34] Zhang W, Zang J, Jing X, *et al.* Identification of candidate miRNA biomarkers from miRNA regulatory network with application to prostate cancer. J Transl Med 2014; 12: 66.
[http://dx.doi.org/10.1186/1479-5876-12-66] [PMID: 24618011]

[35] Yan W, Xu L, Sun Z, *et al.* MicroRNA biomarker identification for pediatric acute myeloid leukemia based on a novel bioinformatics model. Oncotarget 2015; 6(28): 26424-36.
[http://dx.doi.org/10.18632/oncotarget.4459] [PMID: 26317787]

[36] Tang Y, Yan W, Chen J, Luo C, Kaipia A, Shen B. Identification of novel microRNA regulatory pathways associated with heterogeneous prostate cancer. BMC Syst Biol 2013; 7(Suppl. 3):: S6.
[http://dx.doi.org/10.1186/1752-0509-7-S3-S6] [PMID: 24555436]

[37] Shen S, Lin Y, Yuan X, *et al.* Biomarker microRNAs for diagnosis, prognosis and treatment of hepatocellular carcinoma: A functional survey and comparison. Sci Rep 2016; 6: 38311.
[http://dx.doi.org/10.1038/srep38311] [PMID: 27917899]

[38] Burwinkel B, Cuk K, Zucknick M, Madhavan DC. Circulating miRNAs as markers for breast cancer. US20150197812, 2015.

[39] Croce CM, Calin GA, Volina SM. Methods for diagnosing lung cancer using microRNA signatures. US9051618, 2015.

[40] Yinghun H, Yu W, Pingkun Z, Teng M, Qi WA. Application of mRNA-6162 as diagnostic marker of lung cancer. CN106929599, 2017.

[41] Schweiger MR, Lehrach HM. Based method for diagnosis of colorectal tumors and of metastasis. US20150247202, 2015.

[42] Rui C, Na G, Xiaobo Li, Qingtao M, Shenshen WM. Methods and system for detecting rectal cancer related microRNA molecular marker by T (the cancer genome atlas) database resources and application of method and system. CN1066845104, 2017.

[43] Anand S, Tsikitis LC. Compositions and methods used in diagnosing and treating colorectal cancer. WO2018129402, 2018.

[44] Too H, Zhou L, Zou R, *et al.* MicroRNA biomarker for the diagnosis of gastric cancer. WO2016022076, 2016.

[45] Lee A, Shapira IM. MicroRNA biomarkers for ovarian cancer. WO2015095862, 2015.

[46] Leedman PJ, Giles KM, Brown RAMC. Cancer therapy using miRNAs. US20150366895, 2015.

[47] Lee Y, Oh SY. Pharmaceutical composition comprising MicroRNA-30B, MicroRNA-133A or M-20--5P inhibitor for inhibiting cancer. US9295709, 2016.

[48] Yamashiro H, Siomi MC. PIWI-Interacting RNA in *Drosophila*: Biogenesis, transposon regulation, and beyond. Chem Rev 2018; 118(8): 4404-21.
[http://dx.doi.org/10.1021/acs.chemrev.7b00393] [PMID: 29281264]

[49] Lu Y, Li C, Zhang K, *et al.* Identification of piRNAs in Hela cells by massive parallel sequencing. BMB Rep 2010; 43(9): 635-41.
[http://dx.doi.org/10.5483/BMBRep.2010.43.9.635] [PMID: 20846497]

[50] Cichocki F, Lenvik T, Sharma N, Yun G, Anderson SK, Miller JS. Cutting edge: KIR antisense transcripts are processed into a 28-base PIWI-like RNA in human NK cells. J Immunol 2010; 185(4): 2009-12.
[http://dx.doi.org/10.4049/jimmunol.1000855] [PMID: 20631304]

[51]   Yan Z, Hu HY, Jiang X, *et al.* Widespread expression of piRNA-like molecules in somatic tissues. Nucleic Acids Res 2011; 39(15): 6596-607.
[http://dx.doi.org/10.1093/nar/gkr298] [PMID: 21546553]

[52]   Liu X, Sun Y, Guo J, *et al.* Expression of hiwi gene in human gastric cancer was associated with proliferation of cancer cells. Int J Cancer 2006; 118(8): 1922-9.
[http://dx.doi.org/10.1002/ijc.21575] [PMID: 16287078]

[53]   Lee TI, Jenner RG, Boyer LA, *et al.* Control of developmental regulators by Polycomb in human embryonic stem cells. Cell 2006; 125(2): 301-13.
[http://dx.doi.org/10.1016/j.cell.2006.02.043] [PMID: 16630818]

[54]   Zhengdong Z, Meilin W, Haiyan C, Changjun J, Na T, Lin YB. Bladder cancer-related biomarkers and their application piRNA. CN103627705, 2016.

[55]   Stone S, Gutin A, Reid JG. Gene signatures for cancer prognosis. WO2015175692, 2015.

[56]   Stone S, Reid J, Askeland EJ, Brown JAG. Gene signatures for renal cancer prognosis. WO2015085095, 2015.

[57]   Zhu YC. Compositions and methods of using piRNAs in cancer diagnostics and therapeutics. WO2017147594, 2017.

[58]   Fu H, Feng J, Liu Q, *et al.* Stress induces tRNA cleavage by angiogenin in mammalian cells. FEBS Lett 2009; 583(2): 437-42.
[http://dx.doi.org/10.1016/j.febslet.2008.12.043] [PMID: 19114040]

[59]   Yamasaki S, Ivanov P, Hu G-F, Anderson P. Angiogenin cleaves tRNA and promotes stress-induced translational repression. J Cell Biol 2009; 185(1): 35-42.
[http://dx.doi.org/10.1083/jcb.200811106] [PMID: 19332886]

[60]   Etoh T, Shibuta K, Barnard GF, Kitano S, Mori M. Angiogenin expression in human colorectal cancer: The role of focal macrophage infiltration. Clin Cancer Res 2000; 6(9): 3545-51.
[PMID: 10999742]

[61]   Emara MM, Ivanov P, Hickman T, *et al.* Angiogenin-induced tRNA-derived stress-induced RNAs promote stress-induced stress granule assembly. J Biol Chem 2010; 285(14): 10959-68.
[http://dx.doi.org/10.1074/jbc.M109.077560] [PMID: 20129916]

[62]   Badhai J, Fröjmark A-S, J Davey E, Schuster J, Dahl N. Ribosomal protein S19 and S24 insufficiency cause distinct cell cycle defects in Diamond-Blackfan anemia. Biochim Biophys Acta 2009; 1792(10): 1036-42.
[http://dx.doi.org/10.1016/j.bbadis.2009.08.002] [PMID: 19689926]

[63]   Su J, Liao J, Gao L, *et al.* Analysis of small nucleolar RNAs in sputum for lung cancer diagnosis. Oncotarget 2016; 7(5): 5131-42.
[http://dx.doi.org/10.18632/oncotarget.4219] [PMID: 26246471]

[64]   Crea F, Quagliata L, Michael A, *et al.* Integrated analysis of the prostate cancer small-nucleolar transcriptome reveals SNORA55 as a driver of prostate cancer progression. Mol Oncol 2016; 10(5): 693-703.
[http://dx.doi.org/10.1016/j.molonc.2015.12.010] [PMID: 26809501]

[65]   Jha P, Agrawal R, Pathak P, *et al.* Genome-wide small noncoding RNA profiling of pediatric high-grade gliomas reveals deregulation of several miRNAs, identifies downregulation of snoRNA cluster HBII-52 and delineates H3F3A and TP53 mutant-specific miRNAs and snoRNAs. Int J Cancer 2015; 137(10): 2343-53.
[http://dx.doi.org/10.1002/ijc.29610] [PMID: 25994230]

[66]   Youssef OA, Safran SA, Nakamura T, Nix DA, Hotamisligil GS, Bass BL. Potential role for snoRNAs in PKR activation during metabolic stress. Proc Natl Acad Sci USA 2015; 112(16): 5023-8.
[http://dx.doi.org/10.1073/pnas.1424044112] [PMID: 25848059]

[67]   Siprashvili Z, Webster DE, Johnston D, *et al.* The noncoding RNAs SNORD50A and SNORD50B bind K-Ras and are recurrently deleted in human cancer. Nat Genet 2016; 48(1): 53-8.
[http://dx.doi.org/10.1038/ng.3452] [PMID: 26595770]

[68]   Jiang FB. Biomarkers for diagnosis and prognosis of lung cancer. US20180074059, 2018.

[69]   Foster B, Seedhouse SJM. Methods for diagnosing cancer based on small nucleolar RNA hbii-52. US20150354011, 2015.

[70]   Kapranov P, Cheng J, Dike S, *et al.* RNA maps reveal new RNA classes and a possible function for pervasive transcription. Science 2007; 316(5830): 1484-8.
[http://dx.doi.org/10.1126/science.1138341] [PMID: 17510325]

[71]   Fejes-Toth K, Sotirova V, Sachidanandam R, *et al.* Post-transcriptional processing generates a diversity of 5′-modified long and short RNAs. Nature 2009; 457(7232): 1028-32.
[http://dx.doi.org/10.1038/nature07759] [PMID: 19169241]

[72]   Seila AC, Calabrese JM, Levine SS, *et al.* Divergent transcription from active promoters. Science 2008; 322(5909): 1849-51.
[http://dx.doi.org/10.1126/science.1162253] [PMID: 19056940]

[73]   Preker P, Nielsen J, Kammler S, *et al.* RNA exosome depletion reveals transcription upstream of active human promoters. Science 2008; 322(5909): 1851-4.
[http://dx.doi.org/10.1126/science.1164096] [PMID: 19056938]

[74]   Yao J, Li J, Geng P, Li Y, Chen H, Zhu Y. Knockdown of a HIF-2α promoter upstream long noncoding RNA impairs colorectal cancer stem cell properties *in vitro* through HIF-2α downregulation. OncoTargets Ther 2015; 8: 3467-74.
[http://dx.doi.org/10.2147/OTT.S81393] [PMID: 26648739]

[75]   Davicioni E, Erho NG, Vergara CIAC. Cancer diagnostics using non-coding transcripts. WO2013090620, 2013.

[76]   Taft RJ, Simons CS. Small RNA molecules and methods of use. WO2011120101, 2011.

[77]   Lerner MR, Steitz JA. Antibodies to small nuclear RNAs complexed with proteins are produced by patients with systemic lupus erythematosus. Proc Natl Acad Sci USA 1979; 76(11): 5495-9.
[http://dx.doi.org/10.1073/pnas.76.11.5495] [PMID: 316537]

[78]   Wolin SL, Steitz JA. Genes for two small cytoplasmic Ro RNAs are adjacent and appear to be single-copy in the human genome. Cell 1983; 32(3): 735-44.
[http://dx.doi.org/10.1016/0092-8674(83)90059-4] [PMID: 6187471]

[79]   Wolin SL, Steitz JA. The Ro small cytoplasmic ribonucleoproteins: Identification of the antigenic protein and its binding site on the Ro RNAs. Proc Natl Acad Sci USA 1984; 81(7): 1996-2000.
[http://dx.doi.org/10.1073/pnas.81.7.1996] [PMID: 6201849]

[80]   Nicolas FE, Hall AE, Csorba T, Turnbull C, Dalmay T. Biogenesis of Y RNA-derived small RNAs is independent of the microRNA pathway. FEBS Lett 2012; 586(8): 1226-30.
[http://dx.doi.org/10.1016/j.febslet.2012.03.026] [PMID: 22575660]

[81]   Christov CP, Gardiner TJ, Szüts D, Krude T. Functional requirement of noncoding Y RNAs for human chromosomal DNA replication. Mol Cell Biol 2006; 26(18): 6993-7004.
[http://dx.doi.org/10.1128/MCB.01060-06] [PMID: 16943439]

[82]   Christov CP, Trivier E, Krude T. Noncoding human Y RNAs are overexpressed in tumours and required for cell proliferation. Br J Cancer 2008; 98(5): 981-8.
[http://dx.doi.org/10.1038/sj.bjc.6604254] [PMID: 18283318]

[83]   Spindler S, Dhahbi JM. Circulating small noncoding RNA markers. US20160024575, 2016.

[84]   van Zon A, Mossink MH, Houtsmuller AB, *et al.* Vault mobility depends in part on microtubules and vaults can be recruited to the nuclear envelope. Exp Cell Res 2006; 312(3): 245-55.

[PMID: 16310186]

[85]   Kickhoefer VA, Searles RP, Kedersha NL, Garber ME, Johnson DL, Rome LH. Vault ribonucleoprotein particles from rat and bullfrog contain a related small RNA that is transcribed by RNA polymerase III. J Biol Chem 1993; 268(11): 7868-73.
[PMID: 7681830]

[86]   Gopinath SCB, Wadhwa R, Kumar PKR. Expression of noncoding vault RNA in human malignant cells and its importance in mitoxantrone resistance. Mol Cancer Res 2010; 8(11): 1536-46.
[http://dx.doi.org/10.1158/1541-7786.MCR-10-0242] [PMID: 20881010]

[87]   Horos R, Hentze M, Sachse C. Modulators of vault RNAs for use in the treatment of diseases. EP3263704, 2018.

[88]   Khalil AM, Guttman M, Huarte M, *et al.* Many human large intergenic noncoding RNAs associate with chromatin-modifying complexes and affect gene expression. Proc Natl Acad Sci USA 2009; 106(28): 11667-72.
[http://dx.doi.org/10.1073/pnas.0904715106] [PMID: 19571010]

[89]   Huarte M, Guttman M, Feldser D, *et al.* A large intergenic noncoding RNA induced by p53 mediates global gene repression in the p53 response. Cell 2010; 142(3): 409-19.
[http://dx.doi.org/10.1016/j.cell.2010.06.040] [PMID: 20673990]

[90]   Guttman M, Donaghey J, Carey BW, *et al.* lincRNAs act in the circuitry controlling pluripotency and differentiation. Nature 2011; 477(7364): 295-300.
[http://dx.doi.org/10.1038/nature10398] [PMID: 21874018]

[91]   Gupta RA, Shah N, Wang KC, *et al.* Long non-coding RNA HOTAIR reprograms chromatin state to promote cancer metastasis. Nature 2010; 464(7291): 1071-6.
[http://dx.doi.org/10.1038/nature08975] [PMID: 20393566]

[92]   Penny GD, Kay GF, Sheardown SA, Rastan S, Brockdorff N. Requirement for Xist in X chromosome inactivation. Nature 1996; 379(6561): 131-7.
[http://dx.doi.org/10.1038/379131a0] [PMID: 8538762]

[93]   Yoon J-H, Abdelmohsen K, Srikantan S, *et al.* LincRNA-p21 suppresses target mRNA translation. Mol Cell 2012; 47(4): 648-55.
[http://dx.doi.org/10.1016/j.molcel.2012.06.027] [PMID: 22841487]

[94]   Ren D, Li H, Li R, *et al.* Novel insight into MALAT-1 in cancer: Therapeutic targets and clinical applications. Oncol Lett 2016; 11(3): 1621-30.
[http://dx.doi.org/10.3892/ol.2016.4138] [PMID: 26998053]

[95]   Huarte M, Rinn JL. Large non-coding RNAs: Missing links in cancer? Hum Mol Genet 2010; 19(R2): R152-61.
[http://dx.doi.org/10.1093/hmg/ddq353] [PMID: 20729297]

[96]   Zhang Y, He Q, Hu Z, *et al.* Long noncoding RNA LINP1 regulates repair of DNA double-strand breaks in triple-negative breast cancer. Nat Struct Mol Biol 2016; 23(6): 522-30.
[http://dx.doi.org/10.1038/nsmb.3211] [PMID: 27111890]

[97]   Fu J-W, Kong Y, Sun X. Long noncoding RNA NEAT1 is an unfavorable prognostic factor and regulates migration and invasion in gastric cancer. J Cancer Res Clin Oncol 2016; 142(7): 1571-9.
[http://dx.doi.org/10.1007/s00432-016-2152-1] [PMID: 27095450]

[98]   Xiaodong J, Yi Z, Rikao Y, Alin J, Xiaolin Y, Jiajie FA. Applications of targeted H small R in preparation of anti-prostate cancer drugs. CN201510264863, 2015.

[99]   Marsden PA, Das S, Wang JJ, Wu MY. Novel lincRNA and interfering nucleic acid molecules compositions and methods and uses thereof for regulating angiogenesis and related conditions. WO2015042720, 2015.

[100] Esteller M. Non-coding RNAs in human disease. Nat Rev Genet 2011; 12(12): 861-74.

[http://dx.doi.org/10.1038/nrg3074] [PMID: 22094949]

[101]   Bejerano G, Pheasant M, Makunin I, *et al.* Ultraconserved elements in the human genome. Science 2004; 304(5675): 1321-5.
[http://dx.doi.org/10.1126/science.1098119] [PMID: 15131266]

[102]   Calin GA, Liu CG, Ferracin M, *et al.* Ultraconserved regions encoding ncRNAs are altered in human leukemias and carcinomas. Cancer Cell 2007; 12(3): 215-29.
[http://dx.doi.org/10.1016/j.ccr.2007.07.027] [PMID: 17785203]

[103]   Vannini I, Wise PM, Challagundla KB, *et al.* Transcribed ultraconserved region 339 promotes carcinogenesis by modulating tumor suppressor microRNAs. Nat Commun 2017; 8(1): 1801.
[http://dx.doi.org/10.1038/s41467-017-01562-9] [PMID: 29180617]

[104]   Peng JC, Shen J, Ran ZH. Transcribed ultraconserved region in human cancers. RNA Biol 2013; 10(12): 1771-7.
[http://dx.doi.org/10.4161/rna.26995] [PMID: 24384562]

[105]   Lujambio A, Portela A, Liz J, *et al.* CpG island hypermethylation-associated silencing of non-coding RNAs transcribed from ultraconserved regions in human cancer. Oncogene 2010; 29(48): 6390-401.
[http://dx.doi.org/10.1038/onc.2010.361] [PMID: 20802525]

[106]   Olivieri M, Ferro M, Terreri S, *et al.* Long non-coding RNA containing ultraconserved genomic region 8 promotes bladder cancer tumorigenesis. Oncotarget 2016; 7(15): 20636-54.
[http://dx.doi.org/10.18632/oncotarget.7833] [PMID: 26943042]

[107]   Croce CMU. Ultraconserved regions encoding ncRNAs. EP20130175161, 2013.

[108]   Davicioni E, Haddad Z, Wiseman SMT. Thyroid cancer diagnostics. WO2014043803, 2014.

[109]   Karreth FA, Tay Y, Perna D, *et al. In vivo* identification of tumor- suppressive PTEN ceRNAs in an oncogenic BRAF-induced mouse model of melanoma. Cell 2011; 147(2): 382-95.
[http://dx.doi.org/10.1016/j.cell.2011.09.032] [PMID: 22000016]

[110]   Poliseno L, Salmena L, Zhang J, Carver B, Haveman WJ, Pandolfi PP. A coding-independent function of gene and pseudogene mRNAs regulates tumour biology. Nature 2010; 465(7301): 1033-8.
[http://dx.doi.org/10.1038/nature09144] [PMID: 20577206]

[111]   Karreth FA, Reschke M, Ruocco A, *et al.* The BRAF pseudogene functions as a competitive endogenous RNA and induces lymphoma *in vivo*. Cell 2015; 161(2): 319-32.
[http://dx.doi.org/10.1016/j.cell.2015.02.043] [PMID: 25843629]

[112]   Irminger-Finger I. Novel non-coding RNA cancer target and compounds for cancer treatment. US20160319276, 2016.

[113]   Navarro P, Page DR, Avner P, Rougeulle C. Tsix-mediated epigenetic switch of a CTCF-flanked region of the Xist promoter determines the Xist transcription program. Genes Dev 2006; 20(20): 2787-92.
[http://dx.doi.org/10.1101/gad.389006] [PMID: 17043308]

[114]   Yao Y, Ma J, Xue Y, *et al.* Knockdown of long non-coding RNA XIST exerts tumor-suppressive functions in human glioblastoma stem cells by up-regulating miR-152. Cancer Lett 2015; 359(1): 75-86.
[http://dx.doi.org/10.1016/j.canlet.2014.12.051] [PMID: 25578780]

[115]   Schouten PC, Vollebergh MA, Opdam M, *et al.* High XIST and low 53BP1 expression predict poor outcome after high-dose alkylating chemotherapy in patients with a BRCA1-like breast cancer. Mol Cancer Ther 2016; 15(1): 190-8.
[http://dx.doi.org/10.1158/1535-7163.MCT-15-0470] [PMID: 26637364]

[116]   Cusanelli E, Chartrand P. Telomeric repeat-containing RNA TERRA: A noncoding RNA connecting telomere biology to genome integrity. Front Genet 2015; 6: 143.
[http://dx.doi.org/10.3389/fgene.2015.00143] [PMID: 25926849]

[117]   Hirashima K, Seimiya H. Telomeric repeat-containing RNA/G-quadruplex-forming sequences cause genome-wide alteration of gene expression in human cancer cells *in vivo*. Nucleic Acids Res 2015; 43(4): 2022-32.
[http://dx.doi.org/10.1093/nar/gkv063] [PMID: 25653161]

[118]   Birnbaum D, Charafe-Jauffret E, Ginestier C, Salvador MB. Biomarkers for the identification of chemosensitivity. US20160040251, 2016.

[119]   Lee JT, Zhang LM. Methods and compositions for identifying undifferentiated stem cells and assessing cell health. US20110008784, 2011.

[120]   Kohwi-Shigematsu T, Kohwi Y, Ordinario EC, Balamotis MA, Han H-J. Long non-coding RNA expressed in aggressive cancer. US20170067125, 2017.

[121]   Wang H, Liu M, Fang L, *et al.* The cisplatin-induced lncRNA PANDAR dictates the chemoresistance of ovarian cancer via regulating SFRS2-mediated p53 phosphorylation. Cell Death Dis 2018; 9(11): 1103.
[http://dx.doi.org/10.1038/s41419-018-1148-y] [PMID: 30375398]

CHAPTER 2

Taxol To Nanotaxol: A Journey Towards Enhanced Drug Delivery

Tanvi Kaku[1], **Aiswarya Dash**[2] and **Biswa P. Chatterji**[2,*]

[1] *Post Graduate Department of Biotechnology, St. Xavier's College Autonomous Mumbai, Maharashtra 400001, India*

[2] *School of Engineering, Ajeenkya DY Patil University, Pune, Maharashtra 412105, India*

Abstract: Drug delivery in the field of cancer has undergone a continuous revolution over the past few decades. Development of novel chemotherapeutic agents without the method of delivering them to the tumor site would find no practical application in uprooting the fatal disease of uncontrolled cell proliferation, cancer. This makes the development of drug carriers exceedingly essential for diagnostics and therapy alike. Nanotechnological science has gained impetus in the recent past and has found applications in a plethora of fields. It has managed to create an impact in the field of diagnostics, drug delivery and therapy, equally. Taxol®, a chemotherapeutic agent that was initially obtained from the bark of *Taxus brevifolia*, moved on to the semi-synthetic approach for its synthesis to address the shortage of its natural source. This drug is partially soluble in water and its initial formulation with Cremophor EL manifested as anaphylactic reactions. To do away with these problems and others such as lower circulation time in blood and non-specificity, nanotechnology is now being looked at as a promising solution. Nanotechnological carriers aim at enhancing target-specificity by functionalization, drug stabilization and preventing its degradation due to physiological conditions, pH, enzymes, etc., demonstrating an Enhanced Permeability and Retention (EPR) effect, prolonged blood circulation and thus better anti-tumor activity, while the side effects being almost negligible. The patents in this chapter aim to highlight how nanotechnology can find practical applications and how one or more than one drugs could be administered *in vivo* in a sustained fashion. The step-wise development in using this potent anticancer drug (Taxol) involved the use of human serum albumin associated compositions (Abraxane®), cremophor-free formulations (Capxol™, Genexol-PM™), numerous oil-in-water emulsions, liposomes and micelles, use of graphene quantum dots (GQDs) for bioimaging and drug delivery and the use of single-walled and multi-walled carbon nanotubes. It also allows the readers to explore nanodevices that can be turned on and off as and when the need be for localized drug delivery. Enabling the nanocarriers to modulate the pharmacokinetic and pharmacodynamic properties of the drug is another notable feature that some of these nanocarriers possess.

---

* **Corresponding author Biswa P. Chatterji:** School of Engineering, Ajeenkya DY Patil University, Pune, Maharashtra 412105, India; Tel: +91-8686868686; E-mail: biswaprasun@gmail.com

Atta-ur-Rahman and Khurshid Zaman (Eds.)

Keywords: Abraxane®, anti-angiogenic, cancer, carbon nanoparticles, Cremophor-free, devices, drug delivery, emulsions, increased tumor specificity, liposomes, micelles, nanocarriers, paclitaxel, prolonged circulation time, protein associated, reduced hypersensitivity, surface-functionalized, Taxol®, *Taxus brevifolia*, tubulin stabilizing.

1. INTRODUCTION

A normal cell, when developing a neoplastic behaviour, adopts the 6 hallmarks of cancer, turns tumorigenic and may exhibit malignancy. Withstanding cell death signals while sustaining the proliferative ones, eluding growth suppressors, induction of the process of angiogenesis, actuating invasion and promoting metastasis and thus enabling the cells to attain immortal replication ability are the six prominent hallmarks of cancer that the cells adopt [1]. In the developed and the developing countries, cancer is the first and the second leading cause of death, respectively [2]. According to the GLOBOCAN project which is an initiative by The International Agency for Research on Cancer (IARC), the world witnessed 12.7 million cancer cases in the year 2008 [2], while the numbers increased to 14.1 million in the year 2012 [3]. The number of deaths resulting from succumbing to cancer also saw a rise from 7.6 million in the year 2008 [2] to 8.2 million in 2012 [3]. This alarming rate of falling prey to the disease crops up from the present-day sedentary lifestyle, imitation of food and diet fads from the western world and increased tendencies of smoking and alcoholism [2, 4 - 6]. The current modes of treatment available to combat cancer include surgery, employing chemotherapy and radiation therapy in combination or individually, depending on the severity, the type and the stage of cancer [7]. The 1960's witnessed the approval of chemotherapeutic agents like vincristine and vinblastine that were derived from natural sources [8]. The forage for more natural alternatives heightened between the period from 1960-1981, when a collaborative plant screening program was initiated by the National Cancer Institute (NCI) and the U.S. Department of Agriculture (USDA). This program was successful in the collection of about 1,15,000 extracts from 15,000 plant species and their testing which resulted in the identification of a few natural sources for the isolation of molecules that possess potent anticancer activities [9].

Samples from *Taxus brevifolia*, the Pacific yew tree were analyzed by Arthur Barclay, a botanist as USDA. The fruit, needle, twig and bark extracts were tested for their anticancer activity and only the bark extract showed significant cytotoxicity [9, 10]. The bark samples of *Taxus brevifolia* were received in 1964 by two scientists, Mansukh Wani and Monroe Wall, working at the Research Triangle Institute [9, 10]. The bark extract showed potent cytotoxicity against human nasopharynx cancer cell line, 9KB and mouse leukemia cells (*in vitro* cytotoxicity assessment models), while it did not show promising results *in vivo*

[11 - 13]. Following this, attempts to obtain Taxol in its pure crystalline form, begun. In 1966, the active ingredient, that was responsible for the cytotoxic activity, was isolated in its crystalline form. It was named as Taxol in the year 1967 [9, 10], after its source of origin and the presence of hydroxyl groups [9]. Determination of the structure of Taxol required its purified form to be available in large quantities. This was, however, not the case. Twelve kg of stem bark that was air dried could produce only 0.5g of Taxol, the yield being as low as 0.004% [12]. It was also estimated that around 1g of active Taxol could be obtained from three 100-year-old, mature *Taxus brevifolia* trees [11]. With the betterment of the procedures for isolation and purification, the structure of Taxol was elucidated in the year 1971 and reported to be the first compound with a taxane ring possessing antileukemic properties and those capable of tumor inhibition [12, 14]. Although a potential candidate for a chemotherapeutic drug, certain drawbacks of Taxol caused researchers to lose interest in the molecule. Water insolubility of the molecule meant elimination at the formulation stage due to the difficulty in drug delivery [10, 11]. Polyethoxylated castor oil was thus employed for its formulation which leads to various anaphylactic reactions. This was another major cause why the development of Taxol as a chemotherapeutic was looked down at [9]. The inability of total chemical synthesis owing to its complicated structure, complex multistep synthesis procedure, as well as low yields and scarce availability of natural resources for its extraction, further discouraged the drug from reaching advanced development stages [9 - 13, 15]. Also, a low degree of cytotoxicity was identified in P-388 and L-1210 cells and this further dampened the interests [12, 13]. For about a decade, the investigations in this field were at a standstill.

The excellent cytotoxic activity of Taxol against murine B16 melanoma (relatively resistant) and xenografts of human tumors introduced into nude mice when brought to light, furthered its development and it advanced from the preclinical stage to the animal toxicology study stage [10, 12, 13]. Its unique mode of action enthralled the researchers and they were motivated to work towards developing this molecule into a promising chemotherapeutic drug. Taxol promotes the process of microtubule assembly by stabilizing tubulin, thus inhibiting cell division, by preventing the disassembly of the microtubules [9 - 11, 15 - 17]. It does so by causing a shift in the equilibrium towards microtubule assembly by the elimination of the lag period that precedes the process [15, 18]. Taxol interacts with β-tubulin at a specific site (a binding pocket) constituting of β-strands and α-helices [11, 19, 20]. The cells are seen to be arrested in the G2/M phase of the cell cycle, post binding of Taxol to the binding site, not enabling the mitotic spindle to de-construct [11, 15, 18, 20]. Reports on activities of Taxol other than that on microtubules highlight its ability to alter cellular signalling cascades by activation of molecules like Raf-1, nitric oxide synthase and kinases including the tyrosine kinases, c-Jun NH_2 terminal kinase and mitogen-activated protein kinases [21 - 26]. The expression of proteins that are central to apoptosis like the Bcl-2, Bad, Bcl-xL is also regulated by taxol which leads to apoptosis by both caspase-dependent and independent pathways [16, 27 - 33]. Taxol has also been reported to possess anti-angiogenic properties, thereby reducing the chances of survival of neoplastic cells [16, 34 - 36].

Since the total chemical synthesis of this drug would prove to be a herculean task, a semi-synthetic approach was adopted. Needles of *Taxus baccata* were found to be rich in a precursor of taxol, 10-deacetlybaccatin III. These were seen as a potential constant source for the availability of the molecule [10, 11]. Use of endophytic fungi and plant cell suspension culture has also been looked at [8, 11, 37]. Currently, the clinical supply of taxol can be owed to its nursery cultivation and semi-synthetic approach of production [8]. After passing successfully through the Phase II and Phase III clinical trials, Taxol was finally approved by the Food and Drug Administration (FDA) for treatment of ovarian cancer on the 29th December, 1992 [8, 10, 12]. Ever since, Taxol® has found applications in the treatment of numerous cancers and achieved the status of a blockbuster drug [8]. In addition to the use of Taxol® for the treatment of metastatic ovarian, breast and non-small cell lung cancers [8, 9], [11, 15, 37], it also shows activity against cancers of the squamous epithelium such as prostate, gastroesophageal tract, head and neck, endometrium, cervix and the bladder [8, 9, 15]. The drug has also found success in the treatment of AIDS-related Kaposi's sarcoma, restenosis, leukemia, lymphoma, malignant brain tumors, psoriasis and rheumatoid arthritis [8, 9, 11, 15, 37]. Of late, it is being explored for activity against tauopathies including frontotemporal dementia, Alzheimer's disease and Parkinsonism [8, 37]. Although Taxol® has shown great effects in treating numerous disorders, certain drawbacks have restricted its scope. One of the major setbacks is that the drug shows poor solubility in water. This necessitates the use of solvents like Cremophor EL® and ethanol in a 50:50 ratio, that enhance its hydrophilicity and drug delivery [38, 39]. CrEL has been proposed to lead to type I hypersensitivity reactions which are attributed to the release of di(-ethylhexyl)phthalate leaching from standard tubing used for delivering the drug via intravenous routes [11, 15, 38 - 42]. Its infusion causes activation of the complement pathway (alternative and classical pathways can both be involved) by histamine release [11, 15, 40, 43]. The induced hypersensitivity reaction manifests itself in the form of symptoms including hypotension, chest pain, fever, rigors, dyspnea with bronchospasm, abdominal pain, urticaria, pain in the extremities, wheezing, diaphoresis, erythematous rash, flushing and angioedema [11, 15, 40, 43, 44]. Other adverse reactions reported due to Taxol® delivery include neurotoxicity, nephrotoxicity and hepatotoxicity, cardiotoxicity, sinus bradycardia, bigeminy, trigeminy, ventricular arrhythmias, cardiac ischemia, atrioventricular conduction block, mucositis, sensory neuropathy, erythrocyte aggregation, hematologic toxicity mainly neutropenia and leukopenia, myalgias, alopecia, injection site erythema, infections like sepsis, pneumonia, peritonitis, upper respiratory tract infections and urinary tract infections, diarrhoea, fatigue, hyperlipidemia, abnormal patterns of lipoprotein, P-glycoprotein activity being reversed, nausea, vomiting, headache, alterations in taste [11, 15, 38 - 40, 44, 45].

To circumvent the aforementioned problems associated with the vehicle used for drug administration, nanotechnology is being looked at as a propitious, viable solution. While Taxol had hit the markets due to its versatile activity against numerous solid tumors and others, its drawbacks fostered the development of Abraxane®, an albumin-bound form of paclitaxel (generic form of Taxol®), that was approved by the US FDA in January 2005 [46 - 48]. Abraxane® uses human serum albumin, thus reducing hypersensitivity reactions [46, 49, 50]. Infusion of higher doses of the drug with reduced infusion time and volume and improved activity due to the Enhanced Permeability and Retention (EPR) effect in tumors [11, 39, 48, 49] are a few positive aspects of Abraxane® that have helped it gain popularity. A plethora of other nano-carriers have been worked upon and a few have managed to reach the clinical trials to find applications in cancer diagnostics and therapy. For a nano-carrier to be an ideal one, it must inherit the following properties: (i) stabilization of the drug without affecting its pharmacological activity, (ii) preventing the drug from degradation before it can reach its target site, (iii) drug release at the intended tumor site, (iv) decrease the toxicity profile of the drug which helps prevent hypersensitivity reactions [51]. The nanocarriers currently gaining impetus include biodegradable polymeric nanospheres [38], molecular hydrogels [52], liposomes, gold nanoparticles, carbon nanoparticles [39, 40, 51], nanocapsules and microspheres [40]. The advantages that these nanoparticles confer are inclusive of enhanced solubility in aqueous medium, small size and thus increased EPR effect, reduced side-effects, higher Maximum Tolerated Doses (MTD), increased activity and tumor suppression owing to an increased half-life, the possibility of functionalization that enhances specificity [48].

1.1. Methods for Preparation of Paclitaxel Nanoparticles

1.1.1. CN1463969A

The patent describes a method for the synthesis of paclitaxel nanoparticles. 1-10% paclitaxel solution is made in ethanol. A 0.05-5% solution of Tween-80, a surfactant, made in purified water which is 5-500 times that of the mother liquor is then added dropwise into this ethanolic paclitaxel solution while constantly stirring and exposure to ultrasonic vibrations, thus forming the nano-paclitaxel suspension. To obtain the formulation in the form of a nano-powder, it can be subjected to vacuum drying or freeze drying. The average size of the particles thus obtained was 202nm and to increase its bioavailability and target specificity, the nanoparticle can be subjected to surface modifications [53].

1.1.2. CN101829061A

The patent explains the formation of a paclitaxel nanoparticle, ranging from 50-1000nm, formed when a surface stabilizer material binds to paclitaxel without reacting with it. This surface stabilizer may either be nonionic, cationic, anionic or zwitterionic. Along with these, the addition of pharmaceutically acceptable excipients, adjuvants, carriers, anti-freezing agents, fillers, tonicity adjusting agents in combinations or singly to about 30-90% Taxol® is required. Different methods for synthesizing the said nanoparticles have been described. These include the wet grinding method, the high-pressure homogenization method, the emulsification and the microemulsion methods [54].

To reduce the hypersensitivity reactions associated with the cremophor-based formulation of Taxol and to attain increased specificity, protein conjugated Taxol nanoparticles have been developed. Prolonged circulation time in the blood has been achieved by the use of liposomes, micelles and emulsion. Use of carbon-based nanoparticles functionalized with polymers is an upcoming trend in the nanoparticle-based delivery of the drug. GQDs have been shown to find applications in bioimaging and SWCNTs and MWCNTs have been used effectively for delivering Taxol. Conjugation with antibodies has shown to increase tumor-specificity and surface functionalization enhances the circulation time, thereby benefitting the formulation. The three main categories, namely protein conjugated nanoparticles, liposomes and carbon based nanoparticles have been described in Fig. (**1**) [55 - 58].

1.2. Human Serum Albumin (HSA) Associated and Other Protein Associated and Functionalized Taxol® or Paclitaxel Nanoparticles as Drug Delivery Agents

1.2.1. US6506405B1

The said invention, Capxol™ is a cremophor-free lyophilized powder of paclitaxel, which when reconstituted with sodium chloride (0.9%) or dextrose (5%) injections, forms a stable colloidal paclitaxel solution. The size of the suspended particles lies in the range of 20-400nm and its constituents include HSA and paclitaxel, which can be reconstituted to concentrations ranging from as low as 0.1mg/ml to as high as 20mg/ml. This allows smaller volumes to be administered via the parenteral route. Metabolization rates for paclitaxel in this formulation are lower than the metabolization of Taxol®, thus enabling sustained release for longer durations. Lowered chances of infections, hypersensitivity reactions and toxicity allow administration of the drug at higher concentration, thereby increasing its efficacy. Premedication with antihistamines and steroids is also not a requirement for the said formulation. Particles ranging in the early hundreds of nanometres may show target specific activities. Formulations for numerous *in vivo* delivery routes including the oral, intramuscular, intraperitoneal, intrathecal, subcutaneous, intravenous, topical, transdermal, inhalational have been described [56].

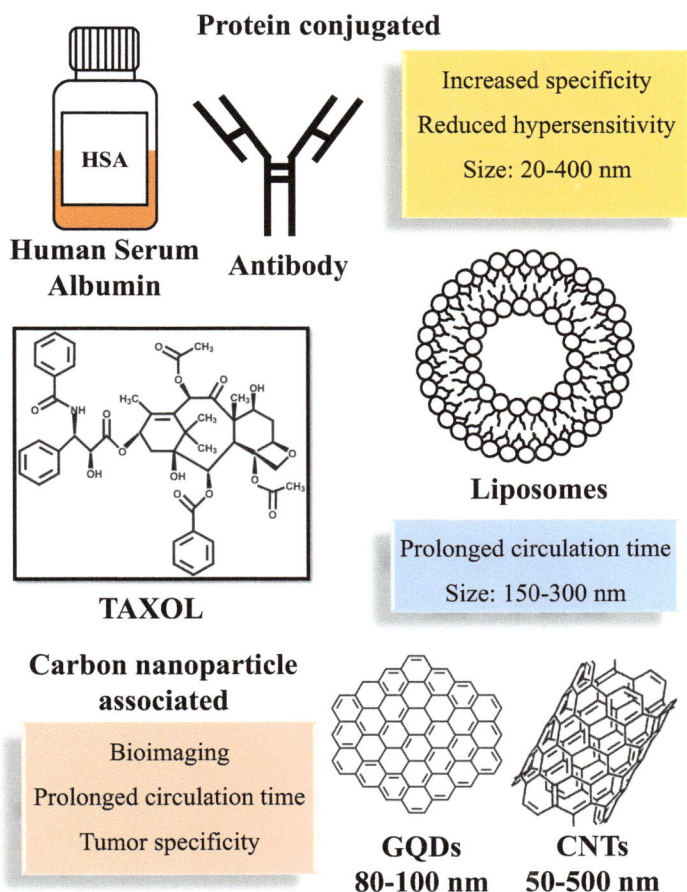

Fig. (1). The figure summarizes the developments in Taxol that led to nanotaxol formulations that are protein-conjugated, entrapped in liposomes and GQDs and SWCNT and MWCNT associated. The benefits associated with the various formulations of nanotaxol have been highlighted [55 - 58]. Sizes specified.

1.2.2. US8268348B2 and US20100112077A1

The scope of these patents describes the use of a combination therapy for cancer treatment which includes administration of taxane in a nanoparticle formulation followed by either surgery or radiation therapy. Albumin-bound paclitaxel nanoparticles, where the ratio of albumin to paclitaxel is 9:1 and lack cremophor for its formulation, are employed. The average size of these nanoparticles is less than or up to 200nm. The prescribed dosage ranges from 50-250mg/m^2 weekly. The patent also highlights the method of administration and enlists why the metronomic system of drug administration is preferred over the maximum drug tolerance one. Reduced cytotoxicity and side effects, antiangiogenic effects and enhanced anti-tumor efficacy are achieved by using the former. The drug dosage prescribed for this approach is 6-10mg/kg. Abraxane™ is seen to possess higher efficacy than Taxol® and reduced side effects [57, 58].

1.2.3. WO1994018954A1

The current patent describes a method for synthesis of protein-walled polymeric shells that contain dissolved Taxol. The Taxol was dissolved in soybean oil at a concentration of 2mg/ml. 5% HSA was overlayered on to this and sonicated vigorously for 30 seconds to give a milky white solution with the particles. These are stable at 4°C, 25°C, 38°C for about 4 weeks and demonstrated a controlled drug release along with no toxicity induced due to the composition of the formulation [59].

1.2.4. US20040092577A1

The patent describes a pharmaceutical powder that contains 50-90% by weight paclitaxel and the remaining constitutes of a water-soluble polymer and either an emulsifier, water-soluble salts, low molecular weight sugars as excipients and can be used as a formulation for an intra-tumoral injection. The polymer is one among hydroxypropyl cellulose, methylcellulose, polyvinylpyrrolidone, hydroxypro-pylmethyl cellulose, sodium carboxymethylcellulose and polysaccharides. The method for synthesis of the microparticles has been described; the solvent evaporation or the solvent extraction techniques were used. When reconstituted, the average size of the particles ranges from 0.5μ to 10μ and achieving concentrations between 20mg/ml to 300mg/ml, released for an extended period in effective amounts. These microparticles demonstrated a zero-order release and the extracellular concentration of the drug can be controlled efficiently by drug load in the microspheres and the drug release from it. The smaller 2μ microspheres were seen to be homogeneously present in the tumors, while the larger 10μ ones would require pre-treatment. The treatment groups when studied, showed smaller tumors and the residual tumor proliferation was either absent or minimal in the no treatment and the sham treatment groups [60].

1.2.5. US20090004118

The patent describes the method of synthesis of a Paclitaxel-Heparin-Folic acid conjugate of around 1200nm in diameter. Activity of this conjugate in normal breast cells (MCF-10A) as well as breast cancer cells (KB) indicated showed that it showed high selectivity towards malignant cells as compared to normal cells and also demonstrated increased cytotoxicity as compared to paclitaxel alone. Studies in mice indicate that the paclitaxel-heparin-folic acid conjugates show reduced tumor growth and angiogenesis in tumors and are relatively non-toxic to normal cells [61].

1.2.6. US20090226393

The scope of this patent describes a pharmaceutical conjugate that consists of poly-(gamma-L-glutamyl glutamine) (PGGA) and paclitaxel (PTX), thus referred to as PGGA-PTX. The molecular weight of the PGGA in the conjugate is about 70,000 and the amount of PTX is 35% and the formulation could also contain a pharmaceutically acceptable carrier, diluent or excipient. The conjugate can be administered intravenously and can be locally administered to the skin, lung, spleen and the kidney. The prescribed dose for patients suffering from melanoma is 40-345mg PTX equivalents/kg and those suffering from cancers of lung, liver, spleen, kidney is 40-550mg PTX equivalents/kg. The conjugate shows an increased half-life at the tumor site and in the plasma and shows an increased efficacy due to a 7.7 fold increase in the amount of paclitaxel delivered to the tumor, which delays its growth. The conjugate is seen to have an antitumor activity better than that of Abraxane™ [62].

1.2.7. US20100015051

Multiple dosing of Taxol® (the cremophor formulation) is required to maintain its therapeutic concentration in the tumor and this may lead to the non-specific hypersensitivity reactions. To circumvent this problem, the current patent introduces a composition capable of enabling its sustained-release in the cell and causes increased intracellular retention, thus increasing its efficacy. The said composition consists of a biodegradable polymer with a functional group that enables conjugation with transferrin. The said nanoparticles can also be used as a carrier for a radionuclide, efficient for treating bulky tumors. The transferrin conjugated nanoparticles showed an increased antiproliferative activity as compared to transferrin non-conjugated and free solutions of paclitaxel in both MCF-7/Adr and PC3 prostate cancer cells [63].

1.2.8. US20100303723

The scope of this patent covers the description of a nanoparticle that has FcRn binding partners (Fc fragment of IgG) that help in cell-specific transcytosis and allows controlled drug release. The other two peptides associated with the polymer include an MMP-2 degradable peptide and CREKA, for binding of collagen IV. The polymer that may be employed would either be PLA-PEG or PLGA-PEG. Targeted nanoparticles showed higher transcytosis (18%) as compared to the non-targeted ones (6%) [64].

1.2.9. WO2007034479

The patent describes a polymer-based nanoparticle that contains a bi-functional linker on its surface. This linker has a hydrophobic region embedded in the nanoparticle and a hydrophilic portion at its surface. The surface coating with the polymer allows increased blood circulation times. A monoclonal antibody, trastuzumab, was used to confer specificity to HER/neu tumor antigen which is seen to show an overexpression in prostate cancer cells. Paclitaxel is encapsulated in the PEG-PLA [65].

1.3. Micelles, Emulsions and Liposomes as Drug Delivery Carriers for Paclitaxel

1.3.1. US20150366806

This patent describes the invention, Genexol-PM™, which is a cremophor free formulation of paclitaxel that is bound to diblock mPEG-PDLLA polymer and can be used for intravenous administration. The nanoparticle is engineered such that the pharmacokinetic parameters of the drug like its area under the curve (AUC), maximum serum concentration that the drug achieves (C_{max}) and its volume of distribution (V_d). The said biodegradable polymeric micelle-type formulation possesses lower AUC and C_{max} values and a higher V_d as compared to the solvent formulated drug. The pharmacokinetics of the said formulation remained dose-proportional up to 435mg/m^2 and showed a higher efficacy as compared to Taxol® and Abraxane™ [66].

1.3.2. WO2009070761

The current patent describes a pharmaceutical composition of nanoparticles or micelles formed from paclitaxel conjugated to either tocopherol or to a phospholipid that is linked via a glycolate linker, where polyethylene glycol and polystyrene act as amphiphilic stabilizers. A low drug/polymer ratio is preferred. Preparation of the micelle involves rapid mixing of the aforementioned while maintaining controlled flow rates. These were seen to be stable for three months when stored at 4°C. The micelles show a longer circulation half-life of about 24 hours due to the presence of diglycolate bound prodrug [67].

1.3.3. EP2494956 and EP2494957

The patents detail two methods for the production of oil-in-water submicron emulsion, used as a carrier for paclitaxel. A natural steroid is selected as the lipid phase and the preferred molar ratio of paclitaxel to steroid is 1:0.33~1. An antioxidant stabilizer is also added along with an appropriate amount of organic solvent. After this, one of the two methods can be employed: a) stirring at a suitable temperature, removal of the organic solvent followed by vacuum drying. b) stirring at a suitable temperature, removal of the organic solvent by either spray drying or using a rotary evaporator followed by vacuum drying. The speculated advantages include lowered production costs, enhanced safety and reduced hypersensitivity, improved efficiency of encapsulation and formation of a stable submicron emulsion [68, 69]. This could find an application in the treatment of head and neck cancer, breast cancer, cervical carcinoma, non-small cell, renal carcinoma, liver carcinoma, esophagus cancer [69].

1.3.4. WO1994007484

The patent describes a pharmaceutically acceptable emulsion for delivery of Taxol. Marine oils rich in lipid ether and terpene hydrocarbons and that have a dipole moment between 0.5-2.0 Debyes is used. Taxol in the concentration of not greater than 5mg/ml is dissolved in an anhydrous alcohol and then mixed with oil. The alcohol is then evaporated completely. This was then added to normal saline and self-emulsifying glass was added to it, which produced droplet size ranging from 2-10μ. Mice with lung tumors were injected with the formulation with and without Taxol and the ones with Taxol showed reduced tumor sizes [70].

1.3.5. WO1996002247

The scope of this patent describes the composition of a stable oil-in-water emulsion that incorporates 5mg Taxol /ml of the emulsion. The oil used for dissolving Taxol is safflower oil, the co-solvent used is a short-chain alcohol and the surfactant is lecithin, a phospholipid. After evaporation of the co-solvent, the mixture was stirred at a high speed and formed stable emulsions of Taxol. The so formed emulsion can be used successfully for intravenous administration of Taxol [71].

1.3.6. CN102772368A

Long-circulating nanoparticles of Taxol are disclosed in this patent. It comprises of paclitaxel, PLGA or PLA as the copolymer, vitamin E (water soluble) as the co-solvent and water for injection. The weight ratio of copolymer to paclitaxel is 10:1 while that of co-solvent to paclitaxel is 30:1. The size of the copolymer is around 200nm and its drug encapsulation rate is as high as 70-95%. The method involves dissolving the copolymer and paclitaxel in the oil phase, dissolving the co-solvent in acetone and dissolving it in the aqueous phase, water. Following this, the oil phase is added in a dropwise controlled fashion to form an emulsion. The ratio of the volume of oil phase to that of the aqueous phase is 1:5. The nanoparticle is seen to be less toxic, shows specific tumor activity, shows the EPR effect owing to its size and the slow and sustained release imparts a better anti-tumor activity [72].

1.3.7. US5424073

The content of this patent explains the formation of liposome encapsulated Taxol, where cardiolipin serves as the liposome-forming material. It is administered along with a pharmaceutically accepted excipient. The so formed liposomes may either be positive, negative or neutral and this depends upon the liposome-forming material employed. These were stable for four days at room temperature and for a month at 4°C as compared to free Taxol in saline, that starts showing degradation within 3 hours at room temperature. It is administered to humans either intravenously or intraperitoneally at a dose of 1.0-3.0mg of compound per kg body weight. The composition has advantages such as increased solubility and stability of Taxol, avoiding hypersensitivity reactions and cardiotoxicity, capability of administering short infusion and increased therapeutic efficacy [73].

1.3.8. KR101612194

The patent introduces an albumin-bound paclitaxel that is encapsulated within a liposome comprising of phospholipids. The first step involves dissolving albumin and paclitaxel in an alcohol buffer solution. The second step involves forming a thin film of phospholipids and the final step constitutes mixing the two followed by stirring and sonication. This is then followed by an extrusion step wherein the amount of polycarbonate, small membrane pore size, higher pressure and larger the number of passes, smaller the particles formed ranging from 150-200nm. *In vitro* drug release shows a prolonged drug release profile, extended serum half-life and shows the EPR phenomenon. When compared to pure paclitaxel and albumin-bound paclitaxel, the liposome encapsulated albumin-bound paclitaxel showed preferential accumulation in the tumor [74].

1.3.9. US8663599B1

The patent discloses pH-sensitive liposomes that are less than 300nm in size and are self-assembled. It contains paclitaxel and is adapted for direct delivery to the tumor site. These are capable of entering cells via receptor-mediated endocytosis. The activity of the nanoparticles coated with galactosamine was comparable to the formulation Phyxol® in inhibiting the growth of HepG2 cells. The scheme for the synthesis of these nanoparticles demonstrates that the terminal hydroxyl group of poly(lactide) (PLA) was activated by use of N,N'-Carbonyldiimidazole. A coupling reaction between poly(γ-glutamic acid) (γ-PGA) with activated PLA yields an amphiphilic block polymer that further self-assembles to form the nanoparticle loaded with paclitaxel. Galactosamine is then conjugated to the nanoparticle using N-(3-dimethylaminopropyl)-N'-ethylcarbodiimide (EDC) in the presence of N-hydroxysuccinimide (NHS) [75].

1.4. Carbon Nanoparticles as Drug Delivery Agents for Cancer Chemotherapy

1.4.1. EP3063091

The said invention describes the procedure for synthesis and application of biocompatible Graphene Quantum Dots (GQDs) for bioimaging and drug delivery applications. The hydrothermal approach was used for the synthesis and GQDs of 5-10nm were embedded in Polyethylene Glycol (PEG) to yield nanoparticles ranging from 80-100nm. The GQDs were embedded into the PEG at a concentration ranging from 1-4mg/ml. To assess the biocompatibility of the material, the PEG-GQDs were tested on HeLa cells and 50% of the cells remained viable at a concentration of 8mg/ml of PEG-GQDs. The method for synthesis of the PEG-GQDs involves electrochemical etching of multi-walled carbon nanotubes at 25°C for a period of 12 hours to yield GODs that are further subjected to a hydrothermal reaction for 24 hours at 160°C in the presence of PEG to yield the final product [76].

1.4.2. US20090087493

The patent describes the use of single-walled Nanotubes (SWNTs) as drug delivery agents. The SWNTs have a length of approximately 50-500nm while they range from 1-2nm in diameter. These are functionalized either functionalized non-covalently using phospholipids-PEG (PL-PEG) that acts as a surfactant or covalently by the process of PEGylation. Paclitaxel was attached to PEG by a cleavable linkage through supramolecular bonding. 4T1 tumors were implanted into female Balb/c mice and were dosed with 5mg/kg of PTX. These mice showed reduced tumor growth rates and side effects and longer circulation time in blood with SWNT-PTX as compared to PEG-PTX or PTX formulation alone [77].

1.4.3. KR20180016231

The current patent describes a method by which GQDs were surface functionalized with amine groups using L-glutamic acid. They were then reacted with β-Cyclodextrin in the presence of 1,1'-carbonyldiimidazole (CDI) to form GQD- βCD complex which is further freeze dried. Trastuzumab (HER) antibodies were then attached to the GQD- βCD complex. The said complex can be employed for cancer cell bioimaging due to the blue fluorescence it inherits. Human epidermal growth factor receptor 2 (HER2) positive (BT-474) and negative (MCF-7) cell lines were treated with βCD-GQD-HER and it was found that the complex exhibited cytotoxicity specifically to the HER2 positive cells, BT-474. Thus, they are concluded to attain tumor-specificity [78].

1.4.4. CN104998261

The scope of the current patent describes a dual drug magnetic microsphere with fluorescent properties where the two drugs are kaempferol and paclitaxel. Fe_3O_4 magnetic fluid was used to dissolve kaempferol and the mixture was dropped in bovine serum albumin to form an emulsion. The second step involves synthesis of amino hydrothermal graphene green quantum dots that is loaded with paclitaxel where the mass ratio of paclitaxel:GQDs is 1:15. An aminocarboxyl reaction then connects the paclitaxel-loaded GQDs to the kaempferol loaded magnetic microsphere. Presence of kaempferol increases the sensitivity of human cervical carcinoma cells to the action of paclitaxel, delay the development of resistance, improves the efficacy of the treatment while managing to reduce the side effects, significantly [79].

1.4.5. WO2014015334

This patent describes a method and a construct of a nanoparticle that allows targeted drug delivery at the tumor site. The said conductive nanostructures are the Carbon Nanotubes (CNTs). The partially soluble or relatively insoluble therapeutic agent is present in the form of a nanoemulsion in the liquid or sol hydrogel at a suitable concentration. The CNTs are aligned in an array and the formulation containing the therapeutic agent (paclitaxel) is filled into the CNTs by applying the formulation to one side of the array and applying vacuum to the other side to draw it in. This prevents the exposure of paclitaxel to the normal tissues and thus protecting it from degradation by body fluids or tissues prevents any adverse effects to them. The size of these nanoparticles is around 50nm in diameter and 200-1000nm in length which makes them ideal for cellular uptake by endocytosis. The nanoparticles may also be surface functionalized so that they are readily taken up by the tumor cells and then subjected to inductive heating that causes the hydrogel to undergo a Phase-transition and it is released at the tumor site inducing localized toxicity. Surface functionalization also ensures prolonged circulation time in the bloodstream [80].

1.5. Nanodevices for Paclitaxel Delivery to Cancer Cells

1.5.1. US20100215724

The patent describes a microcapsule nanotube device consisting of functionalized nanotubes for targeted drug delivery to breast cancer cells. The patent describes the use of SWNT that can be surface functionalized with drug-folate conjugates. Paclitaxel was bound to albumin and surface functionalized on the SWNT that was pre-functionalized with folate, the binding efficiency being 90%. This enables targeted delivery of paclitaxel, intratumorally for breast cancer. These nanotubes post-treatment are cleared by the macrophages [81].

1.5.2. US20100303716

The current patent introduces a switchable nanodevice that can be turned on or off either magnetically, ultrasonically or thermally. The nanodevices are hollow multifunctional nanospheres that are triggerable by one of the aforementioned physical parameters. The nanodevice contains two prodrugs in its amphiphilic membrane which protects them from degradation in the body due to enzymes, pH and other body fluids, until they reach their target tumor sites. This causes an extension in the half-life of the drug *in vivo*, thereby causing its pharmacokinetic and pharmacodynamic properties to be enhanced. Functionalization of these with tumor-specific antibodies and luminescent quantum dots can render specificity and enable tracking [82].

DISCUSSION

The chapter talks about patents that follow different approaches for enhanced drug delivery. Taxol is a drug with a notable history. It was initially extracted from *Taxus brevifolia* and due to its limited natural availability, the chemical synthesis approach was considered. However, the structure of Taxol being complicated, could not be synthesized using this approach leading to employing a semi-synthetic approach. Taxol possessed one major drawback; poor solubility in aqueous medium, which was the prime reason why its development stalled at the formulation stage. Use of solvents like cremophor EL and ethanol in order to solubilize the drug for administration was the next stage in its development. However, hypersensitivity associated with the aforementioned solvents raised alarms. The adverse effects caused by this formulation outnumbered its benefits which lead to the human serum albumin associated formulation, Abraxane®, showing EPR effect. Different protein-conjugated formulations, with reduced cytotoxicity, were developed in due course of time. The next advancement involved imparting tumor specificity by forming conjugates with heparin, folic acid, transferrin, poly-(gamma-L-glutamyl glutamine), Fc fragment of IgG and trastuzumab, as discussed previously. To be able to engineer the pharmacokinetic properties of the nanoparticles, cremophor-free micelles were developed which showed reduced hypersensitivity, longer circulation half-life and increased stability and efficacy. Stable oil-in-water emulsions and liposomes that show tumor specificity, EPR effect, sustained release, increased therapeutic efficacy have also been looked at as viable options for drug delivery. Another path-breaking advancement is the use of carbon nanoparticles that enable simultaneous bioimaging and drug delivery to cancer cells with added specificity. This is achieved by using GQDs, SWCNTs, MWCNTs and the like. These particles are engineered such that they inherit fluorescence capability, can be loaded with drugs and surface functionalized with antibodies that render them tumor specific. To be able to translate these particles for successful use in cancers of all kinds and preventing their recurrence by bioimaging guided surgery is not far-fetched. Translational medicine is advancing at a pace all set to expedite diagnosis, treatment and cure of this life-threatening disease, cancer.

CURRENT & FUTURE DEVELOPMENTS

A variety of polymers, carbon nanoparticles, proteins, carriers, vitamins, natural agents, metals, lipids, steroids and other biological molecules have been employed for the synthesis of nanoparticles capable of delivering paclitaxel (Table **1**) [49, 83 - 93]. These molecules are specifically non-toxic and not hypersensitivity inducing, thus preventing adverse reactions. Research on paclitaxel had halted for a brief period due to its insolubility in aqueous medium and its finite natural availability. Use of a semi-synthetic approach and nanotechnology for the production and smart delivery respectively, of this antitumor drug, have worked wonders and prevented the downfall of this blockbuster drug. The table summarizes well, the forms of paclitaxel available and approved for use, while some are still in the clinal trial phases. Out of these, Abraxane® (approved for use internationally), Cynviloq™ (approved for use in South Korea), Paclical® (approved for use in Russian Federation), Lipusu® (approved for use in China), PICN (approved for use in India) and DHP-107 (approved for use in South Korea) are approved, while, NK105, LEP-ETU and DHP-107 have completed phase II clinical trials. NK105, however, did not show the expected outcomes in phase II clinical trials and Triolimus is still in its preclinical stages. These, and more such drugs, thus form the future of Taxol delivery to different solid tumors and also form an integral part of combination therapy for the treatment of cancer.

Table 1. Different Formulations of Paclitaxel and their Applications in Treating Cancer.

Formulation	Nanoparticles	Size	Type of Cancer Used	Reference
Abraxane®	Albumin-bound	130nm	Metastatic breast cancer (MBC), NSCLC, pancreatic cancer	[49, 83, 84]
Cynviloq™	Polymeric micelle	25nm	MBC, NSCLC, pancreatic, ovarian, bladder cancers	[83, 84]
Paclical®	Micelle	20-60nm	NSCLC, ovarian and breast cancer	[83, 85]
Lipusu®	Liposome	400nm	Breast cancer, NSCLC, oophoron and ovarian metastatic cancer	[83, 86]
PICN	Polymeric-Lipidic	100nm	Biliary, breast, anal, liver cancers, angiosarcoma, melanoma	[83, 87]
NK105	Polymeric micelle	85nm	Colorectal, gastric, ovarian cancer	[83, 88]
SB05	Liposome	200nm	Breast, pancreatic, liver, biliary cancers, angiosarcoma, melanoma	[83, 89]
LEP-ETU	Liposome	150nm	Breast, ovarian, gastric cancers	[83, 90, 91]
DHP-107	Emulsion	10μm	Gastric cancer, NSCLC	[83, 92]
Triolimus	Polymeric micelle	40nm	Breast cancer, NSCLC	[83, 93]

CONSENT FOR PUBLICATION

Not applicable.

CONFLICT OF INTEREST

The authors confirm that this chapter content has no conflicts of interest.

ACKNOWLEDGEMENTS

The authors thank Mr. Rohan Bahadur for critical reading of the chapter and assisting in its revision.

REFERENCES

[1] Hanahan D, Weinberg RA. Hallmarks of cancer: The next generation. Cell 2011; 144(5): 646-74.
[http://dx.doi.org/10.1016/j.cell.2011.02.013] [PMID: 21376230]

[2] Jemal A, Bray F, Center MM, Ferlay J, Ward E, Forman D. Global cancer statistics. CA Cancer J Clin 2011; 61(2): 69-90.
[http://dx.doi.org/10.3322/caac.20107] [PMID: 21296855]

[3] Ferlay J, Soerjomataram I, Dikshit R, *et al.* Cancer incidence and mortality worldwide: Sources, methods and major patterns in GLOBOCAN 2012. Int J Cancer 2015; 136(5): E359-86.
[http://dx.doi.org/10.1002/ijc.29210] [PMID: 25220842]

[4]   Schmid D, Leitzmann MF. Television viewing and time spent sedentary in relation to cancer risk: A meta-analysis. J Natl Cancer Inst 2014; 106(7): dju098.
[http://dx.doi.org/10.1093/jnci/dju098] [PMID: 24935969]

[5]   Pang Q, Qu K, Zhang J, *et al.* Cigarette smoking increases the risk of mortality from liver cancer: A clinical-based cohort and meta-analysis. J Gastroenterol Hepatol 2015; 30(10): 1450-60.
[http://dx.doi.org/10.1111/jgh.12990] [PMID: 25967392]

[6]   Grewal P, Viswanathen VA. Liver cancer and alcohol. Clin Liver Dis 2012; 16(4): 839-50.
[http://dx.doi.org/10.1016/j.cld.2012.08.011] [PMID: 23101985]

[7]   De Souza C, Chatterji BP. HDAC inhibitors as novel anti-cancer therapeutics. Recent Pat Anticancer Drug Discov 2015; 10(2): 145-62.

[8]   Liu WC, Gong T, Zhu P. Advances in exploring alternative Taxol sources. RSC Advances 2016; 6(54): 48800-9.
[http://dx.doi.org/10.1039/C6RA06640B]

[9]   Weaver BA. How Taxol/paclitaxel kills cancer cells. Mol Biol Cell 2014; 25(18): 2677-81.
[http://dx.doi.org/10.1091/mbc.e14-04-0916] [PMID: 25213191]

[10]   Walsh V, Goodman J. From Taxol to Taxol®: The changing identities and ownership of an anti-cancer drug. Med Anthropol 2002; 21(3-4): 307-36.
[http://dx.doi.org/10.1080/01459740214074] [PMID: 12458837]

[11]   Marupudi NI, Han JE, Li KW, Renard VM, Tyler BM, Brem H. Paclitaxel: A review of adverse toxicities and novel delivery strategies. Expert Opin Drug Saf 2007; 6(5): 609-21.
[http://dx.doi.org/10.1517/14740338.6.5.609] [PMID: 17877447]

[12]   Deardon R, Brooks SP, Grenfell BT, *et al.* Inference for individual-level models of infectious diseases in large populations. Stat Sin 2010; 20(1): 239-61.
[PMID: 26405426]

[13]   Oberlies NH, Kroll DJ. Camptothecin and Taxol: Historic achievements in natural products research. J Nat Prod 2004; 67(2): 129-35.
[http://dx.doi.org/10.1021/np030498t] [PMID: 14987046]

[14]   Wani MC, Taylor HL, Wall ME, Coggon P, McPhail AT. Plant antitumor agents. VI. The isolation and structure of Taxol, a novel antileukemic and antitumor agent from *Taxus brevifolia*. J Am Chem Soc 1971; 93(9): 2325-7.
[http://dx.doi.org/10.1021/ja00738a045] [PMID: 5553076]

[15]   Foa R, Norton L, Seidman AD. Taxol (paclitaxel): A novel anti-microtubule agent with remarkable anti-neoplastic activity. Int J Clin Lab Res 1994; 24(1): 6-14.
[http://dx.doi.org/10.1007/BF02592403] [PMID: 7910054]

[16]   Herbst RS, Khuri FR. Mode of action of docetaxel - a basis for combination with novel anticancer agents. Cancer Treat Rev 2003; 29(5): 407-15.
[http://dx.doi.org/10.1016/S0305-7372(03)00097-5] [PMID: 12972359]

[17]   Jordan MA, Wilson L. Microtubules as a target for anticancer drugs. Nat Rev Cancer 2004; 4(4): 253-65.
[http://dx.doi.org/10.1038/nrc1317] [PMID: 15057285]

[18]   Schiff PB, Fant J, Horwitz SB. Promotion of microtubule assembly *in vitro* by Taxol. Nature 1979; 277(5698): 665-7.
[http://dx.doi.org/10.1038/277665a0] [PMID: 423966]

[19]   Nogales E, Wolf SG, Downing KH. Correction: Structure of the αβ tubulin dimer by electron crystallography. Nature 1998; 393(6681): 191.
[http://dx.doi.org/10.1038/30288]

[20]   Snyder JP, Nettles JH, Cornett B, Downing KH, Nogales E. The binding conformation of Taxol in β-

tubulin: A model based on electron crystallographic density. Proc Natl Acad Sci USA 2001; 98(9): 5312-6.
[http://dx.doi.org/10.1073/pnas.051309398] [PMID: 11309480]

[21]   Okano J, Rustgi AK. Paclitaxel induces prolonged activation of the Ras/MEK/ERK pathway independently of activating the programmed cell death machinery. J Biol Chem 2001; 276(22): 19555-64.
[http://dx.doi.org/10.1074/jbc.M011164200] [PMID: 11278851]

[22]   Wolfson M, Yang CP, Horwitz SB. Taxol induces tyrosine phosphorylation of SHC and its association with Grb2 in murine RAW 264.7 cells. Int J Cancer 1997; 70(2): 248-52.
[http://dx.doi.org/10.1002/(SICI)1097-0215(19970117)70:2<248::AID-IJC17>3.0.CO;2-E]   [PMID: 9009167]

[23]   Kim YM, Paik SG. Induction of expression of inducible nitric oxide synthase by Taxol in murine macrophage cells. Biochem Biophys Res Commun 2005; 326(2): 410-6.
[http://dx.doi.org/10.1016/j.bbrc.2004.11.043] [PMID: 15582593]

[24]   Boudny V, Nakano S. SRC tyrosine kinase augments taxotere-induced apoptosis through enhanced expression and phosphorylation of Bcl-2. Br J Cancer 2002; 86(3): 463-9.
[http://dx.doi.org/10.1038/sj.bjc.6600080] [PMID: 11875716]

[25]   Boldt S, Weidle UH, Kolch W. The role of MAPK pathways in the action of chemotherapeutic drugs. Carcinogenesis 2002; 23(11): 1831-8.
[http://dx.doi.org/10.1093/carcin/23.11.1831] [PMID: 12419831]

[26]   Stone AA, Chambers TC. Microtubule inhibitors elicit differential effects on MAP kinase (JNK, ERK, and p38) signaling pathways in human KB-3 carcinoma cells. Exp Cell Res 2000; 254(1): 110-9.
[http://dx.doi.org/10.1006/excr.1999.4731] [PMID: 10623471]

[27]   Ofir R, Seidman R, Rabinski T, et al. Taxol-induced apoptosis in human SKOV3 ovarian and MCF7 breast carcinoma cells is caspase-3 and caspase-9 independent. Cell Death Differ 2002; 9(6): 636-42.
[http://dx.doi.org/10.1038/sj.cdd.4401012] [PMID: 12032672]

[28]   Huang Y, Sheikh MS, Fornace AJ Jr, Holbrook NJ. Serine protease inhibitor TPCK prevents Taxol-induced cell death and blocks c-Raf-1 and Bcl-2 phosphorylation in human breast carcinoma cells. Oncogene 1999; 18(23): 3431-9.
[http://dx.doi.org/10.1038/sj.onc.1202685] [PMID: 10376521]

[29]   Park SJ, Wu CH, Gordon JD, Zhong X, Emami A, Safa AR. Taxol induces caspase-10-dependent apoptosis. J Biol Chem 2004; 279(49): 51057-67.
[http://dx.doi.org/10.1074/jbc.M406543200] [PMID: 15452117]

[30]   von Haefen C, Wieder T, Essmann F, Schulze-Osthoff K, Dörken B, Daniel PT. Paclitaxel-induced apoptosis in BJAB cells proceeds via a death receptor-independent, caspases-3/-8-driven mitochondrial amplification loop. Oncogene 2003; 22(15): 2236-47.
[http://dx.doi.org/10.1038/sj.onc.1206280] [PMID: 12700660]

[31]   Ding AH, Porteu F, Sanchez E, Nathan CF. Shared actions of endotoxin and Taxol on TNF receptors and TNF release. Science 1990; 248(4953): 370-2.
[http://dx.doi.org/10.1126/science.1970196] [PMID: 1970196]

[32]   Tudor G, Aguilera A, Halverson DO, Laing ND, Sausville EA. Susceptibility to drug-induced apoptosis correlates with differential modulation of Bad, Bcl-2 and Bcl-xL protein levels. Cell Death Differ 2000; 7(6): 574-86.
[http://dx.doi.org/10.1038/sj.cdd.4400688] [PMID: 10822281]

[33]   Bhalla KN. Microtubule-targeted anticancer agents and apoptosis. Oncogene 2003; 22(56): 9075-86.
[http://dx.doi.org/10.1038/sj.onc.1207233] [PMID: 14663486]

[34]   Pasquier E, Honoré S, Braguer D. Microtubule-targeting agents in angiogenesis: Where do we stand? Drug Resist Updat 2006; 9(1-2): 74-86.

[http://dx.doi.org/10.1016/j.drup.2006.04.003] [PMID: 16714139]

[35]   Bijman MN, van Nieuw Amerongen GP, Laurens N, van Hinsbergh VW, Boven E. Microtubule-targeting agents inhibit angiogenesis at subtoxic concentrations, a process associated with inhibition of RAC1 and CDC42 activity and changes in the endothelial cytoskeleton. Mol Cancer Ther 2006; 5(9): 2348-57.
[http://dx.doi.org/10.1158/1535-7163.MCT-06-0242] [PMID: 16985069]

[36]   Wang J, Lou P, Lesniewski R, Henkin J. Paclitaxel at ultra low concentrations inhibits angiogenesis without affecting cellular microtubule assembly. Anticancer Drugs 2003; 14(1): 13-9.
[http://dx.doi.org/10.1097/00001813-200301000-00003] [PMID: 12544254]

[37]   Malik S, Cusidó RM, Mirjalili MH, Moyano E, Palazón J, Bonfill M. Production of the anticancer drug Taxol in *Taxus baccata* suspension cultures: A review. Process Biochem 2011; 46(1): 23-34.
[http://dx.doi.org/10.1016/j.procbio.2010.09.004]

[38]   Feng S, Huang G. Effects of emulsifiers on the controlled release of paclitaxel (Taxol) from nanospheres of biodegradable polymers. J Control Release 2001; 71(1): 53-69.
[http://dx.doi.org/10.1016/S0168-3659(00)00364-3] [PMID: 11245908]

[39]   Miele E, Spinelli GP, Miele E, Tomao F, Tomao S. Albumin-bound formulation of paclitaxel (Abraxane ABI-007) in the treatment of breast cancer. Int J Nanomedicine 2009; 4: 99-105.
[PMID: 19516888]

[40]   Gelderblom H, Verweij J, Nooter K, Sparreboom A. Cremophor EL: The drawbacks and advantages of vehicle selection for drug formulation. Eur J Cancer 2001; 37(13): 1590-8.
[http://dx.doi.org/10.1016/S0959-8049(01)00171-X] [PMID: 11527683]

[41]   Szebeni J, Muggia FM, Alving CR. Complement activation by Cremophor EL as a possible contributor to hypersensitivity to paclitaxel: An *in vitro* study. J Natl Cancer Inst 1998; 90(4): 300-6.
[http://dx.doi.org/10.1093/jnci/90.4.300] [PMID: 9486816]

[42]   Michaud LB. Methods for preventing reactions secondary to Cremophor EL. Ann Pharmacother 1997; 31(11): 1402-4.
[http://dx.doi.org/10.1177/106002809703101120] [PMID: 9391700]

[43]   Weiss RB, Donehower RC, Wiernik PH, *et al.* Hypersensitivity reactions from Taxol. J Clin Oncol 1990; 8(7): 1263-8.
[http://dx.doi.org/10.1200/JCO.1990.8.7.1263] [PMID: 1972736]

[44]   Walker FE. Paclitaxel (TAXOL): Side effects and patient education issues. Semin Oncol Nurs 1993; 9(4) (Suppl. 2): 6-10.
[http://dx.doi.org/10.1016/S0749-2081(16)30036-5] [PMID: 7904378]

[45]   Rowinsky EK, McGuire WP, Guarnieri T, Fisherman JS, Christian MC, Donehower RC. Cardiac disturbances during the administration of Taxol. J Clin Oncol 1991; 9(9): 1704-12.
[http://dx.doi.org/10.1200/JCO.1991.9.9.1704] [PMID: 1678781]

[46]   Cucinotto I, Fiorillo L, Gualtieri S, *et al.* Nanoparticle albumin bound Paclitaxel in the treatment of human cancer: Nanodelivery reaches prime-time? J Drug Deliv 2013; 2013: 905091.
[http://dx.doi.org/10.1155/2013/905091] [PMID: 23738077]

[47]   Petrelli F, Borgonovo K, Barni S. Targeted delivery for breast cancer therapy: The history of nanoparticle-albumin-bound paclitaxel. Expert Opin Pharmacother 2010; 11(8): 1413-32.
[http://dx.doi.org/10.1517/14656561003796562] [PMID: 20446855]

[48]   Ma P, Mumper RJ. Paclitaxel nano-delivery systems: A comprehensive review. J Nanomed Nanotechnol 2013; 4(2): 1000164.
[http://dx.doi.org/10.4172/2157-7439.1000164] [PMID: 24163786]

[49]   Zhao M, Lei C, Yang Y, *et al.* Abraxane, the nanoparticle formulation of paclitaxel can induce drug resistance by up-regulation of P-gp. PLoS One 2015; 10(7): e0131429.
[http://dx.doi.org/10.1371/journal.pone.0131429] [PMID: 26182353]

[50]   Williamson SK, Johnson GA, Maulhardt HA, *et al.* A phase I study of intraperitoneal nanoparticulate paclitaxel (Nanotax®) in patients with peritoneal malignancies. Cancer Chemother Pharmacol 2015; 75(5): 1075-87.
[http://dx.doi.org/10.1007/s00280-015-2737-4] [PMID: 25898813]

[51]   Riggio C, Pagni E, Raffa V, Cuschieri A. Nano-oncology: Clinical application for cancer therapy and future perspectives. J Nanomater 2011; 2011: 17.
[http://dx.doi.org/10.1155/2011/164506]

[52]   Wang H, Wei J, Yang C, *et al.* The inhibition of tumor growth and metastasis by self-assembled nanofibers of Taxol. Biomaterials 2012; 33(24): 5848-53.
[http://dx.doi.org/10.1016/j.biomaterials.2012.04.047] [PMID: 22607913]

[53]   Bin Z, Yi'an Z, Liyun Z. Process for the manufacture of paclitaxel nano granules. CN1463969, 2003.

[54]   Bin W. Taxol nanoparticle composition and preparation method thereof. CN101829061, 2010.

[55]   Paclitaxel- Drugbank. Available at: https://www.drugbank.ca/drugs/DB01229 Accessed on: August 1, 2018.

[56]   Desai N, Soon-Shiong P. Methods and formulations of cremophor-free taxanes. US6506405, 1993.

[57]   Desai N, Soon-Shiong P. Combinations and modes of administration of therapeutic agents and combination therapy. US8268348, 2006.

[58]   Desai N, Soon-Shiong P. Nanoparticles of paclitaxel and albumin in combination with bevacizumab against cancer. US20100112077, 2010.

[59]   Grinstaff M, Soon-Shiong P, Wong M, Sanford P, Suslick K, Desai N. Methods for *in vivo* delivery of biologics and compositions useful therefor. WO018954, 1994.

[60]   Lerner E, Flashner-Barak M, Tzafriri A, Parness H, Smith A, Hinchcliffe M. Microparticle pharmaceutical compositions for intratumoral delivery. US20040092577, 2004.

[61]   Nie S, Lee Y, Kim G. Multifunctional nanoparticle conjugates and their us. US20090004118, 2009.

[62]   Wang X, Zhao G, Van S, Yu L. Polymer paclitaxel conjugates and methods for treating cancer. US20090226393, 2009.

[63]   Labhasetwar V, Sahoo S. Transferrin-conjugated nanoparticles for increasing efficacy of a therapeutic agent. US20100015051, 2010.

[64]   Farokhzad O, Alexis F, Kuo T, Pridgen E, Radovic-Moreno A, Langer R. Drug delivery systems using Fc fragments. US20100303723, 2010.

[65]   Benita S, Debetton N, Goldstein D. Nanoparticles for targeted delivery of active agents. WO2007034479, 2007.

[66]   Trieu V. Methods of engineering nanoparticle. US20150366806, 2015.

[67]   Ansell S, Johnstone S, Tardi P, Mayer L. Improved taxane delivery system. WO2009070761, 2009.

[68]   Liu Y, Xia X, Guo R, *et al.* Paclitaxel/steroidal complex. EP2494956, 2012.

[69]   Liu Y, Xia X, Guo R, *et al.* Submicro emulsion of paclitaxel using steroid complex as intermediate carrier. EP2494957, 2012.

[70]   Shively M. Pharmaceutical solutions and emulsions containing Taxol. WO1994007484, 1994.

[71]   Kaufman R, Richard T, Fuhrhop R. Stable oil-in-water emulsions incorporating a taxine (Taxol) and method of making same. WO1996002247, 1996.

[72]   Kingdom Y, Yuan C. Taxol long-circulating nanoparticle preparation and preparation method thereof. CN102772368, 2012.

[73]   Rahman A, Rafaeloff R, Husain S. Liposome encapsulated Taxol and a method of using the same.

US5424073, 1995.

[74]   Yongkak H, Rutala H. Composition for drug delivery comprising liposome encapsulated nanoparticle of drug combined with Albumin. KR101612194, 2014.

[75]   Sung H, Liao Z, Chung M, Cheng K, Cheng P, Tu H. Pharmaceutical composition of nanoparticles. US8663599, 2004.

[76]   Singh N, Chandra A. Biocompatible graphene quantum dots for drug delivery and bioimaging applications. EP3063091, 2017.

[77]   Dai H, Liu Z, Li X, Sun X. Supramolecular functionalization of graphitic nanoparticles for drug delivery. US20090087493, 2009.

[78]   Go K. Graphene quantum dot complex. KR20180016231, 2018.

[79]   Xiaojuan Z, Lingyun H, Zhiying Z, *et al.* A dual drug fluorescent microsphere composite magnetic system and preparation method. CN104998261, 2015.

[80]   Wu C, Kim J, Wu J. System and methods for nanostructure protected delivery of treatment agent and selective release thereof. WO2014015334, 2014.

[81]   Prakash S, Chen H, Raja P, Nalamasu O, Ajayan P. Microcapsule nanotube devices for targeted delivery of therapeutic molecules. US20100215724, 2010.

[82]   Jin S, Oh S, Brammer K, Kong S. Switchable nano-vehicle delivery systems, and methods for making and using them. US20100303716, 2010.

[83]   Sofias AM, Dunne M, Storm G, Allen C. The battle of "nano" paclitaxel. Adv Drug Deliv Rev 2017; 122: 20-30.
[http://dx.doi.org/10.1016/j.addr.2017.02.003] [PMID: 28257998]

[84]   Shin DH, Tam YT, Kwon GS. Polymeric micelle nanocarriers in cancer research. Front Chem Sci Eng 2016; 10(3): 348-59.
[http://dx.doi.org/10.1007/s11705-016-1582-2]

[85]   Khanna C, Rosenberg M, Vail DM. A review of paclitaxel and novel formulations including those suitable for use in dogs. J Vet Intern Med 2015; 29(4): 1006-12.
[http://dx.doi.org/10.1111/jvim.12596] [PMID: 26179168]

[86]   Muthu MS, Feng SS. Nanopharmacology of liposomes developed for cancer therapy. Nanomedicine (Lond) 2010; 5(7): 1017-9.
[http://dx.doi.org/10.2217/nnm.10.75] [PMID: 20874016]

[87]   Ma WW, Lam ET, Dy GK, *et al.* A pharmacokinetic and dose-escalating study of paclitaxel injection concentrate for nano-dispersion (PICN) alone and with carboplatin in patients with advanced solid tumors. J Clin Oncol 2013; 31(15): 2557-7.

[88]   Hamaguchi T, Matsumura Y, Suzuki M, *et al.* NK105, a paclitaxel-incorporating micellar nanoparticle formulation, can extend *in vivo* antitumor activity and reduce the neurotoxicity of paclitaxel. Br J Cancer 2005; 92(7): 1240-6.
[http://dx.doi.org/10.1038/sj.bjc.6602479] [PMID: 15785749]

[89]   Chowdhury P, Nagesh PKB, Khan S, *et al.* Development of polyvinylpyrrolidone/paclitaxel self-assemblies for breast cancer. Acta Pharm Sin B 2018; 8(4): 602-14.
[http://dx.doi.org/10.1016/j.apsb.2017.10.004] [PMID: 30109184]

[90]   Zhang JA, Anyarambhatla G, Ma L, *et al.* Development and characterization of a novel Cremophor EL free liposome-based paclitaxel (LEP-ETU) formulation. Eur J Pharm Biopharm 2005; 59(1): 177-87.
[http://dx.doi.org/10.1016/j.ejpb.2004.06.009] [PMID: 15567316]

[91]   Slingerland M, Guchelaar HJ, Rosing H, *et al.* Bioequivalence of Liposome-Entrapped Paclitaxel Easy-To-Use (LEP-ETU) formulation and paclitaxel in polyethoxylated castor oil: A randomized, two-period crossover study in patients with advanced cancer. Clin Ther 2013; 35(12): 1946-54.

[http://dx.doi.org/10.1016/j.clinthera.2013.10.009] [PMID: 24290734]

[92]   Shin BS, Kim HJ, Hong SH, *et al.* Enhanced absorption and tissue distribution of paclitaxel following oral administration of DHP 107, a novel mucoadhesive lipid dosage form. Cancer Chemother Pharmacol 2009; 64(1): 87-94.
[http://dx.doi.org/10.1007/s00280-008-0849-9] [PMID: 18941747]

[93]   Hasenstein JR, Shin HC, Kasmerchak K, Buehler D, Kwon GS, Kozak KR. Antitumor activity of Triolimus: A novel multidrug-loaded micelle containing paclitaxel, rapamycin, and 17-AAG. Mol Cancer Ther 2012; 11(10): 2233-42.
[http://dx.doi.org/10.1158/1535-7163.MCT-11-0987] [PMID: 22896668]

CHAPTER 3

Advanced Therapy in Cancer: Stimuli-Responsive Nanocarriers for On-Demand Drug Delivery

Azadeh Haeri[*], **Fatemeh Mehryab** and **Hamid R. Moghimi**

Department of Pharmaceutics and Nanotechnology, School of Pharmacy, Shahid Beheshti University of Medical Sciences, Tehran, Iran

Abstract: Cancer is one of the major causes of death worldwide. Most of the conventional anticancer chemotherapeutics have limited efficacy and toxic side effects. During the last decades, nanomedicine has sparked a rapidly growing interest in cancer therapy due to numerous advantages including efficient encapsulation of hydrophilic and hydrophobic drugs, enhanced cargo accumulation at the target site, reduced off-target drug distribution, ease of administration, and minimized side effects. However, application of drug-loaded nanocarriers is restricted by slow and inefficient drug release at the pathological site. A promising approach to address this issue is the development of stimuli-responsive nanocarriers that can be triggered by exogenous physical or endogenous chemical or biochemical stimuli to release the anticancer drug. In this chapter, recent patents published on stimuli-sensitive nanocarriers which are responsive to either external stimuli (such as hyperthermia, magnetic field, light, and ultrasound) or internal stimuli (including acidic pH, certain enzymes, and redox condition) are discussed.

Keywords: Acidic pH, cancer, drug delivery, enzymes, external stimuli, hyperthermia, internal stimuli, light, magnetic field, patent, redox condition, responsive nanocarriers, stimuli-sensitive, ultrasound.

1. INTRODUCTION

Cancer is one of the major causes of death worldwide. Although great efforts have been made to overcome cancer, the current treatments are still far from satisfactory results. Various treatment modalities such as chemotherapy, radiotherapy, surgery, and immunotherapy have been employed for cancer treatment. Systemic chemotherapeutics administration is associated with many problems. To reach the tumor, drugs need to pass through several biological

[*] **Corresponding author Azadeh Haeri:** Department of Pharmaceutics and Nanotechnology, School of Pharmacy, Shahid Beheshti University of Medical Sciences, Tehran, Iran; Tel: + 98 21 88200212: Fax: + 98 21 88665317; E-mail: a_haeri@sbmu.ac.ir

Atta-ur-Rahman and Khurshid Zaman (Eds.)

barriers, such as blood vessels, tissues, cell membranes, or even subcellular membranes. Lack of specificity for the target site, distribution of drugs at off-target sites, and the necessity to administer high doses of drugs to achieve sufficient concentration at the site of action, cause the occurrence of nonspecific toxicity to healthy tissue and serious side effects. Moreover, limited aqueous solubility and cellular uptake of some chemotherapeutics can also hinder their efficacy [1 - 3]. The current chemotherapy drugs are far from Paul Ehrlich's idea of a "magic bullet", that a therapeutic agent would be selectively reached to the target organ.

Nanocarriers provide a number of advantages in cancer therapy including efficient encapsulation of hydrophilic and hydrophobic drugs, enhanced cargo accumulation at the target site, reduced off-target drug distribution, ease of drug administration, maximized therapeutic efficacy and minimized side effects [4, 5]. Following intravascular administration, nanocarriers show longer circulation times, as they are small enough to escape the reticuloendothelial system (RES) and large enough to bypass glomerular filtration [6]. Therefore, long-circulating nanostructures can preferentially extravasate into tumor tissues due to hypervascularity and defective fenestrated vascular architecture and retain in the tumor due to impaired lymphatic drainage. The phenomenon is known as the Enhanced Permeability and Retention (EPR) effect (Fig. **1**) which leads to higher concentration of the anticancer loaded nanocarriers within tumors [7, 8]. In the light of this concept, various nanostructures have been investigated for cancer therapy. Liposomes, polymeric nanoparticles, micelles, and metal nanoparticles are among the most widely studied nanocarriers.

Liposomes are bilayer vesicles composed of amphiphilic phospholipids and other materials, such as cholesterol. Based on vesicle structure and size, there are three main types of liposomes: SUV (Small Unilamellar Vesicles, less than 0.1μm), LUV (Large Unilamellar Vesicles, larger than 0.1 μm), and MLV (Multilamellar Vesicles). Liposomal formulations can be prepared by different techniques such as thin film hydration, dehydration-rehydration, reverse-phase evaporation, and pro-liposome methods [9 - 11].

Polymeric nanoparticles are solid particles with a size in the range of 10-1000nm. They allow incorporation of cargos throughout a polymeric matrix (nanospheres) or encapsulated and protected inside the core (nanocapsules). Polymeric nanoparticles can be prepared by several techniques including nanoprecipitation, emulsion diffusion, solvent displacement, and solvent evaporation from various polymers such as chitosan, gelatin, poly(D,L-lactide-co-glycolide) (PLGA), poly(D,L-lactic acid) (PLA), polycaprolactone, and poly-alkyl-cyanoacrylates [9, 12, 13].

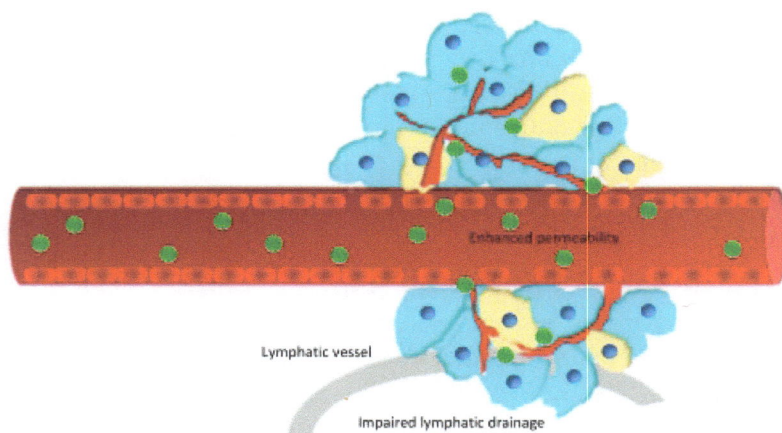

Fig. (1). Schematic representation of Enhanced Permeability and Retention (EPR) effect. The EPR effect causes higher accumulation of nanocarriers in tumor tissues compared to normal tissues by passive targeting. Nanocarriers circulating in the blood vessels can accumulate in a tumor by extravasating through leaky blood vessels at the tumor site. Impaired lymphatic drainage mediates the nanoparticle retention at the tumor site.

Micelles are globular or spherical nanostructures formed by supramolecular self-assembly of amphiphilic copolymers or lipids in aqueous environments, normally as a consequence of hydrophobic or ion pair interaction [14 - 16]. The hydrophobic parts (typically composed of lipids or polymers like PLA and PCL) form the interior core of the sphere while the hydrophilic parts (typically consisting of a polyethylene glycol (PEG) group) locate to the aqueous environment [16]. Film casting, direct dispersion, dialysis, and oil in water emulsion procedures are used for micellar nanocarrier preparation [14].

Nanogels are hydrogels with nanometer-scale, which possess physically or chemically crosslinked three-dimensional network structures consisting of hydrophilic polymers [17, 18]. Controlled drug release, swelling and degradation properties, large surface area, high water content, flexible size, availability of various polymers, ease of alteration of their characteristics, and response to various environmental stimuli have rendered nanogels formulations advantageous for delivery of all biologically active agents [17, 18]. Polymerization of monomers, physical self-assembly of interactive polymers, cross-linking of preformed polymers, and emulsion photopolymerization are some of the nanogel preparation methods [17].

Metal nanoparticles have gained considerable attention for diagnostic, imaging, and therapeutic purposes. Iron oxide and gold nanoparticles are widely investigated for cancer therapy and prepared by various methods including reduction, hydrothermal synthesis, sonolysis, and pyrolysis [19].

2. STIMULI-RESPONSIVE NANOCARRIERS

Stimuli-responsive nanocarriers are nanosized delivery vehicles and their structural composition/conformation can be modified by external or internal signals, thereby promoting cargo release at specific biological environment and make drugs bioavailable for interaction with their targets. Degradation, polymerization, isomerization, vesicles membrane fluidity, hydrolytic cleavage, and activation of supramolecular aggregation, are some of the changes that cause drug release. The major benefits of stimuli-responsive nanocarriers are precise temporal or spatial release patterns that substantially reduce side effects [20 - 23].

Stimuli-responsive nanocarriers can be designed to be sensitive to be applied as exogenous physical stimuli including hyperthermia, magnetic field, light, and ultrasound (Fig. **2**). Specific endogenous stimuli, such as an acidic pH, a higher level of certain enzymes, or an increased glutathione concentration can trigger cargo release as well (Fig. **2**) [20, 21]. In this chapter, we discuss recent patents published mainly during the past seven years in the field of stimuli-responsive nanocarriers.

3. EXTERNAL STIMULI-RESPONSIVE DRUG DELIVERY

3.1. Temperature-Responsive Nanocarriers

Hyperthermia can be applied either as high temperature for short periods (> 50°C for 10 min) often called thermal ablation or lower temperatures just above physiological condition for long periods (39-42°C for ~ 1 hour) referred to as mild hyperthermia. The former is usually used to directly kill cancer cells while the second approach is more often used to trigger drug release from thermosensitive carriers. However, both ablative and mild hyperthermia strategies have been successfully combined with thermosensitive nanoparticles [24 - 28].

Combination of temperature-triggered release nanocarriers and hyperthermia (commonly mild hyperthermia) can improve cancer therapy by various mechanisms including enhanced blood flow, increased tumor perfusion and drug or nanoparticle penetration into the tumor, triggering drug release from heat-triggered nanoformulations within the tumor vasculature and interstitium, increased tumor cell membrane permeability and drug cellular uptake, and increased susceptibility of cancer cells to chemotherapy [25, 29 - 31].

Internal stimuli   **External stimuli**

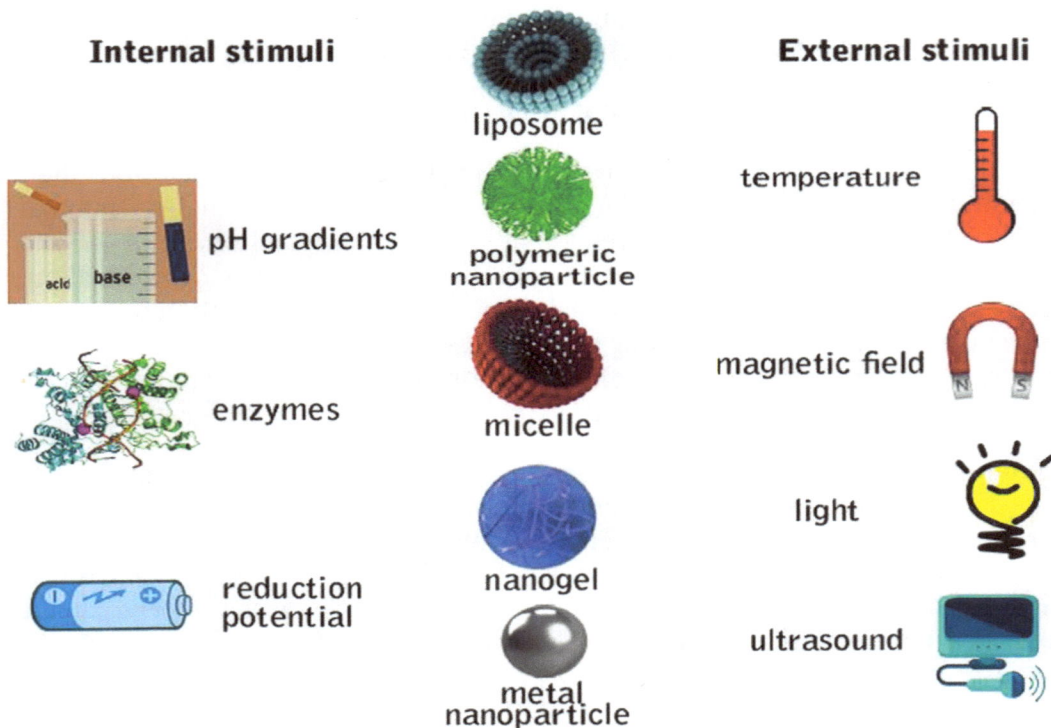

liposome

pH gradients

polymeric
nanoparticle   temperature

enzymes

micelle   magnetic field

reduction
potential   nanogel   light

metal
nanoparticle   ultrasound

Fig. (2). Schematic for stimuli-responsive nanocarriers triggered upon external or internal stimulation and main classes of responsive nanostructures.

The success of thermosensitive nanocarrier researches has beenrelied on the accurate, effective, and safe control of temperature elevations in target tumor tissues. Various modes of heating such as regional hyperthermia with heated water baths (mainly used in preclinical studies), external electromagnetic applicators, localized interstitial hyperthermia electrodes, high-intensity focused ultrasound (FUS), and magnetic resonance-guided FUS have been used to trigger drug release and reviewed elsewhere [24, 29].

Traditional thermosensitive liposomes (TSL) are composed of lipids (mainly dipalmitoylphosphatidylcholine, DPPC) that undergo a gel to liquid phase transition at a few degrees above 37°C. More recently, lysolipids, surfactants (the Brij family of nonionic surfactants), and synthetic temperature-responsive polymers have been used for the design of TSL [29, 32, 33].

One of the most advanced thermosensitive nanoformulations is lysolipid-based

TSL under the trade name of ThermoDox® (Celsion Corp.),which is currently in different clinical trial phases for hepatocellular carcinoma and recurrent breast cancer [34, 35]. A recent invention described the lysolipid enriched TSL that was composed of: i) DPPC (or one/a combination of other phosphatidylcholines, phosphatidylinositols, phosphatidylglycerols, and phosphatidylethanolamines); ii) one or more lysolipids, and iii) one or more phospholipids derivatized with a hydrophilic polymer at a molar ratio of about 80-90:2-18:2-8. The size of nanoliposomes varied from ~50 to ~150nm. It has been claimed that by using the ammonium sulfate buffer for liposomes preparation, long-term stability under storage temperatures of $\leq 8°C$ was achieved [36].

Li's group described an invention of TSL composed of DPPC and a compound with $C_{17}H_{35}(CH_2)_p(CO)_q(OCH_2CH_2)_nOH$ formula (polyethoxylated surfactants), wherein p and q are both selected from 0 or 1; p + q = 1; and n is an integer selected from about 10 to about 100. This compound was reported to be preferably Brij78 and the optimum liposome formulation was prepared by 96:4 molar ratio of DPPC and Brij78 (Fig. **3**). Drug release profiles at normothermic and hyperthermic conditions, intracellular uptake, pharmacokinetic profile, and *in vivo* anticancer efficacy were reported. Compared to lysolipid enriched TSL, this formulation resulted in a 1.4-fold increase in tumor doxorubicin content. Intratumoral cargo release was monitored by Magnetic Resonance Imaging (MRI) contrast agents (Gd^{3+} or Mn^{2+}) [37, 38].

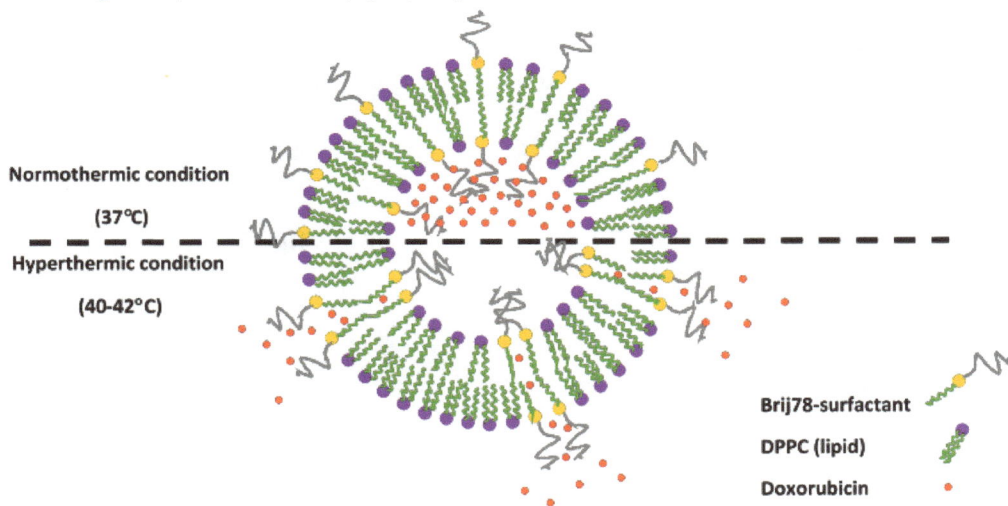

Normothermic condition

(37°C)

Hyperthermic condition

(40-42°C)

Brij78-surfactant

DPPC (lipid)

Doxorubicin

Fig. (3). Schematic of TSL formulated with DPPC and a Brij surfactant (Brij 78) with stability at 37°C and enhanced drug release at mild hyperthermic temperatures (40-42°C). Redrawn with modification from Ref. [38].

Most TSL researches have focused on hydrophilic drugs. Hydrophobic drugs such as paclitaxel, docetaxel, etc. are difficult to encapsulate and retain in the liposomal lumen cavity and modulate cargo release by hyperthermia. A recent invention described rendering of a hydrophobic drug into a hydrophilic prodrug and encapsulation within aqueous medium of TSL or polymersome. In this patent, the hydrophilic prodrug composed of a hydrolysable hydrophilic group can release the active form of the drug. For example, docetaxel modified with N-methy--piperazinyl butanoic acid was encapsulated in TSL or polymersomes [39].

Temperature-sensitive polymers display Lower Critical Solution Temperature (LCST) behavior. Below the LCST, the polymers are soluble, and above the LCST they become insoluble, causing the gel formation [40]. Temperature can either trigger the content release of micelles or facilitate micelles assembly. Poly(N-isopropylacrylamide) (polyNIPAM) has been intensively investigated for this approach. However, polyNIPAM based micelles are not biodegradable. In addition to thermoresponsive behavior, biodegradablity and biocompatibility are among the desirable characteristics of thermoresponsive delivery systems [40]. On the other hand, cationic nature would be beneficial for *in vivo* application as the carrier can electrostatically bind to anionic biological and/or biochemical species. Another invention that addressed the design of cationic, thermoresponsive, biodegradable, and biocompatible carrier was prepared from unsaturated pluronic diacrylate/ unsaturated L-arginine base poly(ester-amide) (PluronicDA/UArg-PEA) hybrid hydrogels by UV-induced photopolymerization of different weight ratios of the two polymers. The hybrid carrier can be used to deliver and/or release various compounds. Thermal responsiveness of this carrier was contributed to PluronicDA. Paclitaxel was successfully loaded into the hydrogel. The thermoresponsive swelling behavior of the hydrogel over a wide range of temperature was due to the inner core structure of Pluronic micelles [41].

There are various patented studies on thermosensitive liposomes, micelles, and polymeric nanoparticles (Table 1) [36, 37, 39, 42 - 52].

Table 1. Summary of Patents on Temperature-Responsive Nanocarriers.

Patent No.	Formulation Type	Drug(s)	*In vivo* Model	Cancer Type	Description	Ref.
US20130230457	Liposome	Doxorubicin			Comprising liposomes consisting of phospholipids and a surfactant (lysolipid)	[36]

(Table 1) cont.....

Patent No.	Formulation Type	Drug(s)	*In vivo Model*	Cancer Type	Description	Ref.
US8642074	Liposome	Docetaxel, Carboplatin	BALB/c mice	Lung cancer	Comprising vesicles composed of phosphatidylcholine, phosphatidylglycerol, and lysolipid	[42]
EP2670394	Liposome				Comprising iron oxide nanoparticles loaded into thermosensitive liposomes	[43]
WO2012055020	Liposome	Doxorubicin, Gemcitabine	EMT-6 tumor-bearing mice	Pancreatic cancer, lung cancer, mammary cancer	Comprising liposomes composed of DPPC and Brij surfactants	[37]
US20110190623	Liposome				Comprising thermoregulatable nanocarriers composed of polymerized and unpolymerized lipids	[44]
EP2667848	Liposome/ polymersome	Docetaxel			Comprising liposomes or polymersomes containing a hydrophilic prodrug of a hydrophobic drug	[39]
US8685382	Micelles	Paclitaxel			Comprising temperature-sensitive and solubility-changeable polymers (particularly poly (hydroxyalkyl(meth) acrylamide mono/di-lactate) by incubation	[45]
WO2011047486	Micelles/hydrogel				Comprising copolymers composed of polyethylene glycol and polycaprolactone	[46]
WO2016090103	Micelles/gel	Gemcitabine			Comprising biodegradable polymers having tunable LCST	[47]

(Table 1) cont.....

Patent No.	Formulation Type	Drug(s)	*In vivo* Model	Cancer Type	Description	Ref.
US8858998	Micelles/hydrogel	Paclitaxel			Comprising hydrogel composed of pluronic and L-arginine base poly(ester-amide)	[41]
WO2016207296	Nanogel	Doxorubicin, Methotrexate	Nude mice	Ovarian cancer	Comprising a semi-interpenetrating or an interpenetrating network formed from a charged component and a conjugated polymer	[48]
US8153612	Nanogel		Rat		Comprising a chitosan composition forming a hydrogel	[49]
US20160303241	Hydrogel/nanogel		Rat		Comprising ROS degradable ABC triblock terpolymer	[50]
EP2813213	Hydrogel containing inorganic nanoparticles				Comprising a dispersion of nanoparticles linked to a copolymer composed of an osmotically active polymer block and a thermoresponsive polymer block	[51]
WO2017020025	Bioconjugate		Male C57BL/6J mice		Comprising an elastin-like peptide, a molecule susceptible to form an oligomer, and a linker part	[52]

3.2. Magnetic Field-Responsive Nanocarriers

Magnetic drug hybrid nanocarrier is another physical approach employed to advance nanoparticle based cancer therapy. By applying external magnetic fields, targeted guidance of the nanocarriers, hyperthermia or magnetic triggered cargo release, and *in vivo* tracking by MRI can be achieved (Fig. **4**). These multifunctional features of magnetic nanostructures make them as a promising theranostic carrier in which diagnostic and therapeutic agents are combined. In the approach of drug delivery, in most researches, polymeric nanoparticles, liposomes, micelles, and silica nanoparticles are merged with magnetic nanocrystals to prepare magnetic nanocarriers [53 - 56]. First, the heat produced by the magnetic nanocrystals under alternating magnetic field promotes drug release triggering and can subsequently enhance therapeutic drug efficacy due to the synergistic effect of dual hyperthermia and chemotherapy application [53]. Second, the magnetic nanoparticles incorporation offers the potential to remotely control and target the nanosystems in the body to tumor by an external magnet [57, 58]. Third, magnetic nanocrystals as T_2 (negative) contrast agents for MRI can make the hybrid system trackable [54].

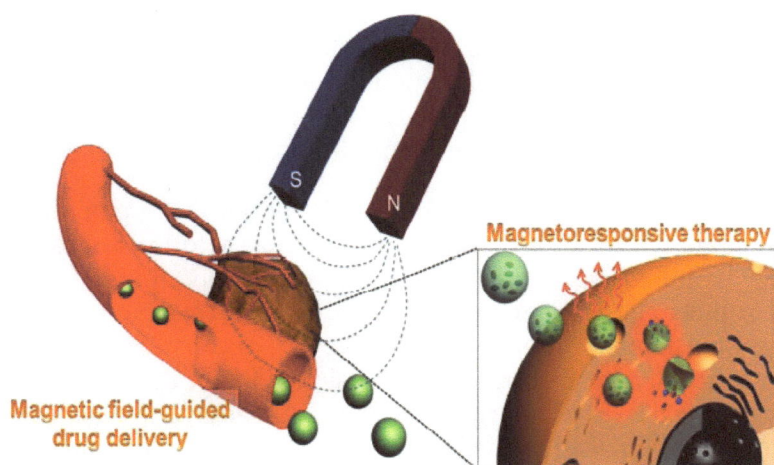

Fig. (4). Schematic of magnetic field-responsive nanocarriers. By applying external magnetic fields, targeted guided delivery, hyperthermia or magnetic triggered cargo release, and *in vivo* imaging can be achieved using magnetic nanoparticles. Figure reproduced with modification from Ref [59]. with permission. Copyright (2015) American Chemical Society.

Numerous materials, such as Fe, Ni, and Co metallic nanoparticles and their oxide, have been studied for their potential use in magnetoresponsive nanosystems [59]. Pure metals and Co metallic nanoparticles showed higher saturation magnetization as well as better magnetic response, however, safety concern, high toxicity, and poor chemical stability (quick oxidation process) have limited their biomedical applications. Gadolinium- or iodine-based contrast agents are hazardous for chronic kidney disease patients. Therefore, a safer replacement is required. Among many types of magnetic nanoparticles, magnetic iron oxides, maghemite (γ-Fe$_2$O$_3$) and magnetite (Fe$_3$O$_4$), are the most used components in magnetoresponsive nanostructures due to good chemical stability, good biocompatibility, low toxicity, Specific Absorption Rate (SAR) values, magnetic properties, and ease of preparation and surface functionalization [56, 57, 60, 61]. Magnetic particles can be divided into two main groups of paramagnetic nanoparticles (> 100nm) and superparamagnetic iron oxide nanoparticles

(SPIONs) (< 100nm). SPIONs show superparamagnetic behavior at size less than 30nm [62].

Various methods have been investigated for magnetic nanoparticle synthesis. The hydrolytic co-precipitation and the non-hydrolytic thermal decomposition are widely used techniques. In the first method, aqueous solutions of metallic ingredients are rapidly mixed with reducing agents in the presence of surfactants. In spite of easy scale-up for industrial production, uncontrollable generation of nanoparticles with inhomogeneous sizes and shapes was a major disadvantage of this method. In the non-hydrolytic thermal decomposition method, heating of a metallic precursor in an organic solvent containing appropriate surfactants caused thermal decomposition of the components and formation of finely tuned crystalline nanoparticles in terms of size, composition, and shape [19, 63].

In parallel with design and characterization of ThermoDox® patented by Celsion company, magnetic liposomes (also called magnetoliposomes) have been introduced by pioneering study of De Cuyper and Joniau in 1988 [64]. Magnetoliposomes can be prepared by either incorporation of hydrophobic magnetic nanoparticles in liposomal bilayer or encapsulation of hydrophilic magnetic nanoparticles in aqueous core of vesicle. One of the main applications of magnetic liposomes is hyperthermia mediated "on-demand" release properties controlled by an externally applied Alternating Current (AC) magnetic field at target site. As the triggered release property relies on a change in permeability of the lipidic membrane rather than the vesicle destruction, repetitive switching on and off can also be achieved [65, 66].

In a very recent patent, a theranostic liposome was composed of phospholipids, magnetic nanoparticles (with 2-10nm in size), a therapeutic agent, an imaging label, and at least one active agent. The lipid bilayer was made of 10-45mol% sphingomyelin. Sphingomyelinase mediated drug release is another possible strategy for specific drug delivery. This enzyme is involved in cell stress response pathways. Elevated activity is often observed in pathologic conditions such as tumors, inflammation, and necrosis. In this study, cargo release was triggered by enzymatic degradation of phospholipids and the release rate was further amplified by applying AC magnetic field. Sphingomyelin liposomes encapsulating 5nm Fe_3O_4 nanoparticles was tested in a mouse model of SCC4 oral squamous cell carcinoma exposed to AC magnetic field [67].

Magnetic nanoparticles can be encapsulated in polymeric nanoparticles. In a recent study, PLGA polymer and hydrophobic drugs (zotarolimus, everolimus, or sirolimus) dissolved in chloroform were mixed with hydrophobic magnetite. The mixture was added to a 2.5% polyvinyl alcohol (PVA) solution. After probe sonication and centrifugation nanosized polymeric magnetic nanoparticles (< 200nm) were prepared [68].

In another patent, magnetic polymeric nanocomposites were prepared from PLGA (39%), human serum albumin (39%), magnetite nanoparticles (1%), 5-FU (20%) and a fluorescent marker,1,6-diphenyl-1,3,5-hexatriene (DPH), (1%). Squamous-cell carcinoma was the tumor model and albumin and magnetic nanoparticles were used as the driving forces for targeted delivery to the tumor site [69].

Micelles can be engineered to be temperature-sensitive via incorporation of a thermoresponsive polymer either in the hydrophobic tail or in the head polar group. Destabilizing the micelle structure by conformational change from hydrophilic state to hydrophobic state can trigger the drug release. Magnetic micelles can be prepared from magnetic nanoparticles embedded micelles. In a recent Chinese patent, a temperature-sensitive core-shell structure was designed from iron magnetic core and co-polymer of N-isopropylacrylamide and hydrophilic allyl monomer on the surface of the magnetic particles to form the shell. The composite showed a monodisperse particle size and within the range of 30-500nm. The proposed synthesis method was simple and the materials can be produced industrially [70].

There were various patented investigations on magnetic field-responsive nanocarriers that are summarized in Table **2** [67 - 69, 71 - 81].

Table 2. Summary of Patents on Magnetic Field-Responsive Nanocarriers.

Patent No.	Formulation Type	Drug(s)	*In vivo* Model	Cancer Type	Description	Ref.
EP3139964	Liposome	Doxorubicin, Cisplatin, Paclitaxel	Nude mice	Orthotopic SCC-4 carcinoma	Comprising liposomes which release their cargo using a phospholipase and an alternating magnetic field	[67]
EP2739291	Ferriliposome	Doxorubicin, Jpm-565	Female FVB/N and MMTV-PyMT mice, rat	Breast cancer	Aqueous colloidal matrix comprising oxide ferrimagnetics with iron oxide nanoparticles having spinel structure	[71]
US9439978	Micelle		C57BL/6 mice	Prostate cancer	Comprising a hydrophobic iron oxide nanoparticle core, a cationic polymer coating and a polynucleotide as the second coating	[72]

(Table 2) cont.....

Patent No.	Formulation Type	Drug(s)	*In vivo* Model	Cancer Type	Description	Ref.
US8303990	Metal nanoparticle				Transporting a magnetically sensitive nanoparticle or a conjugated nanoparticle through the ear membrane	[73]
US8651113	Metal nanoparticle	Paclitaxel	Nude mice	HEY human ovarian carcinoma	Comprising single-domain nanoparticles consisting of magnetite	[74]
US9233163	Metal nanoparticle	Paclitaxel and its derivatives	Male Sprague-Dawley rat, athymic nu/nu mice	Neuroblastoma	Comprising a stent and magnetic nanoparticles	[75]
US20160030724	Metal nanoparticle	Taxol, Paclitaxel, Flutax-2		Ovarian carcinoma, uterine sarcoma	Comprising magneto-electric nanoparticles consisting of some ionic bonds to an active agent, a magnetic field weakened the bonds, and the active agent was released	[76]
US20170128573	Metal nanoparticle	Cisplatin		Neuroblastoma	Tumor cell destruction using photo-magnetic irradiation mediated therapy by drug-containing nanoparticles	[77]
WO2011147926	Metal nanoparticle				A vesicular structure containing stabilized magnetic nanoparticles	[78]
WO2014145573	Metal nanoparticle		BALB/c mice	Breast cancer	Comprising casein coated iron oxide nanoparticles	[79]
US20110196474	Metal nanoparticle	Zotarolimus, Everolimus, Rapamycin	New Zealand white rabbit		Comprising nanoparticles consisting of ferrous oxide, ferrite particles, rare earth particles or a material having magnetic properties, responsive to a magnetic field	[68]
US9211346	Metal nanoparticle				Comprising two carrier-linked magnetic nanoparticles, the first containing a prodrug and the second containing an agent for activating the prodrug	[80]
US20110076767	Metal nanoparticle				Comprising the matrix-forming and the coated magnetically sensitive agents, polyelectrolyte-amphiphilic agent adduct	[81]

(Table 2) cont.....

Patent No.	Formulation Type	Drug(s)	*In vivo* Model	Cancer Type	Description	Ref.
US20120265001	Metal nanoparticle	Fluorouracil, Methotrexate, Cisplatin	Nude mice	Squamous-cell carcinoma, osteosarcoma	Comprising a biodegradable polymer, a magnetic nanoparticle prepared by high shear mixing of oil-in-oil emulsion/solvent evaporation, human serum albumin as the targeting agent, and a therapeutic cargo	[69]

3.3. Photo-Responsive Nanocarriers

Among external stimuli, light offers an attractive and flexible stimulus due to its non-invasiveness and control of the treated site and applied intensity. Light in the ultraviolet (UV), visible, or near-infrared (NIR) regions has been used to illuminate photo-responsive systems. The UV light is absorbed by the skin and tissues and is unable to penetrate deeply in the body, therefore, hampering its *in vivo* application in cancer therapy. On the contrary, NIR light is non-damaging to the cells and can penetrate much deeper (10cm) [82 - 84]. In this section, photo-active nanoparticles for cancer therapy were discussed in 3 parts: i) Photodynamic Therapy (PDT), ii) Photothermal Therapy (PTT), and iii) light-triggered delivery.

PDT is a light-initiated and minimally invasive cancer treatment modality based on photo-mediated excitation of a photoactive drug (so-called a photosensitizer) resulting in localized production of ROS, induced apoptosis, and oxidative damage of nearby unwanted biological agents [85, 86]. Due to nonspecific biodistribution and hydrophobic properties of most photosensitizers, their *in vivo* applications in cancer therapy meet technical challenges. Nanoformulations of photosensitizers are attractive systems for improved and targeted delivery of photosensitizers by solubilizing and controlling their *in vivo* fate [86, 87]. Visudyne is a successful example of photosensitizer (verteporfin) liposomal formulations that is currently clinically used for macular degeneration, wet age-related myopia, and ocular histoplasmosis [88].

One issue in PDT is that most currently used photosensitizers are excited by visible or UV light. NIR, in contrast, is a good alternative owing to not only deeper penetration depths, but also lower toxicity and damage on normal cells and tissues [89].

Owing to minimal invasiveness and high selectivity, PTT is emerging as a powerful technique for cancer therapy that employs heat generated from optical energy. Photothermal agents (dye molecules or nanoparticles) with strong and stable NIR absorbance, ability to effectively convert the absorbed light energy into heat, and low toxicity are favorable. Gold based nanomaterials including gold nanoparticles, gold nanoshells, and gold nanorods are the main nanostructures used in PTT [90, 91]. Other gold-based materials, such as nanostars, nanocubes, nanohexapods, and nanocages are also emerging as photothermal agents [92].

Light is also a promising trigger which can remotely control the cargo release spatially and temporally. Light-triggered nanomaterials have been investigated to release cargoes with various mechanisms including photosensitization, photopolymerization, photocrosslinking, photooxidation, photoisomerization, or photodegradation that have been covered in recent review articles [82, 93, 94].

Azobenzenes and cinnamic acid are chemical compounds with photoisomerization capability of their cis and trans isomers. This isomerization led to nanocarrier disruption and cargo release [95, 96]. Later, the azobenzene derivatives were developed as gatekeepers. For example, tethering on mesoporous silica nanoparticle and irradiating, azobenzene moieties moved back and forward, controlling the release of the drug molecules out of the silica [97]. Photoswitchable drug release was also obtained with spiropyran derivatives [98]. Other chromophores, like pyrenyl methyl esters, coumarin, dithienylethene (DTE), stilbene, and o-nitrobenzyl were activated by UV/visible light or NIR irradiation and phase or structural changes triggered drug release [98 - 100].

In a recent patent, photoactivatable liposomes composed of DPPC and 1,2 bis (tricosa-10,12-diynoyl)-sn-glycero-3-phosphocholine (DC(8,9)PC) encapsulating the anticancer PDT drug, 2-(1-Hexyloxyethyl)-2-devinyl pyropheophorbide-a (HPPH), were prepared and activated by a cw-diode 660nm laser. HPPH was utilized to promote liposome membrane destabilization [101].

A light-activatable polymeric nanoparticle composed of a polycation (e.g. poly(ethyleneimine)), a polyanion (e.g. dextran sulphate), and a photo-sensitive photochrome (an o-nitrobenzyl alcohol derivative or coumarin) attached to the polyanion or the polycation was designed and activated by UV light or a blue laser for use in the leukemia treatment [99].

Targeted and light-activated mesoporous silica nanoparticles were proposed for cytosolic delivery of cell-impermeable molecules to multidrug-resistant cells. Streptavidin-functionalized particles were internalized by endocytosis and then the cells were exposed to green excitation light (520-550nm) that mediated endosomal membrane damage (Fig. **5**) [102, 103].

Various light-sensitive nanostructures have been investigated such as liposomes, silica nanoparticles, polymeric nanoparticles, and gold nanostructures (Table **3**) [97, 99 - 101, 104 - 111].

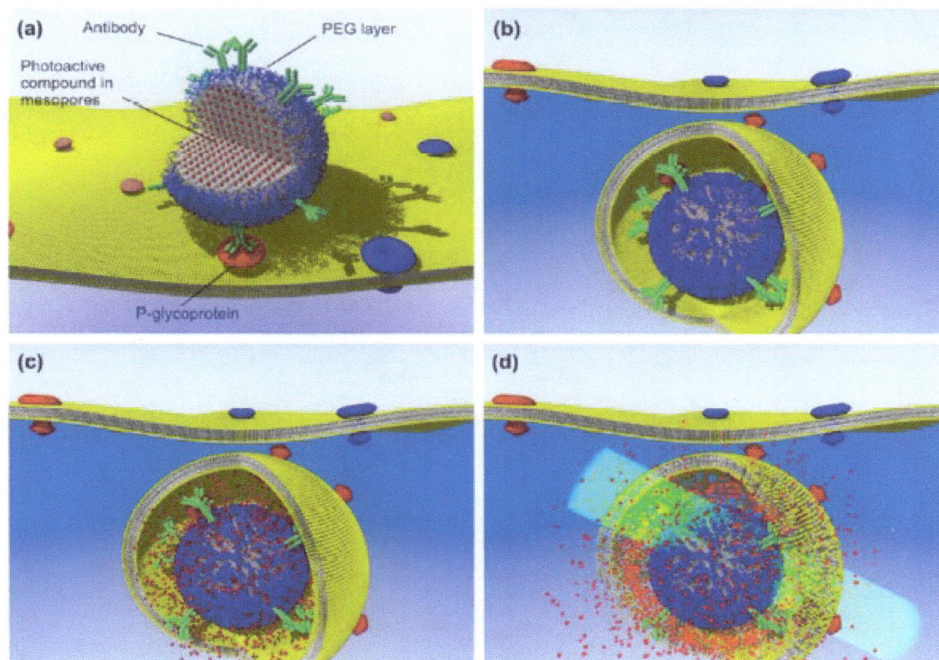

Fig. (5). Schematic of targeted and light-activated nanoparticles proposed for cytosolic delivery of cell-impermeable molecules. (a) Antibody decorated particle is attached to P-glycoprotein expressing cell. (b) The multifunctional nanocarrier is internalized by endocytosis. (c) The cargo is released in the endosome and (d) the cell exposed to green excitation light (520-550nm) which mediates endosomal membrane damage and cargo cytosolic delivery. Figure reprinted from Ref [103]. with permission. Copyright (2010) American Chemical Society.

Table 3. Summary of Patents on Photo-Responsive Nanocarriers.

Patent No.	Formulation Type	Drug(s)	*In vivo* Model	Cancer Type	Description	Ref.
EP3079665	Liposome	Dopamine			Comprising gold nanoshells tethered by femtosecond laser pulses	[104]
US20160136289	Liposome	Chlorin E6, Mitoxantrone, Doxorubicin	Kb xenograft-bearing mice	Nasopharyngeal carcinoma	The lipid-based nanoparticles comprising 1,2-bis(tricosa- 10,12-diynoyl)-sn-glyce-o-3-phosphocholine (DC8,9PC), DPPC, and 2-[1-hexyloxyethyl]-2-devinyl pyropheophorbide-a (HPPH)	[101]
EP3043782	Polymeric nanoparticle		Mice	Leukemia	Comprising a polycation, a polyanion and a light-responsive photochrome	[99]

(Table 3) cont.....

Patent No.	Formulation Type	Drug(s)	*In vivo* Model	Cancer Type	Description	Ref.
US9700620	Polymeric nanoparticle	Paclitaxel			NIR radiation is used to activate thermal plasticization of polymer-based particles to trigger the release of their cargo	[105]
US8652352	Micelle				Comprising a photo-responsive part selected from the group including azobenzene, stilbene, and spiropyran. Cycles of contraction and extension in their molecules can be remoted by UV-visible light	[100]
WO2012039685	Metal nanoparticle	Hypericin		Epidermoid carcinoma, nasopharyngeal carcinoma	Comprising colloidal gold nanoparticles and a light-responsive molecule is adsorbed to their surface	[106]
US20180050077	Gold nanostar	Psoralen, Protoporphyrin IX		Breast cancer	Comprising plasmonics-active nanoparticles excited in the NIR and used for photothermolysis	[107]
WO2016209936	Gold nanostar	PDL1 antibody	iPTQ mice, C57BL/6 mice, white BALB/c mice	Bladder cancer, metastatic triple negative breast cancer, murine sarcoma	Comprising the plasmonicsactive nanoparticles used in localized photothermal therapy by absorbing the photon radiation	[108]
US20170095418	Silica nanoparticle	Camptothecin		Pancreatic cancer, colon cancer	Comprising a nano-device with impellers for capture and release of molecules	[97]
US20170000887	Upconversion nanoparticle		Female BALB/c nude mice	Oral squamous cell carcinoma, mouse leukemia	Comprising the upconversion nanoparticles which upconvert NIR light to different wavelengths and activate the TiO_2 layer to produce ROS	[109]
WO2017029501	Quantum dot nanoparticle				Comprising 5aminolevulinic acid conjugated nanoparticles	[110]
US20130289520	Silica nanoparticle			Glioma	Cytosolic delivery of cell-impermeable compounds	[111]

3.4. Ultrasound-Responsive Nanocarriers

Ultrasound is a promising non-invasive theranostic modality that can be used to track *in vivo* fate of therapeutics carriers, trigger cargo release, enhance permeability of blood-tissue barriers, increase cell membrane permeability, and improve drug delivery to tumors with high spatial precision. Ultrasound wave penetration through a tissue has several physical effects including simple pressure variation, cavitation, acoustic fluid streaming, and hyperthermia which can be used as triggers for ultrasound-responsive carriers. Low-frequency ultrasound refers to frequencies < 1MHz, while the medium and high frequencies refer to 1-5MHz and > 5MHz, respectively. Low-frequency ultrasound may trigger drug release more effectively and penetrate deeper into tissues. A careful balance of acoustic parameters is critical in the design of ultrasound-sensitive carriers to achieve proper stimuli responsiveness without causing damage to tissues and cells. Mostly, nanocarriers are fairly transparent to ultrasound. Therefore, echogenic vesicles and acoustically active carriers containing a gas phase are designed in order to respond to ultrasound [112, 113].

Liposomes are not ultrasound-sensitive unless they contain or link to a gas phase, which makes them responsive to ultrasound stimuli and promotes their content release. To prepare ultrasound-responsive liposomes, various strategies including encapsulating an internal gas bubble, attaching bubbles to the liposomal exterior parts, a liquid phase changeable to a gas bubble upon insonation embedding inside liposomes, and bubbles residing in the close proximity of liposomes have been used (Fig. **6**) that were reviewed by Husseini *et al.* [112]. In a novel strategy, Pitt and Husseini proposed an emulsion-containing liposome (eLiposome) [114]. A nanodroplet phase transforming to a gas at low pressure was encapsulated inside the liposome. eLiposomes were around 600-700nm and encapsulated perfluorohexane emulsion droplets with a size range of ~111-164nm. These vesicles were also decorated with folate to achieve specific delivery to target cells [114].

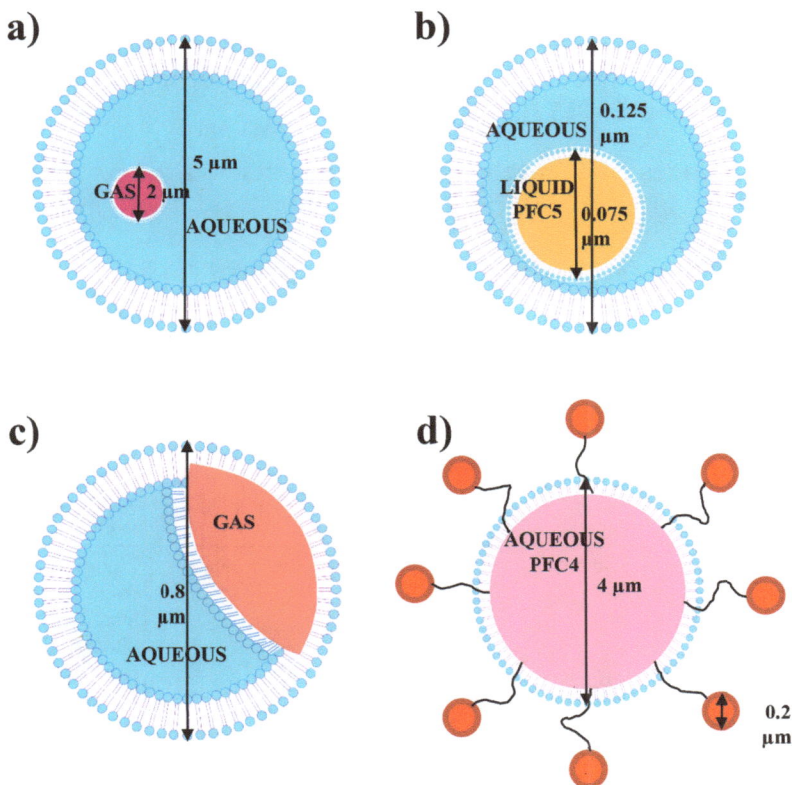

Fig. (6). Schematic of various designs of ultrasound-sensitive liposomes. (a) Liposome encapsulating an internal gas bubble; (b) eLiposome; (c) Echogenic liposome; (d) Liposome loaded microbubble. Relative sizes are not to scale. Redrawn with modification from Ref. [112].

A novel ultrasound-responsive polymeric nanoparticle prepared from suitable polymers such as polystyrene, poly(methyl methacrylate), and poly(2-hydroxyethyl methacrylate) was reported. The vesicle was capable of trapping and stabilizing gas and initiate detectable cavitation activity upon ultrasound exposure. The passive acoustic mapping indicated nanocup accumulation at the tumor following intravascular injection in CT-26 murine colorectal cancer model [115].

Micelles were also studied as ultrasound-sensitive carriers. Pluronic®P105 micellar carriers have been found to be ideal for ultrasound-mediated cargo release since low-frequency ultrasound can perturb the micelles and cause the drug release [116].

A recent patent described drug loaded nanoemulsions that converted into microbubbles upon ultrasound triggering at the tumor site. Nanoemulsions comprising one fluoroether and a block copolymer of hydrophilic block and hydrophobic block were described. Paclitaxel and doxorubicin were loaded into nanoemulsions. This modality showed anticancer efficacy in ovarian and pancreatic tumor models [117].

Table **4** summarizes the recent granted patents on ultrasound-responsive nanocarriers [114, 115, 117 - 129].

Table 4. Summary of Patents on Ultrasound-Responsive Nanocarriers.

Patent No.	Formulation Type	Drug(s)	*In vivo* Model	Cancer Type	Description	Ref.
US20130041311	Liposome		Male CD-1 mice		Comprising liposomes, microbubbles, and hydrogel-forming agents, responsive to ultrasound	[118]
US20150064114	Liposome	Sorafenib		Breast cancer	Liposomes responsive to one or more types of ultrasound such as High-Intensity Focused Ultrasound (HIFU)	[119]

(Table 4) cont.....

Patent No.	Formulation Type	Drug(s)	*In vivo* Model	Cancer Type	Description	Ref.
WO2015200576	Liposome				Comprising a temperature-responsive liposome which is triggered by focused ultrasound for delivery across the blood-brain barrier	[120]
US8999295	eLiposome				Comprising liposomes comprising a phase transforming liquid having vapor pressure which can form a gas at low pressure	[114]
CA2930815	Polymeric nanoparticle		BALB/c mice	Colorectal cancer	Comprising a cup, a gas pocket in its cavity, responsive to ultrasound excitation	[115]
WO2015089154	Polymeric nanoparticle	Doxorubicin		Lung cancer	Localized activation of nanoparticles comprising an inactive form of a therapeutic agent	[121]
WO2012066334	Polymeric nanoparticle				Comprising targeted delivery of nanoparticles and insonating the tissue	[122]
US20130204181	Micelle		BALB/c mice, Sprague-Dawley rat		Comprising ultrasound-triggered micelles containing hydrophobic drug, detectable by magnetic resonance imaging	[123]
WO2018026958	Micelle	Thymoquinone		Lung cancer, breast cancer	Comprising nanoemulsions responsive to the high pressure and short bursts of ultrasound	[124]

(Table 4) cont.....

Patent No.	Formulation Type	Drug(s)	*In vivo* Model	Cancer Type	Description	Ref.
US9427466	Metal nanoparticle		Male NOD/SCID mice	Lung carcinoma, breast adenocarcinoma	Comprising gold or magnetic nanoparticles responsive to a low to medium power ultrasound	[125]
US20170007699	Metal nanoparticle		Mice	Squamous cell carcinoma, liver tumor	A sonosensitizer composition comprising titanium dioxide particles as an active agent	[126]
EP2346996	Nanotube			Breast adenocarcinoma, cervical carcinoma	Comprising magnetic nanoparticles which Low-Intensity Pulsed Ultrasound (LIPUS) can increase their membrane's permeability	[127]
US8709451	Nanoemulsion	Paclitaxel, Doxorubicin	Nu/nu mice	Pancreatic cancer, breast cancer, ovarian cancer	Comprising one or more fluoroether and a copolymer including hydrophilic and hydrophobic blocks	[117]
EP2120722	Microbubble	Trastuzumab			Comprising particles sensitive to an ultrasonic pulse	[128]
US20140046181	Polymeric, metal, and lipidic nanoparticles	Doxorubicin	Mice		Comprising a membrane enveloping an acoustic sensitizer particle	[129]

4. INTERNAL STIMULI-RESPONSIVE DRUG DELIVERY

4.1. pH-Responsive Nanocarriers

pH-sensitive nanocarriers trigger efficient release of cargoes in response to low pH. They have been designed to be stable at neutral pH, but under acidic conditions, they become leaky. They target acidity of tumor tissues or endosomal pH in tumor cells. The pH of bloodstream and extracellular fluid of normal tissues is approximately 7.4 while pH of the extracellular environment in a solid tumor can be reduced as low as 6 [130 - 132]. Uncontrolled cell growth, reduced lymphatic network, abnormal vascularization, and poor tissue perfusion are frequently associated with hypoxia and inadequate nutrient delivery. In this condition, most tumor cells use glycolysis to produce the requested energy and consequently result in high lactate concentration. Reduced tumor blood flow and lack of functional lymphatics lead to increased accumulation and impaired clearance of lactic acid and low extracellular pH in the tumor microenvironment [133, 134]. However, designing nanocarriers to disrupt or destabilize in response to such a narrow pH change (~ 1 unit) are technically challenging [130]. On the other hand, after binding to cancer cells, nanoparticles can be internalized through endocytosis pathways and remain trapped in endosomal and lysosomal compartments with pH ranges from 4.5 to 6.5 (mainly due to the activity of vacuolar-type proton ATPase) [135]. The great potential of pH-responsive drug nanostructures in improving anticancer treatments lies in their ability in destabilization or fusion after cell internalization at the endosomal stage. By cargo delivery into cytoplasm, lysosomal sequestration and degradation, enzymatic instability, and limited intracellular delivery of macromolecules and low permeable drugs can be overcome. The escape process of endocytosed molecules to the cytosol prior to the lysosomal degradation, known as 'endosomal escape', results in enhanced drug bioavailability at intracellular target site. This may also lead to releasing drug payload far from the transmembrane efflux pumps, thereby at least partly circumventing drug resistance development in tumor cells [136 - 138].

pH-sensitive liposomes were most commonly prepared from dioleoylphos-phatidylethanolamine (DOPE). DOPE has a cone shape and by itself cannot form lipid bilayers at neutral pH. To form liposomal bilayer, DOPE is usually combined with amphiphilic molecules with a protonatable acidic group, such as cholesteryl hemisuccinate (CHEMS) and oleic acid. The other approaches to prepare pH-sensitive liposomes are by either incorporation of pH-sensitive polymers such as N-isopropylacrylamide [139, 140], poly(glycidol)s [141, 142], and poly(alkyl acrylic acid)s [143, 144] or fusogenic peptides such as haemagglutinin, gp41, diINF-7, listeriolysin O, diphtheria toxin, ricin, saporin, GALA, KALA, and surfactants [145].

In a recent patent, a novel pH-sensitive polydiacetylene liposome composed of DOPE, 10,12-pentacosadiynoic acid, and N-palmitoyl homocysteine was introduced for anticancer drug delivery. As the pH value decreased, a liposome-liposome fusion caused changes in shape and size of vesicles allowing selective drug release. For example, Transmission Electron Microscopy (TEM) images and size monitoring showed liposome size increased from 110nm to 2047nm while the pH value changes from 7.4 to 3.3 [146].

The anionic character of CHEMS prevented efficient cellular internalization of liposomes. Therefore, CHEMS containing anionic liposomes are barely suitable for the macromolecules transport into cells. Some studies were focused on synthesis of compounds to overcome this problem and prepare cationic pH-sensitive liposomes [147, 148].

Saltzman and his coworkers designed an efficient and safe polymeric gene delivery system. The system was based on quaterpolymers with favorable properties such as acid sensitivity, biodegradability, low cationic charge, and high hydrophobicity. Polymers containing ortho ester groups showed remarkable acid-sensitive degradation at low pH of endosomal compartment, facilitated efficient endosomal escape of its genetic cargo, and gene delivery to a variety of cells. A lyophilized nanoformulation was also developed for improved storage stability [149].

pH-responsive polymeric micelles are prepared by using acid-liable linkages (hydrazone linkage) or attachment of reversible protonation-deprotonation units into the block copolymers [150, 151]. pH-sensitive mixed micelles composed of poly(L-histidine)-poly(ethylene glycol) block copolymer and poly(L-lactic acid)-poly(ethylene glycol) block copolymer were described. The PEG portion had a molecular weight of at least about 2,000 and the poly(L-histidine) portion had a molecular weight of at least about 5,000 [152].

To improve cancer treatment efficacy by combined photothermal/chemotherapy, a pH-responsive nanoparticle was made of PLGA as the hydrophobic cores and a pH-responsive N-acetyl histidine modified D-α-tocopheryl polyethylene glycol succinate shells. The system was used for co-delivery of indocyanine green, a photothermal agent, and doxorubicin The nanocarrier showed surface charge switchable property when pH was changed from 7.4 to 5.0 leading to improve the interaction of the nanoparticle and cancer cells in tumor microenvironment [153]. A polymeric nanoparticle composed of hyperbranched polyglycerol / tri(ethylene glycol) divinyl ether/drug was designed to prepare pH-sensitive carrier [154].

Nanosized hydrogels with fast phase transition and adjustable swelling kinetics can be utilized for drug delivery. A recent patent described combination of pH-responsive characteristics of acrylic based polymers with biodegradable properties of starch. The terpolymer containing poly(methacrylic acid) and Tween 80 was covalently grafted onto starch for co-delivery of anticancer drug and imaging agents. To facilitate brain delivery of the nanocarrier, the Tween 80 content of the nanosystem was optimized. Doxorubicin hydrochloride was loaded into nanoparticles and up to 19-fold decrease in IC50 in drug-resistant cell lines was observed in the invention. The targetability of drug loaded nanoparticles to brain metastasis model of triple negative human breast cancer was investigated using whole body and *ex vivo* fluorescence imaging of the brain. Treatment with the nanosystem reduced tumor growth in murine breast cancer tumor model compared to free drug (Fig. **7**) [155]. A mucoadhesive polymeric delivery device composed of chitosan and PEG for cisplatin targeted delivery to oral locations, such as mouth cancer cells, was developed. The nanoparticle encapsulation masked unpleasant metallic flavor of cisplatin and PEG coating for enhanced penetration through the mucosa as well as attachment of a targeting ligand. High loading (> 30%), efficient drug encapsulation (> 80%), and higher release rate in acidic pH (~5.5) compared to physiological pH (~7) were achieved. The IC_{50} values against hamster cheek pouch carcinoma cells were around 2.3nM for cisplatin-loaded nanoparticles compared to 0.06µM for free drug. The *in vivo* efficacy results showed that the cisplatin loaded nanoparticles reduced tumor size and showed higher drug accumulation [156, 157].

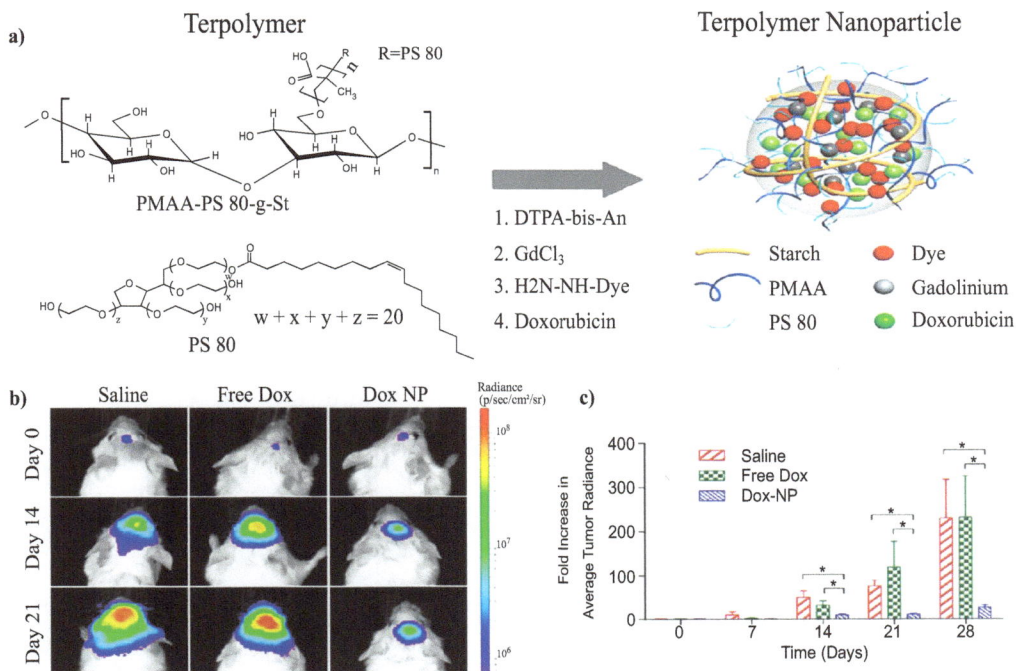

Fig. (7). (**a**) Structures of the terpolymer and Tween 80, and a schematic of the self-assembly into nanoparticles. (**b**) *In vivo* imaging of brain tumor. (**c**) *In vivo* efficacy in murine breast cancer tumor model. Figure reprinted from Ref [157]. with permission. Copyright (2014) American Chemical Society.

A recently published patent described peptide based pH-sensitive nanocarriers. The peptides were composed of pH-sensitive hydrophilic and hydrophobic amino acids in the backbone. The insoluble peptide at a pH of 7.0-8.0 became soluble as the pH environment changes to a weakly acidic (pH 6.5-6.9) releasing the biological substance. The amino acid sequence was composed of one or more nonpolar amino acids and one or more histidines [158].

To date, various nanoparticles including liposomes, micelles, and polymeric nanoparticles have been developed to respond to either low extracellular pH in tumors or acidic endosomal compartments (Table **5**) [146, 149, 152 - 156, 158 - 169].

Table 5. Summary of Patents on pH-Responsive Nanocarriers.

Patent No.	Formulation Type	Drug(s)	*In vivo* Model	Cancer Type	Description	Ref.
US20110027171	Liposome				Liposomes with targeting ligands having the ability of becoming 'hidden' or 'exposed' responding to the pH change	[159]
US20140220115	Liposome	Cisplatin, Rituxan		Breast cancer, cervical cancer, lymphoma, multiple myeloma, breast adenocarcinoma, ovary adenocarcinoma, nasopharyngeal epidermal carcinoma	Co-encapsulation of arsenic-based and platinum-based drugs	[160]
EP2870959	Liposome	Ampicillin			Comprising a polydiacetylene liposome composed of 10,12-pentacosadiynoic acid (PCDA), 1,2-dioleoyl-sn-glycero-3-phospho-ethanolamine (DOPE), and N-palmitoyl homocysteine (PHC)	[146]
CA2865925	Polymeric nanoparticle	Doxorubicin, Omniscan	BALB/c mice, EMT6/WT tumor bearing mice	Breast cancer	Comprising starch based nanoparticles	[155]
WO2014130866	Polymeric nanoparticle	Cisplatin	Golden Syrian hamster, Nude mice	Hamster cheek pouch carcinoma, hypopharyngeal carcinoma	A mucoadhesive matrix such as chitosan nanoparticles containing various agents	[156]
US20160367489	Polymeric nanoparticle	Doxorubicin	Male C57BL/6J mice	Prostate cancer	Comprising a pH-sensitive polymer and a poly(lactic-glycolic acid)	[153]
US8945629	Polymeric nanoparticle	Cisplatin	Mice	Adenocarcinoma, ovarian cancer	Comprising water-soluble polymers and co-polymers	[161]

(Table 5) cont.....

Patent No.	Formulation Type	Drug(s)	*In vivo* Model	Cancer Type	Description	Ref.
US9687563	Polymeric nanoparticle	Lonidamine, Paclitaxel	Mice	Ovarian carcinoma	Comprising peptides having hydrophilic and hydrophobic amino acids which are pH-sensitive	[158]
US9532956	Polymeric nanoparticle			Oral cancer, prostate cancer, prostate adenocarcinoma, nasopharyngeal epidermoid carcinoma	Comprising particles having a cleavable bond component and a fluorescence resonance energy transfer moiety which are responsive to pH and redox changes	[162]
US9895451	Polymeric nanoparticle			Glioblastoma	Comprising a polymeric formulation which low pH can trigger its fast degradation	[149]
WO2012070033	Polymeric implant	Methotrexate, Folic acid			Comprising a polymer composition consisting of poly(methyl vinyl ether), an inorganic salt and the particles formed from chitosan and Eudragit	[163]
US20120003322	Micelle				A polyion complex type micelle made by electrostatic interaction between two polymers having opposite charges	[164]
WO2013127949	Micelle	Docetaxel		Cervix carcinoma	Polylactide-poly (ethylene glycol) copolymers for drug delivery and imaging	[165]
US7951846	Micelle	Doxorubicin	BALB/c nude mice	Breast cancer, lung carcinoma	Mixed micelles comprising poly(L-histidine)- poly(ethylene glycol) and poly(L-lactic acid)-poly(ethylene glycol) block copolymers	[152]
US8911775	Micelle			Breast carcinoma	Copolymerization of polyethylene glycol, poly(amino acid) and heterocyclic alkyl amine compounds inducing the ionic complex formation	[166]
US9080049	Micelle				Comprising micelles prepared by inducing a copolymer of poly (β-amino ester) composites	[167]
US20130217789	Liquogel	Fulvestrant, Camptothecin		Breast cancer	Comprising hyperbranched polyglycerols	[154]
EP2559429	Metal nanoparticle	Doxorubicin		Murine melanoma, breast cancer	Metal nanoparticles which aggregate to release the agent	[168]
US9675629	Metal nanoparticle	Doxorubicin		Cervical cancer	Metal-catechol derivative nanoparticle based on a mussel adhesive protein	[169]

4.2. Enzyme-Responsive Nanocarriers

Enzymes have major roles in all biological and metabolic processes, and therefore are important targets in therapeutics and drug development. In some pathological conditions, such as cancer, inflammation, and infection, the concentrations of different extracellular and intracellular enzymes are elevated. In some cases, enzymatic activity is associated with a specific tissue. Enzyme-responsive nanocarriers can be designed to undergo structural transformation and programmed to release the encapsulated cargoes by the biochemical abnormality or the specific enzyme activity [170 - 172]. Under these conditions, enzyme-responsive cargo delivery is achieved mainly by either nanocarrier degradation and disruption or nanomaterial surface changes [173].

Enzyme-responsive nanomaterials have a number of advantages: i) controlling the payload release achieved by an enzyme with exceptional selectivity for substrates at the target site with no need for any external equipment for triggering; ii) most enzymes catalyze chemical reactions under mild conditions (buffered aqueous solutions, neutral pH, and physiological temperature); iii) the severity of the pathological condition is usually proportional to the concentration of active enzymes and consequently affects the amount of drug released in the targeted tissue; iv) some bioactive molecules produced by enzyme digestion may facilitate the drug uptake or have synergistic therapeutic effects [170 - 172].

Hydrolases, including proteases, lipases, and glycosidases, are the most widely studied enzymes for drug delivery. Matrix metalloproteinases (MMPs), disintegrin metalloproteinases, phospholipase A2, urokinase plasminogen activator, elastase, and prostate-specific antigen are extracellular enzymes and cathepsin B is an intracellular enzyme used as triggers for drug release from various nanocarriers [170 - 172] including liposomes, micelles, and polymeric nanoparticles (Table **6**).

MMPs are probably the most widely group of enzymes used as triggers for content release of nanocarriers. MMPs are zinc dependent proteolytic enzymes that regulate various cell behaviors, including cancer cell growth, migration, differentiation, apoptosis, invasion, and tumor angiogenesis. Two important members of the family, MMP2 and MMP9 are type IV collagenases which are involved in the tumor angiogenesis, progression, and metastasis mainly through the ability to degrade extracellular matrix. Therefore, they are used as biomarkers for various types of cancers [174 - 176].

In a recent patent, increased concentrations of glutathione (GSH) and MMP-9 in the extracellular matrix of tumor tissues were used to trigger contents release from liposomal nanocarriers. An MMP-9-cleavable collagen mimetic lipopeptide was synthesized and in combination with CHEMS, 1-palmitoyl-2-oleolyl-sn-glcero-3-phosphocholine (POPC), and pH-sensitive PEGylated 1-palmitoyl-2-oleoyl-sn-glycero-3-phosphoethanolamine lipid (POPE-SS-PEG) formed responsive nanovesicles. The shielding effect of PEG shells prevented the lipopeptides hydrolysis by MMP-9. However, the PEG groups were reductively detached in the presence of elevated glutathione levels, exposing the lipopeptides to MMP-9. The resultant peptide bond cleavage destabilized the lipid bilayer, leading to the release of encapsulated contents. The effectiveness of the delivery strategy was observed in the xenograft model of human pancreatic cancer (Fig. **8**) [177, 178].

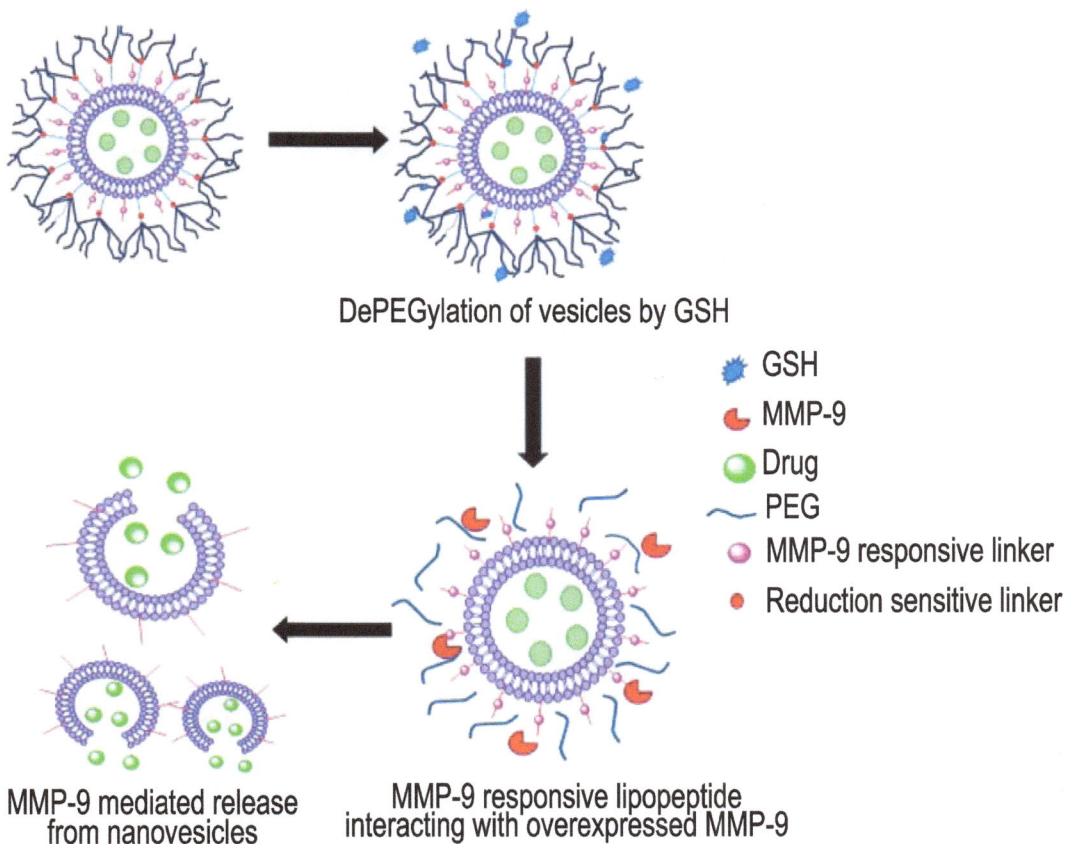

DePEGylation of vesicles by GSH

* GSH
* MMP-9
* Drug
~ PEG
* MMP-9 responsive linker
* Reduction sensitive linker

MMP-9 mediated release from nanovesicles

MMP-9 responsive lipopeptide interacting with overexpressed MMP-9

Fig. (8). Schematic of MMP-9 responsive PEG cleavable nanocarrier for efficient drug delivery. A responsive nanovesicle composed of MMP-9-cleavable lipopeptides and cleavable PEGylated lipid (POPE-SS-PEG) formed. The PEG groups are reductively detached in the presence of elevated glutathione levels, exposing the lipopeptides to MMP-9 leading to the release of encapsulated contents. Figure reproduced with modification from Ref [178]. with permission. Copyright (2014) American Chemical Society.

A nanocapsule was composed of a calcium carbonate core surrounded by a polystyrene sulfonate and poly(allylamine hydrochloride) layer. MMP-2/ MMP-9 cleavable substrate was embedded into the multilayer architecture, which was designed for targeted enzyme-triggered release of anticancer therapies [179].

Secreted phospholipase A_2 (sPLA$_2$) are excreted at the extracellular side of the plasma membrane and their increased expression and activity in prostate, pancreatic, and breast cancers make them good targets to control therapeutics release [180, 181]. In a patent, Vikbjerg and his coworkers designed liposomal carriers composed of an anionic lipid (25-45%), cholesterol ($\leq$ 10%), and a therapeutic agent capable of delivering their payload at sites of increased sPLA2 due to lipid hydrolysis [182].

High levels of cathepsin B, a lysosomal protease belonging to the papain family, are found in a wide variety of human cancers including prostate, breast, brain, lung, and colorectal cancer. Its overexpression is correlated with invasive and metastatic cancers [183, 184]. A peptide-based nanofiber delivery system was made of multiple β-sheet peptides stack parallel to each other with a high aspect ratio (0.5 x 5 x 100nm^3). These nanosystems could respond to activation by cathepsin B. The nanocarriers can be designed either to degrade by cathepsin B and rapidly release the payload or to deshield by hydrophilic PEG removal and form aggregate (storage reservoir) delaying the payload release. When the rapid release carrier was used as a drug delivery system, it showed enhanced cytotoxicity compared to a free drug. On the other hand, the reservoir carrier with slow release profile remained inside the lysosomes after cellular uptake displaying lower cytotoxicity [185].

Table **6** describes various patents on enzyme-responsive nanocarriers [177, 179, 185 - 196].

Table 6. Summary of Patents on Enzyme-Responsive Nanocarriers.

Patent No.	Formulation Type	Drug(s)	*In vivo Model*	Cancer Type	Description	Ref.
US8808733	Liposome	Doxorubicin			Comprising liposomes having an enzyme for the release process and an enzyme activator which is bound in a molecular cage	[186]

(Table 6) cont.....

Patent No.	Formulation Type	Drug(s)	*In vivo* Model	Cancer Type	Description	Ref.
US8318206	Polymeric nanoparticle			Prostate cancer	Comprising a peptide linker which is sensitive to proteases	[187]
US20100010102	Polymeric nanoparticle				Comprising a network cross-linked by peptides to a polymer having proteolytic cleavage sites	[188]
US20140193342	Micelle		Nude mice	Breast cancer, fibrosarcoma	A hydrophilic polymer comprising an enzyme-sensitive part and an imaging label	[189]
EP3191137	Micelle				Comprising amphiphilic PEG-dendron hybrid	[190]
WO2017011618	Conjugate	Gefitinib, Cetuximab	Mice	Lung cancer, adenocarcinoma	Gelatin nanoparticle conjugate which has a siRNA-linked antibody on its surface	[191]
US20140161884	Conjugate		SCID mice	Fibrosarcoma	Comprising nanoparticles which are cleavable, sensitive to enzymes and/or hydrolysis condition	[192]
CA2947895	Conjugate	Gefitinib, I-131		Bronchoalveolar carcinoma	Silica-based nanoparticle having covalently attached drug molecules	[193]
WO2013043812	Polymeric nanoparticle	Paclitaxel		Breast cancer	Comprising a calcium carbonate core and bi-layers of polystyrene sulfonate and poly(allylamine hydrochloride)	[179]

(Table 6) cont.....

Patent No.	Formulation Type	Drug(s)	*In vivo* Model	Cancer Type	Description	Ref.
WO2013033717	Polymeric nanoparticle		Female BALB/c mice		Comprising a polymeric nanoparticle encapsulating polypeptides and components of the shell have cross-linked parts comprising amino acid sequences which are sensitive to proteases	[194]
US9457041	Micelle, liposome, nonoemulsion	Gemcitabine	Nude mice	Pancreatic ductal carcinoma	Comprising a lipoprotein containing a trigger protein having a peptide bond which is cleaved by a protease or a gelatinase	[177]
US20140162966	Polymeric nanoparticle	Paclitaxel	BALB/c mice	Mammary carcinoma, colon carcinoma, prostate cancer	A dipicolylamine/Zn nanoparticle having an artificial phosphate receptor	[195]
WO2017059338	Nanofiber	Mertansine	Nude mice	Breast cancer, ovarian cancer, prostate cancer	A peptide-based nanofiber which is sensitive to cathepsin B	[185]
WO2014120804	Dendrimer	PDD/ovaDNA (Vaccine), Amphotericin B	Female C57BL mice	B16/ova melanoma	Comprising the combination of Major Histocompatibility Complex (MHC) targeting peptides and charged particles	[196]

4.3. Redox-Responsive Nanocarriers

Another efficient internal stimulus to enhance drug and gene delivery is the reducing potential of the intracellular compartments (especially in cytosol, mitochondria, and cell nucleus) compared to the extracellular compartment or in the tumor tissues versus normal tissues. Higher level of the glutathione, a thiol (sulfhydryl) containing tripeptide (L-γ-glutamyl-L-cysteinyl-glycine), is the main reason of this redox potential. GSH level in the cytosol (~ 2-10mM) is 100 to 1000-fold higher than the extracellular fluids (~ 2-20μM) where GSH is rapidly and enzymatically degraded. Furthermore, in some cancer tissues, GSH concentration could be 4-fold higher than normal tissues [197, 198]. These high redox potential differences open up an opportunity to design reduction-responsive tumor selective therapeutic delivery system. Generally, reduction-sensitive carriers have cleavable/reversible disulfide linkages in their structures. These systems are stable at oxidizing extracellular conditions, but in the presence of reducing agents like GSH, they undergo thiol-disulfide interconversion or rapid breakdown [21, 199].

McCarley and Ong proposed redox-gated liposomes composed of quinone-dioleoyl phosphatidylethanolamine (Q-DOPE) lipids. The key component of reduction-responsive liposomes was reduction induced cleavage of a "trimethyl-locked" quinone conjugated to the N-terminus of DOPE [200]. Some liposomal formulations were designed based on redox-sensitive PEG detachment. In an environment with reducing potential, the cleavage of PEG chain from the surface of the liposome facilitates carrier uptake [201].

O(6)-Benzylguanine was used to inhibit O(6)-methylguanine-DNA methyl-transferase in glioblastoma multiforme. In order to improve its efficacy, nanoparticles were designed with superparamagnetic iron oxide core and redox-responsive biocompatible chitosan-PEG copolymer surface coating. While nanoparticles were stable in solutions similar to blood conditions, cargo was rapidly released under conditions mimicking intracellular compartments (pH 5 and 100mM glutathione). By using tumor-targeting peptide, chlorotoxin; nanoparticles showed high tumor accumulation and improved *in vivo* efficacy (Fig. **9**) [202, 203].

Most studies on preparation of reduction-responsive polymers used disulfide bonds for their design. In a recently published patent, a novel cationic redox-sensitive polymer was designed based on diselenide bonds as a gene delivery carrier. Diselenide conjugated oligoethylenimine (800Da) was synthesized, formed nanoparticles with DNA, and had the same reduction sensitivity as disulfide bonds cross-linked oligoethylenimine [204].

A dual responsive (acidic pH and high glutathione level) nanogel was designed by poly[(2-(pyridin-2-yldisulfanyl)-co-[poly(ethylene glycol)]] polymer containing both disulfide and ester bonds. The polymer was then decorated with cyclo(Arg-Gly-Asp-D-Phe-Cys) (cRGD) peptide, an $\alpha_v\beta_5$ integrin targeting ligand. The system with an average particle size of ~130nm and slightly negative surface charge was used for co-delivery of paclitaxel and doxorubicin. The nano-cocktail showed much stronger synergism than its free drug counterpart against colon cancer cells [205].

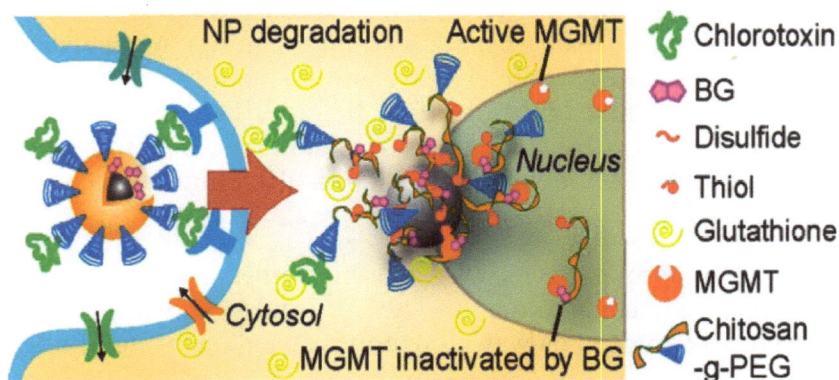

Fig. (9). Schematic of a redox-responsive nanocarrier and mechanism of action. Nanoparticles are designed with superparamagnetic iron oxide core, redox-responsive biocompatible chitosan-PEG copolymer surface coating, and tumor targeting peptide, chlorotoxin. The O(6)-benzylguanine (BG) is rapidly released under conditions mimicking intracellular compartments (pH 5 and 100mM glutathione) and inhibits O(6)-methylguanine-DNA (MGMT) methyltransferase in glioblastoma multiforme. Figure reproduced with modification from Ref [203]. with permission. Copyright (2014) American Chemical Society.

Although PEG-modification is critical for *in vivo* stability as well as pharmacokinetic and biodistribution properties of nanocarriers, it may adversely affect drug loading and cellular uptake. In a recent patent, a redox-responsive nanoparticle based on drug-polymer complex was prepared by surface conjugation of PEG chains with disulfide bonds [206].

Various patented investigations on redox-responsive nanocarriers has been described in Table **7** [200, 202, 204, 207-218].

Table 7. Summary of Patents on Redox-Responsive Nanocarriers.

Patent No.	Formulation Type	Drug(s)	*In vivo* Model	Cancer Type	Description	Ref.
US20110104250	Liposome				Comprising redox-gated Liposomes	[200]
US9707303	Polymeric nanoparticle		Mice	Skin cancer, liver carcinoma	Comprising the cationic polymer material and the plasmid DNA which form complex particles	[204]
WO2015074762	Polymeric nanoparticle	Doxorubicin, Leuprolide	SCID mice	Cervical carcinoma	Comprising organic and inorganic polymeric spheres	[207]

(Table 7) cont.....

Patent No.	Formulation Type	Drug(s)	*In vivo* Model	Cancer Type	Description	Ref.
US7893177	Polymeric nanoparticle				Comprising nanoparticles and nanoparticle conjugates consisting of redox-active species having a disubstituted metallocene	[208]
US9603944	Polymeric nanoparticle		Mice	Melanoma, metastatic lung tumor	Comprising proteins crosslinked to each other, protected by a polymeric or silica-based nanoshell	[209]
US20140286872	Polymeric nanoparticle	O6-benzylguanine, Chlorotoxin	Mice	Glioblastoma	Comprising nanoparticles consisting of a chitosan-polyethylene oxide oligomer copolymer	[202]
EP3177668	Polymeric nanoparticle	Doxorubicin		Cervical carcinoma, breast cancer	Comprising polyesteramides consisting of different chemical groups and disulphide linkages	[210]
EP3193831	Nanogel			Breast cancer	Comprising pH- or redox-responsive and charge-neutral nanogels	[211]
US9149535	Nanogel	Doxorubicin, Paclitaxel	Mice	Colon carcinoma, ovarian cancer	Comprising nanogels consisting of 2-(pyridin-2-yldisulfanyl)ethyl acrylate and poly(ethylene glycol)methacrylate	[205]
US9283281	Nanogel		Male Nu/J mice	Head and neck squamous carcinoma	Comprising poly[(2-(pyridin-2-yldisulfanyl)- co-[poly(ethylene glycol)]-co--N-isopropyl methacrylamide] which is sensitive to high redox potential, temperature and acidic pH	[212]
WO2016179189	Nanogel	Staurosporine		Cervical carcinoma	Comprising a crosslinked nanogel-protein conjugate	[213]
US9585840	Metal nanoparticle		CD-1 mice	Squamous tumor	Comprising a crystalline structure of cerium oxide which is dextran-coated	[214]
WO2014008503	Metal nanoparticle				Comprising redox-active nanoparticles potentiating innate immunity	[215]
WO2012142410	Nanocapsule				Comprising a polymer shell for delivering polypeptides	[216]
US20160067354	Hybrid nanoparticle	Doxorubicin	Female FVB mice	Melanoma, metastatic lung tumor	Comprising gold/mesoporous silica nanoparticles	[217]
US8198368	Micelle, film				Comprising disulfide-coupled block copolymers	[218]

5. OTHER STIMULI-RESPONSIVE NANOCARRIERS

A few other triggers have also been used for targeting solid tumors by nanotherapeutics. Electric field [219, 220], hypoxia [221, 222], and ionic strength [223, 224] have been proposed as triggers for drug delivery in cancer therapy. Electrical signals are easy to generate and control. Zare and Ge have recently proposed a dual stimulus-sensitive nanosystem for programmed drug delivery. Nanoparticles composed of conducting polymer (polypyrrole) served as a cargo nanoreservoir. Drug-loaded nanoparticles were suspended in a temperature-responsive hydrogel, which was liquid at low temperatures and turned to gel in the body temperature. After subcutaneous injection, the application of a small external electric field, triggered drug release and diffusion through the hydrogel to the surroundings [219].

Hypoxia is a condition found in cancer and emerging as a target in the development of therapeutic and diagnostic agents. Compositions and methods for targeting hypoxic tumor areas for detection or treatment of cancer by polymeric micelles were proposed. A hypoxia targeting moiety was conjugated to nanoparticles containing imaging agents or therapeutic agents [221]. Torchilin and his co-workers investigated hypoxia-induced siRNA uptake and silencing using a nanosystem composed of azobenzene, polyethyleneimine (PEI), PEG, and DOPE units where azobenzene mediates hypoxia sensitivity and specificity [222].

CONCLUSION

Design of stimuli-sensitive nanocarriers being responsive to exogenous or endogenous stimuli may represent an attractive area of research in cancer therapy. The diversity of stimuli (hyperthermia, magnetic field, light, ultrasound, acidic pH, enzymes, and chemical reactions such as redox condition) as well as the variety of nanostructures (liposomes, polymeric nanoparticles, micelles, nanogels, dendrimers, etc.) allows great flexibility in the design of appropriate stimuli-responsive nanosystems. In spite of numerous researches and proposed ideas, few responsive nanocarriers reach the clinical stage that is probably due to complexity of the preparation of nanocarriers compositions or difficulties in the scaling-up processes which are both good targets for future in-depth studies.

CURRENT & FUTURE DEVELOPMENTS

Cancer is a complex disease with high inter- and intratumoral heterogeneity that limits the effectiveness of current chemotherapeutics. Therefore, development of advanced therapies is in great demand. Design of more site-specific drug nanocarriers with long circulation residence time, minimum premature drug release, high accumulation in tumor tissues, and controlled on-demand drug release behavior could greatly improve the therapeutic response.

In this chapter, we reviewed different external and internal stimuli that can trigger changes in the properties of drug nanocarriers and stimulate drug release. Although many advancements have been made in the lab-scale design and preclinical evaluation of stimuli-responsive nanocarriers, numerous key challenges remain, especially in their scalable fabrication, industrial production, reproducibility, quality control, and clinical application.

The next generations will be stimuli-responsive nanocarriers for simultaneous tumor diagnosis and therapy (stimuli-responsive theranostic nanocarriers), dual and multi-stimuli-responsive carriers, stimuli-responsive multi-drug nanomedicines for targeting both cancer cells and cancer stem cells, stimuli-responsive nanomedicines for resistant cancers, stimuli-responsive nanocarriers with precise intracellular drug delivery, and combined targeted and triggered release drug carriers. Moreover, in-depth studies in more realistic *in vitro* models (such as tumor spheroids or 3D cell cultures) as well as in large animals with more similarity to the complex human cancers are required. Testing the responsive nanomedicines behavior by using microfluidic-based models would be another promising field of study. A comprehensive understanding of fate and the Absorption, Distribution, Metabolism, and Excretion (ADME) pathways and mechanisms of stimuli-responsive nanomaterials are needed. Specific drug delivery to deep tumor tissues with poor vascularization and therapeutics bioavailability at subcellular targets (mitochondria or nucleus) can boost efficacy and minimize the adverse toxicity of current and future therapeutic agents.

CONSENT FOR PUBLICATION

Not applicable.

CONFLICT OF INTEREST

The authors declare no conflict of interest, financial or otherwise.

ACKNOWLEDGEMENTS

This work was supported by Shahid Beheshti University of Medical Sciences.

REFERENCES

[1]   Bahrami B, Hojjat-Farsangi M, Mohammadi H, *et al.* Nanoparticles and targeted drug delivery in cancer therapy. Immunol Lett 2017; 190: 64-83.
[http://dx.doi.org/10.1016/j.imlet.2017.07.015] [PMID: 28760499]

[2]   Pérez-Herrero E, Fernández-Medarde A. Advanced targeted therapies in cancer: Drug nanocarriers, the future of chemotherapy. Eur J Pharm Biopharm 2015; 93: 52-79.

[http://dx.doi.org/10.1016/j.ejpb.2015.03.018] [PMID: 25813885]

[3]   Narvekar M, Xue HY, Eoh JY, Wong HL. Nanocarrier for poorly water-soluble anticancer drugs-
        -barriers of translation and solutions. AAPS PharmSciTech 2014; 15(4): 822-33.
        [http://dx.doi.org/10.1208/s12249-014-0107-x] [PMID: 24687241]

[4]   Guo S, Huang L. Nanoparticles containing insoluble drug for cancer therapy. Biotechnol Adv 2014;
        32(4): 778-88.
        [http://dx.doi.org/10.1016/j.biotechadv.2013.10.002] [PMID: 24113214]

[5]   Jain V, Jain S, Mahajan SC. Nanomedicines based drug delivery systems for anti-cancer targeting and
        treatment. Curr Drug Deliv 2015; 12(2): 177-91.
        [http://dx.doi.org/10.2174/1567201811666140822112516] [PMID: 25146439]

[6]   Ernsting MJ, Murakami M, Roy A, Li SD. Factors controlling the pharmacokinetics, biodistribution
        and intratumoral penetration of nanoparticles. J Control Release 2013; 172(3): 782-94.
        [http://dx.doi.org/10.1016/j.jconrel.2013.09.013] [PMID: 24075927]

[7]   Baetke SC, Lammers T, Kiessling F. Applications of nanoparticles for diagnosis and therapy of
        cancer. Br J Radiol 2015; 88(1054): 20150207.
        [http://dx.doi.org/10.1259/bjr.20150207] [PMID: 25969868]

[8]   Maeda H, Nakamura H, Fang J. The EPR effect for macromolecular drug delivery to solid tumors:
        Improvement of tumor uptake, lowering of systemic toxicity, and distinct tumor imaging *in vivo*. Adv
        Drug Deliv Rev 2013; 65(1): 71-9.
        [http://dx.doi.org/10.1016/j.addr.2012.10.002] [PMID: 23088862]

[9]   Jeevanandam J, Chan YS, Danquah MK. Nano-formulations of drugs: Recent developments, impact
        and challenges. Biochimie 2016; 128-129: 99-112.
        [http://dx.doi.org/10.1016/j.biochi.2016.07.008] [PMID: 27436182]

[10]   Akbarzadeh A, Rezaei-Sadabady R, Davaran S, *et al.* Liposome: Classification, preparation, and
        applications. Nanoscale Res Lett 2013; 8(1): 102.
        [http://dx.doi.org/10.1186/1556-276X-8-102] [PMID: 23432972]

[11]   Haeri A, Sadeghian S, Rabbani S, Anvari MS, Boroumand MA, Dadashzadeh S. Use of remote film
        loading methodology to entrap sirolimus into liposomes: Preparation, characterization and *in vivo*
        efficacy for treatment of restenosis. Int J Pharm 2011; 414(1-2): 16-27.
        [http://dx.doi.org/10.1016/j.ijpharm.2011.04.055] [PMID: 21554939]

[12]   Kumari A, Yadav SK, Yadav SC. Biodegradable polymeric nanoparticles based drug delivery systems.
        Colloids Surf B Biointerfaces 2010; 75(1): 1-18.
        [http://dx.doi.org/10.1016/j.colsurfb.2009.09.001] [PMID: 19782542]

[13]   Zhao F, Yao D, Guo R, Deng L, Dong A, Zhang J. Composites of polymer hydrogels and
        nanoparticulate systems for biomedical and pharmaceutical applications. Nanomaterials (Basel) 2015;
        5(4): 2054-130.
        [http://dx.doi.org/10.3390/nano5042054] [PMID: 28347111]

[14]   Gill KK, Kaddoumi A, Nazzal S. PEG-lipid micelles as drug carriers: Physiochemical attributes,
        formulation principles and biological implication. J Drug Target 2015; 23(3): 222-31.
        [http://dx.doi.org/10.3109/1061186X.2014.997735] [PMID: 25547369]

[15]   Haeri A, Sadeghian S, Rabbani S, *et al.* Sirolimus-loaded stealth colloidal systems attenuate
        neointimal hyperplasia after balloon injury: A comparison of phospholipid micelles and liposomes. Int
        J Pharm 2013; 455(1-2): 320-30.
        [http://dx.doi.org/10.1016/j.ijpharm.2013.07.003] [PMID: 23867987]

[16]   Reddy BP, Yadav HK, Nagesha DK, Raizaday A, Karim A. Polymeric micelles as novel carriers for
        poorly soluble drugs--A review. J Nanosci Nanotechnol 2015; 15(6): 4009-18.
        [http://dx.doi.org/10.1166/jnn.2015.9713] [PMID: 26369007]

[17]   Sharma A, Garg T, Aman A, *et al.* Nanogel-an advanced drug delivery tool: Current and future. Artif

Cells Nanomed Biotechnol 2016; 44(1): 165-77.
[http://dx.doi.org/10.3109/21691401.2014.930745] [PMID: 25053442]

[18] Zhang H, Zhai Y, Wang J, Zhai G. New progress and prospects: The application of nanogel in drug delivery. Mater Sci Eng C 2016; 60: 560-8.
[http://dx.doi.org/10.1016/j.msec.2015.11.041] [PMID: 26706564]

[19] Sharma H, Mishra PK, Talegaonkar S, Vaidya B. Metal nanoparticles: A theranostic nanotool against cancer. Drug Discov Today 2015; 20(9): 1143-51.
[http://dx.doi.org/10.1016/j.drudis.2015.05.009] [PMID: 26007605]

[20] Mura S, Nicolas J, Couvreur P. Stimuli-responsive nanocarriers for drug delivery. Nat Mater 2013; 12(11): 991-1003.
[http://dx.doi.org/10.1038/nmat3776] [PMID: 24150417]

[21] Fleige E, Quadir MA, Haag R. Stimuli-responsive polymeric nanocarriers for the controlled transport of active compounds: Concepts and applications. Adv Drug Deliv Rev 2012; 64(9): 866-84.
[http://dx.doi.org/10.1016/j.addr.2012.01.020] [PMID: 22349241]

[22] Liu M, Du H, Zhang W, Zhai G. Internal stimuli-responsive nanocarriers for drug delivery: Design strategies and applications. Mater Sci Eng C 2017; 71: 1267-80.
[http://dx.doi.org/10.1016/j.msec.2016.11.030] [PMID: 27987683]

[23] Zhou M, Wen K, Bi Y, *et al.* The application of stimuli-responsive nanocarriers for targeted drug delivery. Curr Top Med Chem 2017; 17(20): 2319-34.
[http://dx.doi.org/10.2174/1568026617666170224121008] [PMID: 28240179]

[24] Frazier N, Ghandehari H. Hyperthermia approaches for enhanced delivery of nanomedicines to solid tumors. Biotechnol Bioeng 2015; 112(10): 1967-83.
[http://dx.doi.org/10.1002/bit.25653] [PMID: 25995079]

[25] May JP, Li SD. Hyperthermia-induced drug targeting. Expert Opin Drug Deliv 2013; 10(4): 511-27.
[http://dx.doi.org/10.1517/17425247.2013.758631] [PMID: 23289519]

[26] McDaniel JR, Dewhirst MW, Chilkoti A. Actively targeting solid tumours with thermoresponsive drug delivery systems that respond to mild hyperthermia. Int J Hyperthermia 2013; 29(6): 501-10.
[http://dx.doi.org/10.3109/02656736.2013.819999] [PMID: 23924317]

[27] Chu KF, Dupuy DE. Thermal ablation of tumours: Biological mechanisms and advances in therapy. Nat Rev Cancer 2014; 14(3): 199-208.
[http://dx.doi.org/10.1038/nrc3672] [PMID: 24561446]

[28] Li L, ten Hagen TL, Haeri A, *et al.* A novel two-step mild hyperthermia for advanced liposomal chemotherapy. J Control Release 2014; 174: 202-8.
[http://dx.doi.org/10.1016/j.jconrel.2013.11.012] [PMID: 24269966]

[29] Ta T, Porter TM. Thermosensitive liposomes for localized delivery and triggered release of chemotherapy. J Control Release 2013; 169(1-2): 112-25.
[http://dx.doi.org/10.1016/j.jconrel.2013.03.036] [PMID: 23583706]

[30] Haeri A, Pedrosa LR, Ten Hagen TL, Dadashzadeh S, Koning GA. A novel combined approach of short-chain sphingolipids and thermosensitive liposomes for improved drug delivery to tumor cells. J Biomed Nanotechnol 2016; 12(4): 630-44.
[http://dx.doi.org/10.1166/jbn.2016.2199] [PMID: 27301190]

[31] Haeri A, Zalba S, Ten Hagen TL, Dadashzadeh S, Koning GA. EGFR targeted thermosensitive liposomes: A novel multifunctional platform for simultaneous tumor targeted and stimulus responsive drug delivery. Colloids Surf B Biointerfaces 2016; 146: 657-69.
[http://dx.doi.org/10.1016/j.colsurfb.2016.06.012] [PMID: 27434152]

[32] Kneidl B, Peller M, Winter G, Lindner LH, Hossann M. Thermosensitive liposomal drug delivery systems: State of the art review. Int J Nanomedicine 2014; 9: 4387-98.
[PMID: 25258529]

[33] Manzoor AA, Lindner LH, Landon CD, *et al.* Overcoming limitations in nanoparticle drug delivery: Triggered, intravascular release to improve drug penetration into tumors. Cancer Res 2012; 72(21): 5566-75.
[http://dx.doi.org/10.1158/0008-5472.CAN-12-1683] [PMID: 22952218]

[34] ClinicalTrials.gov. https://clinicaltrials.gov/ct2/show/NCT006179812017.

[35] ClinicalTrials.gov. https://clinicaltrials.gov/ct2/show/NCT008260852017.

[36] Reed RA, Su D. Thermosensitive nanoparticle formulations and method of making the same. US20130230457, 2013.

[37] Li SD, Tagami T, Ernsting MJ. Thermosensitive liposomes. WO2012055020, 2012.

[38] Tagami T, Ernsting MJ, Li SD. Optimization of a novel and improved thermosensitive liposome formulated with DPPC and a Brij surfactant using a robust *in vitro* system. J Control Release 2011; 154(3): 290-7.
[http://dx.doi.org/10.1016/j.jconrel.2011.05.020] [PMID: 21640149]

[39] Gruell H, Langereis S. Carriers for the local release of hydrophilic prodrugs. EP2667848, 2013.

[40] Matanović MR, Kristl J, Grabnar PA. Thermoresponsive polymers: Insights into decisive hydrogel characteristics, mechanisms of gelation, and promising biomedical applications. Int J Pharm 2014; 472(1-2): 262-75.
[http://dx.doi.org/10.1016/j.ijpharm.2014.06.029] [PMID: 24950367]

[41] Chu CC, Song H. Thermoresponsive arginine-based hydrogels as biologic carriers. US8858998, 2014.

[42] Mei X, Jiang Q, Yu W. Thermosensitive liposomes containing therapeutic agents. US8642074, 2014.

[43] Pottier A, Levy L, Meyre ME, Germain M. Nanoparticles delivery systems, preparation and uses thereof. EP2670394, 2013.

[44] Li KC, Li Z, Qin G. Thermally-activatable liposome compositions and methods for imaging, diagnosis and therapy. US20110190623, 2011.

[45] Hennink WE, Van Nostrum CF, Van Steenbergen MJ, Soga O, Rijcken CJF. Temperature sensitive polymers. US8685382, 2014.

[46] Lavasanifar A, Safaei-Nikouei N. Biodegradable thermoresponsive hydrogels. WO2011047486, 2011.

[47] Kobertstein JT, Samanta S, De SC. Biodegradable thermo-responsive polymers and uses thereof. WO2016090103, 2016.

[48] Calderón M, Molina M, Wedepohl S. Nanogel compound. WO2016207296, 2016.

[49] Ben-Shalom N, Nevo Z, Patchornik A, Robinson D. Injectable chitosan mixtures forming hydrogels. US8153612, 2012.

[50] Duvall CL, Gupta MK, Martin JR, Dollinger BR. Ros-degradeable hydrogels. US20160303241, 2016.

[51] Papen-Botterhuis NE. Injectable hydrogel composition, method for the preparation and uses thereof. EP2813213, 2014.

[52] Kick K, Luo T. Thermoresponsive bioconjugates and their controlled delivery of cargo. WO2017020025, 2017.

[53] Mertz D, Sandre O, Bégin-Colin S. Drug releasing nanoplatforms activated by alternating magnetic fields. Biochim Biophys Acta 2017; 1861(6): 1617-41.
[http://dx.doi.org/10.1016/j.bbagen.2017.02.025] [PMID: 28238734]

[54] Gobbo OL, Sjaastad K, Radomski MW, Volkov Y, Prina-Mello A. Magnetic nanoparticles in cancer theranostics. Theranostics 2015; 5(11): 1249-63.
[http://dx.doi.org/10.7150/thno.11544] [PMID: 26379790]

[55] Nandwana V, De M, Chu S, *et al.* Theranostic magnetic nanostructures (MNS) for cancer. Cancer

Treat Res 2015; 166: 51-83.
[http://dx.doi.org/10.1007/978-3-319-16555-4_3] [PMID: 25895864]

[56]   Zhu L, Zhou Z, Mao H, Yang L. Magnetic nanoparticles for precision oncology: Theranostic magnetic iron oxide nanoparticles for image-guided and targeted cancer therapy. Nanomedicine (Lond) 2017; 12(1): 73-87.
[http://dx.doi.org/10.2217/nnm-2016-0316] [PMID: 27876448]

[57]   Kandasamy G, Maity D. Recent advances in superparamagnetic iron oxide nanoparticles (SPIONs) for *in vitro* and *in vivo* cancer nanotheranostics. Int J Pharm 2015; 496(2): 191-218.
[http://dx.doi.org/10.1016/j.ijpharm.2015.10.058] [PMID: 26520409]

[58]   Polyak B, Friedman G. Magnetic targeting for site-specific drug delivery: Applications and clinical potential. Expert Opin Drug Deliv 2009; 6(1): 53-70.
[http://dx.doi.org/10.1517/17425240802662795] [PMID: 19236208]

[59]   Lee N, Yoo D, Ling D, Cho MH, Hyeon T, Cheon J. Iron oxide based nanoparticles for multimodal imaging and magnetoresponsive therapy. Chem Rev 2015; 115(19): 10637-89.
[http://dx.doi.org/10.1021/acs.chemrev.5b00112] [PMID: 26250431]

[60]   Felton C, Karmakar A, Gartia Y, Ramidi P, Biris AS, Ghosh A. Magnetic nanoparticles as contrast agents in biomedical imaging: Recent advances in iron- and manganese-based magnetic nanoparticles. Drug Metab Rev 2014; 46(2): 142-54.
[http://dx.doi.org/10.3109/03602532.2013.876429] [PMID: 24754519]

[61]   Ho D, Sun X, Sun S. Monodisperse magnetic nanoparticles for theranostic applications. Acc Chem Res 2011; 44(10): 875-82.
[http://dx.doi.org/10.1021/ar200090c] [PMID: 21661754]

[62]   Thomsen LB, Thomsen MS, Moos T. Targeted drug delivery to the brain using magnetic nanoparticles. Ther Deliv 2015; 6(10): 1145-55.
[http://dx.doi.org/10.4155/tde.15.56] [PMID: 26446407]

[63]   Lee JH, Kim JW, Cheon J. Magnetic nanoparticles for multi-imaging and drug delivery. Mol Cells 2013; 35(4): 274-84.
[http://dx.doi.org/10.1007/s10059-013-0103-0] [PMID: 23579479]

[64]   De Cuyper M, Joniau M. Magnetoliposomes. Formation and structural characterization. Eur Biophys J 1988; 15(5): 311-9.
[http://dx.doi.org/10.1007/BF00256482] [PMID: 3366097]

[65]   Bakandritsos A, Fatourou AG, Fatouros DG. Magnetoliposomes and their potential in the intelligent drug-delivery field. Ther Deliv 2012; 3(12): 1469-82.
[http://dx.doi.org/10.4155/tde.12.129] [PMID: 23323563]

[66]   Soenen SJ, Hodenius M, De Cuyper M. Magnetoliposomes: Versatile innovative nanocolloids for use in biotechnology and biomedicine. Nanomedicine (Lond) 2009; 4(2): 177-91.
[http://dx.doi.org/10.2217/17435889.4.2.177] [PMID: 19193184]

[67]   Glüet CC, Penate MT, Penate MO. Magnetoenzymatic carrier system for imaging and targeted delivery and release of active agents. EP3139964 2017.

[68]   Davalian D, Hossainy SFA, Bright R, Wan J, Ludwig FN. Magnetically sensitive drug carriers for treatment or targeted delivery. US20110196474, 2011.

[69]   Asmatulu R, Misak H, Yang S, Wooley P. Composite magnetic nanoparticle drug delivery system. US20120265001, 2012.

[70]   University T. Method for preparing magnetic temperature-sensitive composite microsphere with nuclear shell structure by adopting *in situ* grafting technique. CN101559343, 2011.

[71]   Vasiljeva O, Itin VI, Psakhie SG, Mikhaylov GA, Mikac MU, Turk B, *et al.* Oxide ferrimagnetics with spinel structure nanoparticles and iron oxide nanoparticles, biocompatible aqueous colloidal systems

comprising nanoparticles, ferriliposomes, and uses thereof. EP2739291, 2014.

[72]   Mohapatra S, Wang C. Multilayered magnetic micelle compositions and methods for their use. US9439978, 2016.

[73]   Dyer RK, Hough JVD. Otologic nanotechnology. US8303990, 2012.

[74]   Seeney CE, Klostergaard J, Yuill WA, Gibson DD. Magnetically responsive nanoparticle therapeutic constructs and methods of making and using. US8651113, 2014.

[75]   Alferiev I, Chorny M, Levy RJ. Hydrolytically releasable prodrugs for sustained release nanoparticle formulations. US9233163, 2016.

[76]   Khizroev S, Guduru R, Liang P. On-demand drug release using magneto-electric nanoparticles. US20160030724, 2016.

[77]   Ghosh S. Multimodal therapy for cancer cell destruction. US20170128573, 2017.

[78]   Amstad E, Reimhult E, Textor M. Magnetically responsive membrane structures. WO2011147926, 2012.

[79]   Mao H, Yang L, Huang J. Coated magnetic nanoparticles for imaging enhancement and drug delivery. WO2014145573, 2014.

[80]   Weaver JB. Carrier-linked magnetic nanoparticle drug delivery composition and method of use. US9211346, 2015.

[81]   Chrony M, Polyak B, Fishbein I, Alferiev I, Levy RJ. Magnetically-driven biodegradable gene delivery nanoparticles formulated with surface-attached polycationic complex. US20110076767, 2011.

[82]   Bansal A, Zhang Y. Photocontrolled nanoparticle delivery systems for biomedical applications. Acc Chem Res 2014; 47(10): 3052-60.
[http://dx.doi.org/10.1021/ar500217w] [PMID: 25137555]

[83]   Menon JU, Jadeja P, Tambe P, Vu K, Yuan B, Nguyen KT. Nanomaterials for photo-based diagnostic and therapeutic applications. Theranostics 2013; 3(3): 152-66.
[http://dx.doi.org/10.7150/thno.5327] [PMID: 23471164]

[84]   Yu J, Chu X, Hou Y. Stimuli-responsive cancer therapy based on nanoparticles. Chem Commun (Camb) 2014; 50(79): 11614-30.
[http://dx.doi.org/10.1039/C4CC03984J] [PMID: 25058003]

[85]   Allison RR. Photodynamic therapy: Oncologic horizons. Future Oncol 2014; 10(1): 123-4.
[http://dx.doi.org/10.2217/fon.13.176] [PMID: 24328413]

[86]   Voon SH, Kiew LV, Lee HB, *et al. In vivo* studies of nanostructure-based photosensitizers for photodynamic cancer therapy. Small 2014; 10(24): 4993-5013.
[PMID: 25164105]

[87]   Lucky SS, Soo KC, Zhang Y. Nanoparticles in photodynamic therapy. Chem Rev 2015; 115(4): 1990-2042.
[http://dx.doi.org/10.1021/cr5004198] [PMID: 25602130]

[88]   Bobo D, Robinson KJ, Islam J, Thurecht KJ, Corrie SR. Nanoparticle-based medicines: A review of FDA-approved materials and clinical trials to date. Pharm Res 2016; 33(10): 2373-87.
[http://dx.doi.org/10.1007/s11095-016-1958-5] [PMID: 27299311]

[89]   Idris NM, Jayakumar MK, Bansal A, Zhang Y. Upconversion nanoparticles as versatile light nanotransducers for photoactivation applications. Chem Soc Rev 2015; 44(6): 1449-78.
[http://dx.doi.org/10.1039/C4CS00158C] [PMID: 24969662]

[90]   Guerrero AR, Hassan N, Escobar CA, Albericio F, Kogan MJ, Araya E. Gold nanoparticles for photothermally controlled drug release. Nanomedicine (Lond) 2014; 9(13): 2023-39.
[http://dx.doi.org/10.2217/nnm.14.126] [PMID: 25343351]

[91]   Jaque D, Martínez Maestro L, del Rosal B, *et al.* Nanoparticles for photothermal therapies. Nanoscale 2014; 6(16): 9494-530.
[http://dx.doi.org/10.1039/C4NR00708E] [PMID: 25030381]

[92]   Wang Y, Black KC, Luehmann H, *et al.* Comparison study of gold nanohexapods, nanorods, and nanocages for photothermal cancer treatment. ACS Nano 2013; 7(3): 2068-77.
[http://dx.doi.org/10.1021/nn304332s] [PMID: 23383982]

[93]   Fomina N, Sankaranarayanan J, Almutairi A. Photochemical mechanisms of light-triggered release from nanocarriers. Adv Drug Deliv Rev 2012; 64(11): 1005-20.
[http://dx.doi.org/10.1016/j.addr.2012.02.006] [PMID: 22386560]

[94]   Karimi M, Sahandi Zangabad P, Baghaee-Ravari S, Ghazadeh M, Mirshekari H, Hamblin MR. Smart nanostructures for cargo delivery: Uncaging and activating by light. J Am Chem Soc 2017; 139(13): 4584-610.
[http://dx.doi.org/10.1021/jacs.6b08313] [PMID: 28192672]

[95]   Naciri J, Zhou JC, Ratna BR. Photoresponsive nanoparticles as light-driven nanoscale actuators. US8557140, 2013.

[96]   Akashi M, Matsusaki M, Shi D, Onishi M, Fujita Y. Hydrophilic material, medical material and sustained drug release material. US20110257338, 2011.

[97]   Zink JI, Tamanoi F, Choi E, Angelos SA, Kabehie S, Nel AE, *et al.* Nano-devices having impellers for capture and release of molecules. US20170095418, 2017.

[98]   Erdmann FD, Zhang YD, Fischer GD. Reversibly light-switchable drug-conjugates. EP2116263, 2009.

[99]   Da SFL, Samuel MBC. das Neves Ricardo Neves P. Light-activatable polymeric nanoparticles. EP3043782, 2016.

[100]   Naciri J, Zhou JC, Ratna BR. Photoresponsive nanoparticles as light-driven nanoscale actuators. US8652352, 2014.

[101]   Puri A, Blumenthal RP, Joshi A, Tata DB. Photoactivatable lipid-based nanoparticles as vehicles for dual agent delivery. US20160136289, 2016.

[102]   Febvay S, Marini DM, Clapham DE. Targeted and light-activated cytosolic drug delivery. WO2011133925, 2012.

[103]   Febvay S, Marini DM, Belcher AM, Clapham DE. Targeted cytosolic delivery of cell-impermeable compounds by nanoparticle-mediated, light-triggered endosome disruption. Nano Lett 2010; 10(6): 2211-9.
[http://dx.doi.org/10.1021/nl101157z] [PMID: 20446663]

[104]   Dani KM, Wickens JR, Nakano T. Method for controlled release with femtosecond laser pulses. EP3079665, 2016.

[105]   Almutairi A, Lessard-Viger M, Sheng W. Polymeric nanocarriers with light-triggered release mechanism. US9700620, 2017.

[106]   Praveen N, Thoniyot P, Olivo M. A nanoprobe comprising gold colloid nanoparticles for multimodality optical imaging of cancer. WO2012039685, 2012.

[107]   Vo-Dinh T, Yuan H, Fales A. Plasmonics-active metal nanostar compositions and methods of use. US20180050077, 2018.

[108]   Vo-Dinh T, Inman BA, Maccarini P, Palmer G, Liu Y, Weitzel D. Synergistic nanotherapy systems and methods of use thereof. WO2016209936, 2016.

[109]   Zhang Y. Uniform core-shell TiO_2 coated upconversion nanoparticles and use thereof. US20170000887, 2017.

[110]   Naasani I. 5-Aminolevulinic acid conjugated quantum dot nanoparticle. WO2017029501, 2017.

[111] Febvay S, Marini DM, Clapham DE. Targeted and light-activated cytosolic drug delivery. US20130289520, 2013.

[112] Husseini GA, Pitt WG, Martins AM. Ultrasonically triggered drug delivery: Breaking the barrier. Colloids Surf B Biointerfaces 2014; 123: 364-86.
[http://dx.doi.org/10.1016/j.colsurfb.2014.07.051] [PMID: 25454759]

[113] Ahmed SE, Martins AM, Husseini GA. The use of ultrasound to release chemotherapeutic drugs from micelles and liposomes. J Drug Target 2015; 23(1): 16-42.
[http://dx.doi.org/10.3109/1061186X.2014.954119] [PMID: 25203857]

[114] Pitt WG, Husseini G. Technique for drug and gene delivery to the cell cytosol. US8999295, 2015.

[115] Kwan J, Myers R, Coussios CC, Shah A. Cavitation-inducing polymeric nanoparticles. CA2930815, 2015.

[116] Rapoport N, Pitt WG. Stabilization and acoustic activation of polymeric micelles for drug delivery. US6649702, 2003.

[117] Nam KH, Rapoport NY. Stable nanoemulsions for ultrasound-mediated drug delivery and imaging. US8709451, 2014.

[118] Kohane DS, Epstein-Barash H, Borden MA. Methods, devices, and systems for on-demand ultrasound-triggered drug delivery. US20130041311, 2013.

[119] Park SM, Park K, Kim HR, Park ES. Liposome including hydrophobic material and imaging agent and use of the liposome. US20150064114, 2015.

[120] Arvanitis C. Systems and methods for controlling focused ultrasound to target release of a therapeutic agent from temperature-sensitive liposomal carriers. WO2015200576, 2015.

[121] Esener SC, Schutt IC, Ibsen S, Zahavy E. Regionally activated drug delivery nanoparticles. WO2015089154, 2015.

[122] Wagstaffe SJ, Schiffter-Weinle HA, Molinari MB, Arora M, Coussios CC. Sonosensitive nanoparticles. WO2012066334, 2012.

[123] Liu TY. Dual-modal imaging-guided drug vehicle with ultrasound-triggered release function. US20130204181, 2013.

[124] Malik MT, Kopechek JA, Bates P. Targeted nanodroplet emulsions for treating cancer. WO2018026958, 2018.

[125] Kosheleva OK, Lai P, Chen NG, Hsiao M, Chen CH. Nanoparticle-assisted ultrasound for breast cancer therapy. US9427466, 2016.

[126] Park JH, You DG, Deepagan VG, Lee MC. Sonosensitizer composition containing titanium oxide nanoparticle as active ingredient, composition for preventing or treating cancer comprising the same, and the preparation thereof. US20170007699, 2017.

[127] Xing J, Lu W. Transfection with magnetic nanoparticles and ultrasound. EP2346996, 2011.

[128] Dimitrova N, Hall CS, Chin CT. Controlling release of a material carried by ultrasound sensitive particles. EP2120722, 2014.

[129] Benchimol M, Esener SC, Simberg D, Ibsen S. Acoustically responsive particles with decreased cavitation threshold. US20140046181, 2014.

[130] Ferreira DdosS, Lopes SC, Franco MS, Oliveira MC. pH-sensitive liposomes for drug delivery in cancer treatment. Ther Deliv 2013; 4(9): 1099-123.
[http://dx.doi.org/10.4155/tde.13.80] [PMID: 24024511]

[131] He X, Li J, An S, Jiang C. pH-sensitive drug-delivery systems for tumor targeting. Ther Deliv 2013; 4(12): 1499-510.
[http://dx.doi.org/10.4155/tde.13.120] [PMID: 24304248]

[132] Liu J, Huang Y, Kumar A, *et al.* pH-sensitive nano-systems for drug delivery in cancer therapy. Biotechnol Adv 2014; 32(4): 693-710.
[http://dx.doi.org/10.1016/j.biotechadv.2013.11.009] [PMID: 24309541]

[133] Peppicelli S, Bianchini F, Calorini L. Extracellular acidity, a "reappreciated" trait of tumor environment driving malignancy: Perspectives in diagnosis and therapy. Cancer Metastasis Rev 2014; 33(2-3): 823-32.
[http://dx.doi.org/10.1007/s10555-014-9506-4] [PMID: 24984804]

[134] Al-Zoughbi W, Huang J, Paramasivan GS, *et al.* Tumor macroenvironment and metabolism. Semin Oncol 2014; 41(2): 281-95.
[http://dx.doi.org/10.1053/j.seminoncol.2014.02.005] [PMID: 24787299]

[135] Hernández A, Serrano G, Herrera-Palau R, Pérez-Castiñeira JR, Serrano A. Intraorganellar acidification by V-ATPases: A target in cell proliferation and cancer therapy. Recent Patents Anticancer Drug Discov 2010; 5(2): 88-98.
[http://dx.doi.org/10.2174/157489210790936216] [PMID: 19941463]

[136] Varkouhi AK, Scholte M, Storm G, Haisma HJ. Endosomal escape pathways for delivery of biologicals. J Control Release 2011; 151(3): 220-8.
[http://dx.doi.org/10.1016/j.jconrel.2010.11.004] [PMID: 21078351]

[137] Shete HK, Prabhu RH, Patravale VB. Endosomal escape: A bottleneck in intracellular delivery. J Nanosci Nanotechnol 2014; 14(1): 460-74.
[http://dx.doi.org/10.1166/jnn.2014.9082] [PMID: 24730275]

[138] Yang X, Yi C, Luo N, Gong C. Nanomedicine to overcome cancer multidrug resistance. Curr Drug Metab 2014; 15(6): 632-49.
[http://dx.doi.org/10.2174/1389200215666140926154443] [PMID: 25255871]

[139] Bertrand N, Simard P, Leroux JC. Serum-stable, long-circulating, pH-sensitive PEGylated liposomes. Methods Mol Biol 2010; 605: 545-58.
[http://dx.doi.org/10.1007/978-1-60327-360-2_36] [PMID: 20072905]

[140] Simard P, Leroux JC. *In vivo* evaluation of pH-sensitive polymer-based immunoliposomes targeting the CD33 antigen. Mol Pharm 2010; 7(4): 1098-107.
[http://dx.doi.org/10.1021/mp900261m] [PMID: 20476756]

[141] Yoshizaki Y, Yuba E, Sakaguchi N, Koiwai K, Harada A, Kono K. Potentiation of pH-sensitive polymer-modified liposomes with cationic lipid inclusion as antigen delivery carriers for cancer immunotherapy. Biomaterials 2014; 35(28): 8186-96.
[http://dx.doi.org/10.1016/j.biomaterials.2014.05.077] [PMID: 24969637]

[142] Yuba E, Harada A, Sakanishi Y, Kono K. Carboxylated hyperbranched poly(glycidol)s for preparation of pH-sensitive liposomes. J Control Release 2011; 149(1): 72-80.
[http://dx.doi.org/10.1016/j.jconrel.2010.03.001] [PMID: 20206654]

[143] Naziris N, Pippa N, Meristoudi A, Pispas S, Demetzos C. Design and development of pH-responsive HSPC:$C_{12}H_{25}$-PAA chimeric liposomes. J Liposome Res 2017; 27(2): 108-17.
[http://dx.doi.org/10.3109/08982104.2016.1166512] [PMID: 27558454]

[144] Pippa N, Chountoulesi M, Kyrili A, Meristoudi A, Pispas S, Demetzos C. Calorimetric study on pH-responsive block copolymer grafted lipid bilayers: Rational design and development of liposomes. J Liposome Res 2016; 26(3): 211-20.
[http://dx.doi.org/10.3109/08982104.2015.1076464] [PMID: 26364717]

[145] Hoffman AS, Stayton P, Press OW, Murthy N, Reed CL, Crum LA, *et al.* Enhanced transport using membrane disruptive agents. US8003129, 2011.

[146] Sim SJ, Won SH, Lee JU. pH sensitive fluorescent polydiacetylene liposome and drug delivery vehicle comprising same. EP2870959, 2017.

[147] Essler F, Panzner S, Endert G. Components for producing amphoteric liposomes. US8580297, 2013.

[148] Essler F, Panzner S, Endert G. pH-sensitive cationic lipids, and liposomes and nanocapsules containing the same. US20060002991, 2006.

[149] Saltzman WM, Zhang J, Zhou J, Jiang Z. Formulations for targeted release of agents to low pH tissue environments or cellular compartments and methods of use thereof. US9895451, 2018.

[150] Gao GH, Li Y, Lee DS. Environmental pH-sensitive polymeric micelles for cancer diagnosis and targeted therapy. J Control Release 2013; 169(3): 180-4.
[http://dx.doi.org/10.1016/j.jconrel.2012.11.012] [PMID: 23195533]

[151] Liu Z, Zhang N. pH-Sensitive polymeric micelles for programmable drug and gene delivery. Curr Pharm Des 2012; 18(23): 3442-51.
[http://dx.doi.org/10.2174/138161212801227122] [PMID: 22632817]

[152] Bae YH, Na K, Lee ES. H-sensitive polymeric micelles for drug delivery. US7951846, 2011.

[153] Chiu HC, Chiang WH, Hung CC, Yu TW. Preparation of pH-responsive nanoparticles and promoted delivery of anticancer drugs into deep tumor tissues and application thereof. US20160367489, 2016.

[154] Taylor DK, Ochieng MA. Biodegradable liquogel and pH sensitive nanocarriers. US20130217789, 2013.

[155] Wu XY, Shalviri A, Cai P. Polymeric nanoparticles useful in theranostics. CA2865925, 2013.

[156] Goldberg MN, Alonso MJ, Chen KJ. Targeted buccal delivery of agents. WO2014130866, 2014.

[157] Li J, Cai P, Shalviri A, *et al.* A multifunctional polymeric nanotheranostic system delivers doxorubicin and imaging agents across the blood-brain barrier targeting brain metastases of breast cancer. ACS Nano 2014; 8(10): 9925-40.
[http://dx.doi.org/10.1021/nn501069c] [PMID: 25307677]

[158] Chen IW, Choi H, Zhou R. pH-sensitive peptides and their nanoparticles for drug delivery. US9687563, 2017.

[159] Stavroula S. pH sensitive liposome composition. US20110027171, 2011.

[160] O'Halloran TV, Chen H, Mazar A. Nanoparticle arsenic-platinum compositions. US20140220115, 2014.

[161] Radosz M, Xu P, Shen Y. Nanoparticles for cytoplasmic drug delivery to cancer cells. US8945629, 2015.

[162] Radovic-Moreno AF, Gao W, Swami A, Golomb G, Langer RS, Farokhzad OC. Farokhzad OC. pH sensitive biodegradable polymeric particles for drug delivery. US9532956, 2017.

[163] Choonara YE, Du TLC, Pillay V, Wadee A. An implant for the controlled release of pharmaceutically active agents. WO2012070033, 2012.

[164] Sousa-Herves A, Fernandez-Megia E, Riguera VR. Fernandez-Megia E, Riguera VR. pH-sensitive dendritic polymeric micelles. US20120003322, 2011.

[165] Bazile D, Couvreur P, Lakkireddy HR, Mackiewicz N, Nicolas J. Functional PLA-PEG copolymers, the nanoparticles thereof, their preparation and use for targeted drug delivery and imaging. WO2013127949, 2013.

[166] Lee DS, Kim BS, Lee JH, Gao G. pH-sensitive block copolymer forming polyionic complex micelles and drug or protein carrier using the same. US8911775, 2014.

[167] Lee DS, Kim MS, Kim BS. pH-sensitive graft copolymer, manufacturing method for same, and polymer micelles using method. US9080049, 2015.

[168] Kim S, Nam J. Anticancer drug delivery system using pH-sensitive metal nanoparticles. EP2559429, 2013.

[169]   Cha HJ, Kim BJ, Cheong H. pH-responsive nanoparticle using mussel adhesive protein for drug delivery and method for preparing the same. US9675629, 2017.

[170]   Fouladi F, Steffen KJ, Mallik S. Enzyme-responsive liposomes for the delivery of anticancer drugs. Bioconjug Chem 2017; 28(4): 857-68.
[http://dx.doi.org/10.1021/acs.bioconjchem.6b00736] [PMID: 28201868]

[171]   Hu J, Zhang G, Liu S. Enzyme-responsive polymeric assemblies, nanoparticles and hydrogels. Chem Soc Rev 2012; 41(18): 5933-49.
[http://dx.doi.org/10.1039/c2cs35103j] [PMID: 22695880]

[172]   Hu Q, Katti PS, Gu Z. Enzyme-responsive nanomaterials for controlled drug delivery. Nanoscale 2014; 6(21): 12273-86.
[http://dx.doi.org/10.1039/C4NR04249B] [PMID: 25251024]

[173]   de la Rica R, Aili D, Stevens MM. Enzyme-responsive nanoparticles for drug release and diagnostics. Adv Drug Deliv Rev 2012; 64(11): 967-78.
[http://dx.doi.org/10.1016/j.addr.2012.01.002] [PMID: 22266127]

[174]   Yadav L, Puri N, Rastogi V, Satpute P, Ahmad R, Kaur G. Matrix metalloproteinases and cancer - roles in threat and therapy. Asian Pac J Cancer Prev 2014; 15(3): 1085-91.
[http://dx.doi.org/10.7314/APJCP.2014.15.3.1085] [PMID: 24606423]

[175]   Hadler-Olsen E, Winberg JO, Uhlin-Hansen L. Matrix metalloproteinases in cancer: Their value as diagnostic and prognostic markers and therapeutic targets. Tumour Biol 2013; 34(4): 2041-51.
[http://dx.doi.org/10.1007/s13277-013-0842-8] [PMID: 23681802]

[176]   Tauro M, McGuire J, Lynch CC. New approaches to selectively target cancer-associated matrix metalloproteinase activity. Cancer Metastasis Rev 2014; 33(4): 1043-57.
[http://dx.doi.org/10.1007/s10555-014-9530-4] [PMID: 25325988]

[177]   Kulkarni PS, Haldar MK, Mallik S, Srivastava DK. Controlled release nanoparticles and methods of us. US9457041, 2016.

[178]   Kulkarni PS, Haldar MK, Nahire RR, *et al.* MMP-9 responsive PEG cleavable nanovesicles for efficient delivery of chemotherapeutics to pancreatic cancer. Mol Pharm 2014; 11(7): 2390-9.
[http://dx.doi.org/10.1021/mp500108p] [PMID: 24827725]

[179]   Appleford M, Kelley MM. Logical enzyme triggered (let) layer-by-layer nanocapsules for drug delivery system. WO2013043812, 2013.

[180]   Scott KF, Sajinovic M, Hein J, *et al.* Emerging roles for phospholipase A2 enzymes in cancer. Biochimie 2010; 92(6): 601-10.
[http://dx.doi.org/10.1016/j.biochi.2010.03.019] [PMID: 20362028]

[181]   Kokotou MG, Limnios D, Nikolaou A, Psarra A, Kokotos G. Inhibitors of phospholipase A_2 and their therapeutic potential: An update on patents (2012-2016). Expert Opin Ther Pat 2017; 27(2): 217-25.
[http://dx.doi.org/10.1080/13543776.2017.1246540] [PMID: 27718763]

[182]   Vikbjerg AF, Petersen SA, Melander F, Henriksen JR, Jørgensen K. Liposomes for drug delivery and methods for preparation thereof. WO2009141450, 2009.

[183]   Gondi CS, Rao JS. Cathepsin B as a cancer target. Expert Opin Ther Targets 2013; 17(3): 281-91.
[http://dx.doi.org/10.1517/14728222.2013.740461] [PMID: 23293836]

[184]   Aggarwal N, Sloane BF. Cathepsin B: Multiple roles in cancer. Proteomics Clin Appl 2014; 8(5-6): 427-37.
[http://dx.doi.org/10.1002/prca.201300105] [PMID: 24677670]

[185]   Law SHB, Tung CH, Bellat V. Enzyme-responsive peptide nanofiber compositions and uses thereof. WO2017059338, 2017.

[186]   Fologea D, Salamo G, Henry R, Borrelli MJ, Corry PM. Method of controlled drug release from a

liposome carrie. US8808733, 2014.

[187]   Stevens MM, Ulijn R, Laromaine AS, Koh L. Particles. US8318206, 2012.

[188]   Roy K, Wanakule P, Singh A. Triggered release of drugs from polymer particles. US20100010102, 2010.

[189]   Gianneschi NC, Hahn M, Mattrey R. Enzyme directed assembly of particle theranostics. US20140193342, 2014.

[190]   Amir RJ, Buzhor M, Harnoy AJ, Rosenbaum I, Frid L. Micelar delivery system based on enzyme-responsive amphiphilic peg-dendron hybrid. EP3191137, 2017.

[191]   Kannan R, Raman S, Upendran A, Suresh D. Targeted nanoparticle conjugate and method for co-delivery of siRNA and drug. WO2017011618, 2017.

[192]   Wong CR, Bawendi MG, Fukumura D, Jain RK. Multistage nanoparticle drug delivery system for the treatment of solid tumors. US20140161884, 2014.

[193]   Yoo B, Bradbury MS, Wiesner U, Ma K. Nanoparticle drug conjugates. CA2947895, 2015.

[194]   Segura T, Zhu S, Wen J, Lu Y. Enzyme responsive nanocapsules for protein delivery. WO2013033717, 2013.

[195]   Chen X, Lee S, Choi KY, Liu G. Nanoparticles for delivery of ligands. US20140162966, 2014.

[196]   Daftarian P, Daunert S, Fukata M. Enteric coated nanoparticles for oral vaccine and drug delivery and methods of production and use thereof. WO2014120804, 2014.

[197]   Sun H, Meng F, Cheng R, Deng C, Zhong Z. Reduction-sensitive degradable micellar nanoparticles as smart and intuitive delivery systems for cancer chemotherapy. Expert Opin Drug Deliv 2013; 10(8): 1109-22.
[http://dx.doi.org/10.1517/17425247.2013.783009] [PMID: 23517599]

[198]   Jhaveri A, Deshpande P, Torchilin V. Stimuli-sensitive nanopreparations for combination cancer therapy. J Control Release 2014; 190: 352-70.
[http://dx.doi.org/10.1016/j.jconrel.2014.05.002] [PMID: 24818767]

[199]   Lee Y, Thompson DH. Stimuli-responsive liposomes for drug delivery. Wiley Interdiscip Rev Nanomed Nanobiotechnol 2017; 9(5): e1450.
[http://dx.doi.org/10.1002/wnan.1450] [PMID: 28198148]

[200]   McCarley RL, Ong WZ. Redox-gated liposomes. US20110104250, 2011.

[201]   University S. Reductive sensitivity tumor target lipidosome based on cholesterol modification. CN102266288, 2012.

[202]   Zhang M, Ellenbogen RG, Kievit F, Silber JR, Stephen Z, Veiseh O. Nanoparticle for targeting brain tumors and delivery of o6-benzylguanine. US20140286872, 2014.

[203]   Stephen ZR, Kievit FM, Veiseh O, *et al.* Redox-responsive magnetic nanoparticle for targeted convection-enhanced delivery of O6-benzylguanine to brain tumors. ACS Nano 2014; 8(10): 10383-95.
[http://dx.doi.org/10.1021/nn503735w] [PMID: 25247850]

[204]   Gu Z, Nie Y, He Y, Cheng G, Xie L. Reduction stimulus-responsive gene delivery system and preparation and application thereof. US9707303, 2017.

[205]   Xu P. Polymers and the preparation of nanogel drug cocktails. US9149535, 2015.

[206]   University P. Preparation method and application of reduction-response-type pegylation (PEG) nanomedicine composition. CN103705943, 2014.

[207]   Kordas G, Efthimiadou E. 2015.Multi-responsive targeting drug delivery systems for controlled-release pharmaceutical formulation. WO2015074762

[208] Porter MD, Granger JH. Redox polymer nanoparticles. US7893177, 2011.

[209] Tang L, Irvine DJ. Carrier-free biologically-active protein nanostructures. US9603944, 2017.

[210] Dias AJAA, Zhong Z, Sun H, Wang W, Meng F, Feijen J. Reduction sensitive biodegradable polyesteramides. EP3177668, 2017.

[211] Sankaran T, Molla MR, Garman SC. Polymers and polymeric nanogels with hydrophilics encapsulation and release capabilities and methods thereof. EP3193831, 2017.

[212] Xu P, He H. Preparation of triple responsive nanogel system and its application. US9283281, 2016.

[213] Thayumanavan S, Hardy JA. Polymers and polymeric assemblies for peptide and protein encaosulation and release, and methods thereof. WO2016179189, 2016.

[214] Brenneisen P, Seal S, Karakoti A. Redox active cerium oxide nanoparticles and associated methods. US9585840, 2017.

[215] Schanen B, Warren W, Self W, Seal S, Drake D. Methods of using CeO$_2$ and TiO$_2$ nanoparticles in modulation of the immune system. WO2014008503, 2014.

[216] Tang Y, Gu Z, Zhao M. responsive polymeric nanocapsules for protein delivery. WO2012142410, 2012.

[217] Xu P, Cheng B, He H. Preparations of gold/mesoporous silica hybrid nanoparitcle and applications. US20160067354, 2016.

[218] Thayumanavan S, Klaikherd A, Ghosh S. Cleavable block copolymers, functionalized nanoporous thin films and related methods of preparation. US8198368, 2012.

[219] Zare RN, Ge J. Methods of electric field induced delivery of compounds, compositions used in delivery, and systems of delivery. US9713702, 2017.

[220] Khizroev S, Guduru R, Liang P. On-demand drug release using magneto-electric nanoparticles. US9724503, 2017.

[221] Giri BP, Gregg K, Singh P, Dagli DJ, Giri A. Hypoxia-targeted polymeric micelles for cancer therapy and imaging. US20140010760, 2014.

[222] Torchilin V, Biswas S. Hypoxia-targeted delivery system for pharmaceutical agents. WO2015061321, 2015.

[223] Moslemy P, Wang H, Patane M. Positively-charged poly (d,l-lactide-co-glycolide) nanoparticles and fabrication methods of the same. US20120177741, 2012.

[224] Sharma P, Brown SC, Bengtsson N, *et al.* Near-IR indocyanine green doped multimodal silica nanoparticles and methods for making the same. US20130108552, 2013.

CHAPTER 4

The Regulation and the Function of Autophagy in the Development and Behavior of Esophageal Cancers

Erdem Ayik* and **Gulsum O. Elpek**

Department of Pathology, Medical School, Akdeniz University, Antalya 07070, Turkey

Abstract: Autophagy (AP) is a cell recovery programme that plays a critical role by degrading dysfunctional organelles and misfolded proteins. Besides its position to maintain homeostasis, the contribution of AP to the development and progression of several pathological conditions, including cancer has been denoted. A significant number of findings indicate the involvement of AP-mediated cell survival in the progression of many tumors. However, the data in esophageal cancer (EC) appears to be less initiated. In this chapter, first definition, types and mechanisms of AP are described, and the following sections are focused on giving a clear view of the findings that communicate AP with oncogenesis and tumor progression in EC. Moreover, the use of several drugs, which are known to modulate AP (inhibitors [3-MA, Bafilomycin etc.] and inducers [Nimotuzumab etc.]) in the treatment of EC, is discussed.

The current data indicated that although the role of AP in carcinogenesis, tumor behavior and response to treatment in EC is non-negligible, the first problem to be resolved is to determine whether AP should be stimulated or inhibited because it seems that both strategies are encouraging. Another problem is the identification of the patient who will benefit from the manipulation of AP. Finally; the use of existing drugs that may have off-target effects warrants the development of specific AP modulating compounds suitable for use in patients with EC. The potential role of AP in EC chemoresistance necessitates further investigations not only with AP related proteins but also their related pathways into open up new corners for therapeutic intervention.

Keywords: Apoptosis, autophagosome, autophagy, Beclin-1, cancer, carcinogenesis, cell survival, chemoresistance, esophageal carcinoma, esophagus, inhibition of autophagy, LC3 protein, pathway, regulation of autophagy, treatment.

---

* **Corresponding author Erdem Ayik:** Department of Pathology, Medical School, Akdeniz University, Antalya 07070, Turkey; Tel: +902422496389; E-mail: erdemayik@hotmail.com

Atta-ur-Rahman and Khurshid Zaman (Eds.)

1. INTRODUCTION

First introduced as a term by Christian de Duve in 1963, "autophagy" (literally meaning "self-eating") [1] is an evolutionary cell survival program that plays a critical role by degrading dysfunctional organelles and misfolded proteins. Since its first description, much evidence has been obtained to date that autophagy is not a simple cell survival mechanism and might play opposite roles depending on the cellular microenvironment [2, 3]. Indeed, autophagy is also a pattern of programmed cell death that is entitled "programmed cell death type II" [4]. This type of cell death is not related to the morphological and molecular characteristics of either apoptosis (programmed cell death type I, APT) or necroptosis. However, recent data indicates that the autophagic and apoptotic cell death pathways are interrelated [5]. This relation involves many pathways, the interactions between these events occur at several points, and the fine-tuned balance between them defines the morphology of cell death (see below).

Since the contribution of autophagy to the occurrence and progression of various diseases, including cancer, has been indicated, in the last decade, the dual function of autophagy and its relationship with APT has been one of the most investigated phenomena in carcinogenesis and anticancer treatment. Although several findings suggest the association of autophagy-related cell survival in carcinogenesis and the behavior of many malignancies [6], the data on esophageal cancer (EC) still appears to be more limited.

In this chapter, first, the general characteristics of autophagy and its role in cancer development and tumor behavior will be briefly presented. The next section will address the significant features that communicate autophagy with carcinogenesis and tumor behavior in EC. We suggest that interested readers consult more extensive articles on the involvement of autophagy in other forms of cancer involving the gastrointestinal system.

2. GENERAL ASPECTS OF AUTOPHAGY

Basically, together with the Ubiquitin-Proteasome System (UPS), autophagy is one of the two major degradative pathways in mammalian cells [5]. In contrast to the UPS, autophagy does not necessitate protein labeled with ubiquitin and does not take place in the proteasome. It is a self-digestive event, which occur in the lysosome. Constitutive AP is a pivotal element of the quality control program in cells and the basal turnover of proteins and organelles [7]. On the other hand, induced AP is activated by various stimuli, such as cellular stress [3].

There are three basic forms of autophagy: microautophagy, chaperone-mediated autophagy, and macroautophagy. Although these types share a common terminus, the lysosome, the delivery of the cytosolic components to the lysosome is different. Additionally, their regulation, their targeted substrates, and the conditions in which each of them are activated are also different [8 - 10]. Microautophagy is a simple event necessitating GTP hydrolysis and Ca^{++} [11 - 13]. As the name implies, in chaperone-mediated autophagy, the translocation of cellular protein to the lysosomal membrane depends on chaperone-mediated (Hsc70) transport [14, 15]. This type of autophagy is selective, and only proteins with a KFERQ-like motif are sequestrated [14, 15]. Macroautophagy is a well-characterized form of autophagy [16]. It involves the degradation of cytoplasmic components into lysosomes in a nonselective manner. This form of autophagy has two main purposes: the generation of principal macromolecules and energy in conditions of starvation or as a mechanism for the eradication of altered cellular constituents [16]. Macroautophagy, hereafter referred to as AP, proceeds through the generation of autophagosomes that are constituted from double-membrane vesicles [17, 18]. The autophagosome expands to engulf neighboring cytosolic components and organelles, which are degraded after fusion with lysosomes [18].

AP is a multistep process consisting of eight steps: Initiation, nucleation, membrane elongation, closure, maturation and degradation [19 - 35]. The mechanism of AP was not fully understood before the detection of a group of AP-related genes (ATGs) and the proteins (Atgs) encoded by them [20, 21]. Recently, it has been demonstrated that the harmonious action of these proteins is required for autophagosome formation. For this reason, Atgs are termed the "core" molecular mechanism. These proteins are composed of four broad groups: (1) the unc-51-like kinase complex (ULK1/ULK2); (2) Beclin-1-the class III phosphatidylinositol 3-kinase complex (PI3K); (3) two ubiquitin-like proteins, Atg12 and microtubule-associated protein 1 light chain 3 (LC3); and (4) transmembrane proteins Atg 9 [22]. The main properties and functions of these proteins are summarized in Table **1** [23 - 35].

Table 1. Proteins that are Involved in AP.

Proteins	Properties	Role	References
ULK-1	Binds with ATG13, ATG101, and FIP200	Phosphorylates and activates the Beclin-1/Vps34 complex	[23]
Atg13	Enables the interaction of ULK1 and FIP200	Provides the localization and stability of ULK1 and stimulates its activity	[24]
Atg101	Interacts with ULK1	Stabilization and phosphorylation of ATG13 and ULK1	[23]
FIP200	Binds with ULK1 and ATG13	Proper localization, stabilization and kinase activity of ULK1	[23]
Beclin-1	BH3-only protein	Interacts with Bcl-2	[23, 25]

(Table 1) cont.....

Proteins	Properties	Role	References
Vps34	PI3K	Forms PI3P for autophagosome	[25]
Atg14L	Barkor	Enhances Vps34 lipid kinase activity	[25]
hVps15	Ser/Thr protein kinase	Vps34 membrane association depends on it	[25]
Atg5	-	Forms isopeptide (with ATG12)	[23]
Atg12	Ubiquitin-like protein	Forms isopeptide (with Atg5 conjugation)	[26]
Atg7	E1-like enzyme	ATG12–ATG5 and LC3-II-PE conjugation	[23, 27, 28]
Atg10	E2-like enzyme	ATG12–ATG5 conjugation	[23]
ATG16L1	E2-like conjugating enzyme analog	Catalyzes LC3-II-PE conjugation	[23, 29]
LC3	Ubiquitin-like protein	Conjugates to PE and interact with proteins that recruit cargo (p62/SQSTM1). Closure of autophagosome	[26, 30, 31]
Atg4	Cysteine protease	Regulates the level LC3-I	[32 - 34]
Atg7	E1-like activating enzyme	ATG12–ATG5 and LC3-II-PE conjugation	[23, 27, 35]
ATG3	E2-like conjugating enzyme analog	LC3-II-PE conjugation	[31, 35]
Atg9	A transmembrane protein	Contributes to membrane recruitment	[23, 27, 35]
Atg2	-	Late step of autophagosome formation	[23, 35]
WIPI	PI3P-binding protein	Binds with PI3P, Facilitates LC3 lipidation	[35]

ULK-1: Unc-51-like kinase; **FIP200:** Focal adhesion kinase family-interacting protein of 200 kD; **Bcl-2:** B-Cell lymphoma 2; **PI3K:** Phosphoinositide-3 kinase; **PI3P:** Phosphatidylinositol 3-phosphate; **LC3:** Microtubule-associated protein 1 light chain 3; **PE:** Phosphatidylethanolamine; **p62/SQSTM1:** p62/Sequestosome cytoplasm 1; **WIPI:** WD-repeat protein interacting with phosphoinositides1

The molecular events involved in AP are presented in Fig. (**1**). Briefly, AP initiation is induced by the activation of ULK1/2 to form a complex with Atg13, Atg 101, and the focal adhesion kinase family-interacting protein of 200 kD (FIP200) [23]. Two signal pathways regulate the ULK1/2 activation; while the mechanistic target of rapamycin (mTOR) acts as an inhibitor, the AMP-activated protein kinase (AMPK) pathway stimulates ULK1/2 [24]. The ULK1 complex phosphorylates and activates the Beclin-1/Vps34 complex (Table **1** and Fig. (**1**)) [23 - 25]. Both the initiation and nucleation proteins promote the formation of the autophagic vesicle membrane termed the "phagophore" (a cup-shaped structure). The primary function of the Beclin-1/Vps34 complex is the formation of phosphatidylinositol 3-phosphate (PI3P) in the areas of phagophore nucleation. Subsequently, the accumulation of PI3Ps constitutes a platform for the linkage of proteins such as WD-repeat protein interacting with phosphoinositides 1 (WIPI) [23 - 25]. This platform is fundamental for the aggregation of assembly for the "elongation" of the phagophore [23 - 25]. Atg9 and its cycling system also provide lipid delivery to the membrane, leading to its expansion [17, 27]. During the maturation step, two protein conjugation systems are necessary: The first system is the conjugation of Atg12; the other is the conjugation of LC3 to phosphatidylethanolamine (Table **1** and Fig. (**1**)) [17, 23, 27 - 35].

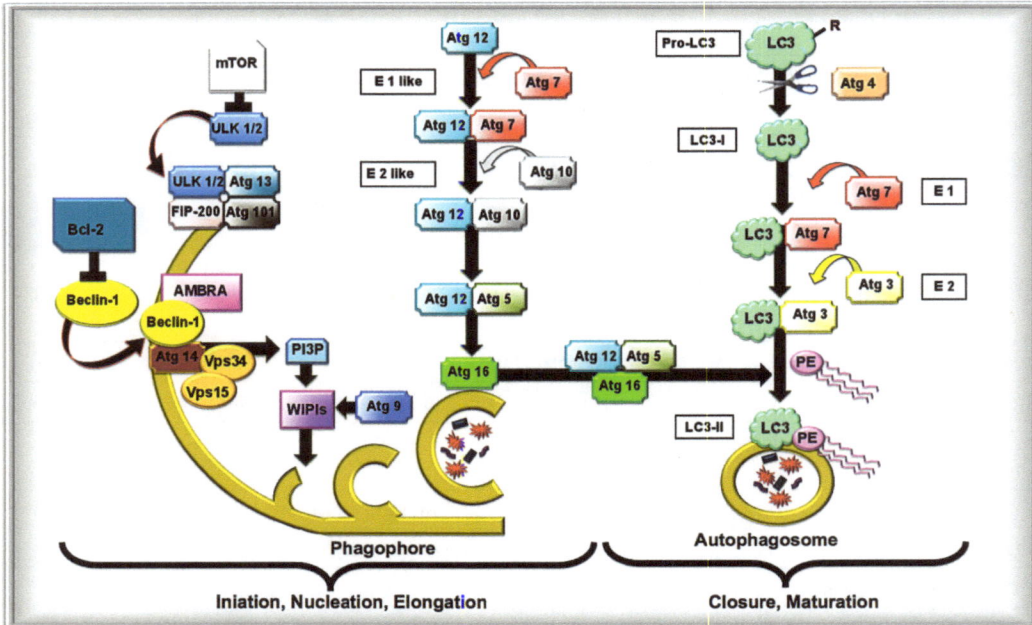

Fig. (1). The molecular events participating AP.

Another vital role of LC3 is its interference with adaptor proteins that recruit cargo from the cytoplasm (e.g. p62/Sequestosome cytoplasm 1 [SQSTM1]) [26, 35]. As recent data indicates that LC3 is a critical AP protein, it is used as an autophagosomal marker in many AP studies [26, 35]. Following closure, autophagolysosomes are generated by the fusion of the autophagosome with lysosomes. Subsequently, the contents that are degraded by hydrolases are released into the cytoplasm [36, 37].

The regulation of AP involves various signaling pathways and small molecules. Many of these pathways also contribute to cell growth, proliferation survival, and death. More detailed information about the effect of these pathways on AP and the underlying mechanisms are presented in previous comprehensive reviews [2, 5, 6, 38 - 45].

As noted earlier, despite the differences between AP and APT, the apoptotic functions of Atgs and the influences of caspases on AP constitute an overlap between AP and APT [46 - 52]. Moreover, recent evidence indicates that several signaling mediators regulate both AP and APT [53 - 59]. At present, it is possible that the relationship between AP and APT is not as simple as it seems and highly dependent on the microenvironment. While in some conditions, AP counteracts APT, in others, it acts synergistically with APT. From this point of view, it is reasonable to suggest that AP can function as a "friend" or "foe" of APT depending on the surrounding milieu.

3. AUTOPHAGY IN CANCER

AP plays dual roles in malignant transformation. Although AP acts as a tumor suppressor, after malignant transformation, it promotes tumor growth.

3.1. AP in Malignant Transformation

Although the relationship between AP and oncogenesis is not fully understood, many studies indicate that failures in this event are related to the development of various tumors [60 - 64]. The adaptive role AP in the protection of cells from malignant transformation has been suggested [62]. AP can act as a barrier to the prevention of oncogenesis through several mechanisms: It can facilitate the preservation of genetic permanency and energy balance [64].

One of the critical initiators of AP, Beclin-1 also acts as a tumor suppressor [65 - 70]. It helps to preserve chromosomal stability and prevent the increased frequency of extra mutations [65]. Accordingly, Beclin-1 has been found to be deleted in many cancers (such as prostate, ovarian, breast, brain, and lung cancers) [66 - 68]. Furthermore, the monoallelic deletion of Beclin-1 in animals has promoted tumor development [69]. Its inadequacy was also found to be related with angiogenesis, an event that can be exploited by transformed cells during tumor development and progression [70].

Other evidence for the role of AP in the prevention of tumor formation is the activation of AP by tumor suppressor genes and its inhibition by oncogenes [71, 72]. Members of the Bcl-2 protein family (anti-apoptotic proteins) prevent AP by inhibiting Beclin-1 function [67]. Additionally, activated receptor tyrosine kinases can hinder AP through their influences on mTOR1 and Akt signaling [72].

Accumulated evidence indicating the involvement of AP in the reduction of oxidative stress also highlights its preventive effect on tumor formation [73 - 75]. For instance, the loss of Atg7 leads to elevated oxidative stress (via ROS) in cells and causes genomic instability, resulting in neoplastic transformation [75, 76]. As AP induces the expression of antioxidant proteins, the defects in AP might induce oncogenesis [77, 78].

Additionally, the deterioration of AP together with APT causes necrosis and inflammation [79]. Indeed, the recruitment of the pro-inflammatory cytokines is strongly related to this phenomenon. It is noteworthy that some of these cytokines are related to carcinogenesis, such as TNF-α, IL-1β, and IL-6 [79]. Taken together, these data suggest a protective role of AP in the early phase of oncogenesis.

3.2. AP in Cancer Behavior and Treatment

As noted earlier, in normal cells, constitutive AP helps to maintain homeostasis by suppressing cancer initiation and progression [80]. However, after malignant transformation, AP is recognized as an important cell survival mechanism [81].

Additionally, recent studies indicate that AP is involved in cellular mechanisms that promote invasion and metastasis [82 - 87]. AP also regulates the coordinated secretion of cytokines that favor invasion, supporting the hypothesis that AP may possess autonomous functions in tumor cells and stromal elements by influencing their secretory capacity [84, 88]. Recently, the relation of AP-related genes to tumor behavior has been investigated in many cancers, demonstrating the relation of AP with aggressive behavior and poor survival [6].

As AP is an important part of cancer cell survival, it also contributes to the escape of tumor cells from chemotherapy and radiotherapy-induced cell death. In many cancers, interplay between AP and APT in the settings of targeted therapies also suggests that the inhibition of APT by AP is more relevant for the survival of tumor cells than the potential apoptotic effects of AP or the selective inhibition of AP by apoptotic mechanisms. Indeed, the influence of AP in drug resistance has been established in cell lines. AP facilitates chemoresistance development by blocking APT [89 - 94], and the induction of AP is involved in the development of resistance to many drugs [92 - 94]. Nevertheless, the molecular machinery of AP in drug resistance is complicated and not yet clear. In this event, many factors or signaling pathways are involved, including the PI3K/protein kinase/mTOR axis, p53, EGFR, and Mitogen-Activated Protein Kinases/p38 signaling [95]. Although the influence of AP in drug resistance together with its underlying mechanisms needs to be confirmed by further studies, all findings described above suggest that the modification of AP may be an essential therapeutic strategy in the treatment of established cancer. Evidence indicates that it is possible to manipulate AP for cancer therapy in two ways. The first way is the inhibition of cytoprotective AP, which leads to cell death other than programmed cell death II. The other way is to stimulate excessive AP, which leads to PCD II [96]. As the modulation of AP in both directions can be performed by the interference of multiple pathways in cancer therapy, many compounds that modulate AP have been discovered [97 - 115] (see Table **2**). On the other hand, to avoid the side effects of the therapy, it is important to demonstrate whether the manipulation of AP affects normal cells. In a genetically engineered mouse model, cancer cells are more dependent on AP than normal cells, suggesting that there may be a therapeutic window for AP modulation for therapy.

Table 2. AP Inhibitors and Inducers and Most Recent Patent About These Products.

Drugs	EtA	Inventors	Title	Patent Number	Ref.
3-MA	inh	Chengyu, J., *et al.*	Use of cell autophagy (type II cell apoptosis) inhibitors	WO2010124618	[97]
Proton pump inhibitors	ind	Matsui, M., Yarosh, D.	Small molecule inhibitors of p-type atpases	WO2013130407	[98]
Bafilomycin	inh	Korur, S., *et al.*	Combination of lysosomotropic or autophagy modulating agents and a gsk-3 inhibitor for treatment of cancer	WO2013182519	[99]
OBX (MG-132)	ind	Levy, N., *et al.*	Proteasome inhibitors for treating a disorder related to an accumulation of non-degraded abnormal protein or a cancer	WO2016113357	[100]
Nimotuzumab	ind	Zaupa, C., *et al.*	Combination product with autophagy modulator	WO2016131945	[101]
Estradiol analogue	ind	Amaravadi, R.K., Winkler, J.	Dimeric quinacrine derivatives as autophagy inhibitors for cancer therapy	WO2016168721	[102]
BEZ235	ind	Deckwerth, T., *et al.*	Autophagy-inhibiting compounds and uses thereof	WO2016196393	[103]
Navitoclax (ABT-263)	ind	Spada, A.P.	Caspase inhibitors for use in the treatment of liver cancer	WO2017079566	[104]
Rapamycin	ind	Faraci, W.S., *et al.*	Particle delivery of rapamycin to the liver	WO2017139212	[105]
CDDO-Me	ind	Siegelin, M.D., Altieri, D.C.	Combination therapies with mitochondrial-targeted anti-tumor agents	US20110268722	[106]
Metformin	ind	Cho, M.-L., *et al.*	Composition using metformin for preventing or treating immune diseases including lupus	US20150238445	[107]
ISG-15	inh	Desai, S.D.	Therapeutic and diagnostic method for ataxia-telangiectasia	US20170196871	[108]
UBE2L6/UBCH8	inh	Desai, S.D.	Therapeutic and diagnostic method for ataxia-telangiectasia	US20170196871	[108]

(Table 2) cont.....

Drugs	EtA	Inventors	Title	Patent Number	Ref.
Chloroquine	inh	Espina, V., Liotta, L.	Methods of treating pre-malignant ductal cancer with autophagy inhibitors	US9096833	[109]
Lithium	ind	McKenna, S., *et al.*	Method for the treatment of cancer	US9155761	[110]
HA14-1	ind	McKenna, S., *et al.*	Method for the treatment of cancer	US9155761	[110]
DHA	ind	Huijun, Z., *et al.*	Application of dihydroartemisinin to preparation of tumor cell autophagy induction medicament	CN102038678	[111]
Tunicamycin	ind	Zhenghong, Q., *et al.*	Application of tunicamycin in preparing medicament for treating ischemic cerebral apoplexy	CN102119935	[112]
Ginsenoside Ro	inh	Zhang, S., *et al.*	20(R)-Ginsenoside Rg3/cationic lipid/cholesterol/folic acid liposome medicine as well as preparation method and application thereof	CN105534911	[113]
Dichloroacetate	ind	Yu, D., *et al.*	Application of diisopropylamine dichloroacetate in treating tumors	CN105748455	[114]
Gambogic acid	ind	Peng, Y., *et al.*	Tumor-targeting gambogic acid compound, and preparation method and application thereof	CN106083898	[115]

Abbreviations: **EtA:** Effect to autophagy; **Ref:** Referance; **3-MA**: 3-Methyladenine; **Gsk3**: Glycogen Synthase Kinase-3; **ISG-15**: Interferon Stimulated Gene 15; **OBX**: Obatoclax (GX15-070); **CDDO-Me**: 2-Cyano-3,12-dioxoolean-1,9- dien-28-oic acid methyl ester (Bardoxolone methyl); **inh:** Inhibition; **ind:** Induction

4. AUTOPHAGY IN ESOPHAGEAL CANCER

Esophageal cancer is the eighth most common cancer worldwide, with a high mortality rate [116, 117]. Indeed, it is the sixth most common cause of cancer death with a 5-year survival rate of 18.4% [116]. There are two predominant histologic types of primary esophageal cancers: squamous cell carcinoma (ESCC) and adenocarcinoma (EAC) [118]. Although both tumors have some overlap, they are different with regard to epidemiologic distribution, risk factors, and pathogenesis [118]. Moreover, the profiles of genomic alterations in both tumors differ widely. For these reasons, in this section, the role of AP in oncogenesis, tumor behavior, and therapeutic response will be delineated in EAC and ESCC separately. The demographical and pathologic findings of both tumors are summarized in Table **3**.

Table 3. Clinicopathological Findings of EAC and ESCC.

Parameters	ESCC	EAC
Incidence	Frequent in Asian/Eastern countries	Frequent in Western World
Age	6 - 7th decade	6 - 7th decade
Gender	Male > Female	Male > Female
Most common localization	Middle third > Lower third > Upper Third	Lower Third > Middle and Upper third
Risk factors	Smoking, Chewing tobacco Alcohol consumption Dietary factors HPV* Tylosis, Achalasia	GERD Male sex Caucasian race, Tobacco smoking Obesity
Premalignant precursor lesion	Squamous dysplasia/Intraepithelial neoplasia	BE
Special stains	TP63, CK5/6, CK7, CK14	CK7, CK20, CDX2
Molecular	TP53 mutation Cyclin D1 overexpression EGFR overexpression mTOR (PIK3CA and PTEN), NOTCH1	TP53 mutation HER2 amplification EGFR amplification KRAS

ESCC: Squamous cell carcinoma; **EAC:** Adenocarcinoma; **GERD:** Gastroesophageal reflux disease; **HPV**: Human papilloma virus; * Still debated; **BE:** Barrett esophagus; **CK:** Cytokeratin; **CDX2:** Caudal-type homeobox transcription factor 2

4.1. Autophagy in the Development of EAC

Although many different risk factors have emerged, the role of AP in EAC development has been barely investigated. As Barrett's esophagus (BE) is an indisputable premalignant lesion and a standard model for investigating early events that take place in the evolution of esophageal adenocarcinoma (EAC), many of these studies are focused on BE and EAC. Multiple complementary techniques demonstrate the contribution of AP to the oncogenesis of EAC: In biopsies from patients with BE and EAC, Beclin-1 positivity is more frequent in normal squamous epithelium and nondysplastic BE when compared to areas of BE with dysplasia and EAC [78, 119, 120]. The same observations were also noted in rat tissues [78, 119]. Parallel with these findings, significantly high levels of Beclin-1 expression have been identified in cell lines derived from normal epithelium when compared to the low expression of Beclin-1 in BE and EAC [78, 119, 120]. The quantitation of AP levels across the BE-EAC spectrum revealed that the mean levels of AP in normal squamous cells were 1.5 times lower than in BE cells [78]. Moreover, in an animal model, immunohistochemical (IHC) staining for LC3 revealed that LC3 expression in the epithelium was higher when compared to that of the control group [120].

The induction of BE by the bile reflux that provokes tissue injury, leading to the secretion of pro-inflammatory cytokines, is well documented [121, 122]. In BE, the role of bile acids in the induction of oxidative stress, activation of STAT3, alteration in cytokine expression, and damage to DNA has been demonstrated [121 - 123]. It is suggested that during esophageal inflammation, the activation of the immune system allows for the stimulation of metaplasia and cancer by means of the upregulation of reactive free-radical species, including ROS [123]. Therefore, the bile reflux can increase ROS in the esophagus [124 - 127]. In an L2-IL-1β transgenic mouse model of BE, a positive correlation between the increase of AP and oxidative stress has been demonstrated [78]. In cell cultures, the pharmacologic inhibition of AP by chloroquine (CQ) following acidic stress has increased ROS production and diminished cell viability in the squamous epithelium and non-dysplastic BE [78]. However, any additional increase in ROS levels has not been observed in either dysplastic BE or EAC cells. Similar findings have been observed in cell lines exposed to acute and chronic deoxycholic acid [78, 119]. Acute exposure has increased Beclin-1 expression and AP. On the other hand, chronic exposure to deoxycholic acid has not resulted from such an alteration. With all of these findings, it is possible to conclude that AP can be observed in the normal esophagus epithelium and its levels increase evenly in inflammation as well as in BE. On the other hand, these levels decrease during neoplastic progression. In other words, in the acute phase of cellular stress, AP plays a protective role against neoplastic transformation [78, 119]. In contrast, in the chronic phase of cellular stress, such as chronic exposure to bile acids, a decline in AP may result in an increased genetic transformation and the progression of cancer. Although the reasons for this event are not fully understood, this pattern has been extensively detected in the neoplastic-cancer transition of other organ tumors [128, 129]. In conclusion, during the development of EAC, acid stress and inflammation induce AP, which is frequently observed as a cellular response leading to the reduction of intracellular oxidative stress and increase in cell survival. However, additional studies are required to completely clarify the mechanisms of AP in the transition of BE to EAC.

4.2. Autophagy in the Development of ESCC

In esophageal squamous cell carcinoma (ESCC), some observations point out that AP might play a role in oncogenesis. While ULK-1 expression is weak or negative in normal epithelial cells or areas adjacent to the tumors, the expression level is higher in ESCC tissues [130, 131] Sirtuin 6 (a member of the sirtuin family) is considered a tumor suppressor as it contributes to the inhibition of aerobic glycolysis and cell growth. However, its expression has recently been reported to be highly elevated in many tumors, indicating that sirtuin 6 plays dual roles in oncogenesis [132]. In addition, sirtuin 6 interacts explicitly with ULK1 and positively regulates its activity by inhibiting its upstream factor mTOR. Although the biological functions of sirtuin 6 in ESCC are still underestimated, its overexpression has been shown in ESCC when compared to the normal epithelium [132].

Similar to EAC, in Beclin-1, expression was found to be significantly increased in normal epithelial cells surrounding ESCC tissues [133]. Additionally, the LC3 expression has been investigated in multistage carcinogenesis in ESCC. Despite the absence of LC3 expression in the normal epithelium, the expression was found to be gradually increased from low-grade dysplasia to high-grade dysplasia with the highest expression in ESCC [134]. In a previous interesting study, Ren et al. [135] demonstrated that miR-638 could regulate AP as well as the malignant behavior of cells by targeting tumor suppressor DACT3 (a key regulator of Wnt/β-catenin signaling) in ESCC. The expression of miR-638 was observed to be significantly higher in ESCC than that of normal epithelial cells, suggesting the oncogenic role of the AP-related miR-638-DACT3 axis. Taken together, all of these findings support the contribution of AP in the development of ESCC.

Unfortunately, AP has not been studied concerning other accepted risk factors for EC, such as tobacco, alcohol consumption, and dietary factors. Recent evidence suggests that tobacco consumption induces AP. Cigarette smoking stimulates AP in an SIRT-1-PARP-1-dependent manner [136]. It is also suggested that cigarette smoking acts via ROS and activates AP, as evidenced by LC3II accumulation [137, 138]. Indeed, the oxidative stress induced by tobacco consumption results in both the prolonged induction of AP and stimulation of pathways that are involved in extrinsic APT [137, 138]. Tobacco consumption also induces AP through HO-1 (a 32kDa heat-shock protein that protects against tobacco-induced APT), a protein that shows its influence by inducing LC3B [139, 140]. However, there is no such data on esophageal carcinogenesis.

Another important hallmark of AP is its use as a potential therapeutic target, especially in cancer and several drugs that have been introduced to regulate AP are approved for humans (inhibitors and inducers), and many others are under investigation [141, 142] (Table **2**). Therefore, the disclosure of the mechanisms of AP in esophageal oncogenesis may lead to the potential utilization of novel therapeutics to prevent the onset of BE as well as its progression to EAC. More recently, a cranberry proanthocyanidin-rich extract (C-PAC), which induces cell death by AP either in APT and AP-resistant cancer cells, was shown to reduce ROS in BE cell lines, suggesting an anti-oxidant role of C-PAC in premalignant lesions [143]. In contrast, proton-pump inhibitors (PPIs), which also induce AP as a survival mechanism following oxidative stress, exerted this effect in BE cells [144]. However, these findings should be supported by additional studies.

4.3. Autophagy in EAC Behavior and Treatment

In EAC, the role of AP in tumor behavior and resistance to therapy has been explored in a limited number of studies. Among them, *in vitro* studies outnumber clinical studies. The findings of these reports are included in Tables **4** and **5**, respectively.

4.3.1. AP-Related Findings on Tumor Behavior and Progression in Patients with EAC

In patients with EAC, Beclin-1 was found to be frequently inactivated, and this inactivation was inversely correlated with tumor stage and grade, supporting the role of AP via Beclin-1 in aggressive tumor behavior [133] (Table **4**). In an elegant study, El-Mashed *et al.* [134] investigated AP utilizing LC3B expression in resection specimens from patients who had been operated on after neoadjuvant therapy (Cisplatin/5-fluorouracil [5-FU]) and from patients who had not been treated before surgery. LC3B expression was detected in three patterns: diffuse cytoplasmic staining, crescent or ring-like, and large globular staining. Although the origin of these different staining patterns of LC3 is obscure, it has been suggested that cytoplasmic staining might reflect a less stressed state of tumor cells that do not tend to aggregate LC3B into larger structures. In patients who had not received neoadjuvant therapy, positive cytoplasmic reactivity was found to be related to the predictability of a favorable outcome when compared to negative staining. In the same group, the existence of LC3B crescent or ring-like structures was related to an adverse outcome. However, in both groups, a positive correlation was observed between the incidence of LC3B-positive globular structures and decreased survival. Moreover, the presence of these structures was more frequently related to lymph node metastasis and a later tumor stage. In patients who had not been treated before surgery, negative cytoplasmic reactivity was found to be associated with a higher grade, perineural invasion, metastasis, and an advanced stage. In patients who had been treated before surgery, no relationship was detected among the LC3B staining patterns and histopathological parameters (Table **4**). In contrast to the survey of El-Mashed *et al.* [134], in another study performed with a different antibody to identify LC3B in patients with EAC [145], low LC3B dot-like structures were found to be related to shorter survival, highlighting the importance of the optimization of LC3B staining before its application as a marker of AP (Table **4**).

Table 4. Results of the Studies that Investigated AP in Patients with EAC.

Ref/Year	Markers	Normal		BE		LGD	HGD	EAC		HP Parameters, Survival
Weh, 2016 [133]	**Beclin-1 IHC**	High		NI		NI	NI	Low		Beclin-1 loss correlates with high stage and high grade
El-Mashed, 2015 [134]	**LC3B**	**GR 1**	**GR 2**	NI		NI	NI	GR 1	GR 2	
	Cytoplasmic	(–)	Low	NI		NI	NI	43%	52.1%	GR 1: Absence correlates with low grade, LNM, high stage, PNI, poor outcome
	Crescent-ring	(–)	(–)	NI		NI	NI	34.6%	72.9%	GR 1: Absence correlates with better outcome
	Globular structure	(–)	(–)	NI		NI	NI	47.1%	77.1%	GR 1: Presence correlates with LNM, high stage, poor outcome In GR 2: Poor outcome
Adams, 2016 [145]	**LC3B and p62**	High	Low	High	Low	NI	NI	High	Low	NP
	LC3B dots	↓	↑	↓	↑	NI	NI	83.6%	16.4%	NP
	p62 dots	↓	↑	↓	↑	NI	NI	41.4%	58.6%	NP
	p62 cytoplasmic	↓	↑	↓	↑	NI	NI	10.3%	89.7%	High staining correlates with early stage, poor outcome
	p62 nuclear	↓	↑	↓	↑	NI	NI	50%	50%	Low staining correlates with high grade, LN met, high stage, poor outcome
	p62 sum	↓	↑	↓	↑	NI	NI	19%	81%	A low score was associated with stage I tumors. Poor outcome

Abbreviations: **Ref**: Reference; **IHC**: Immunohistochemistry; **NI**: Not investigated; **LC3**: Microtubule-associated protein 1 light chain; **GR**: Grade; **LNM**: Lymph node metastasis; **PNI**: Perineural invasion; **NP**: Not predictive

In the same study, LC3B and p62 expression were significantly higher in earlier tumor stages. The prognosis was better in patients with tumors that expressed high nuclear and cytoplasmic p62 staining. The worst prognosis was observed in tumors with low total p62 or low LC3B/low p62 expression, and these tumors also exhibited the most aggressive behavior [145]. Although the role of AP in tumor behavior and prognosis is non-negligible, future investigations are warranted to unveil the underlying mechanism of AP in the progression of EAC.

4.3.2. In Vitro Investigation of AP in EAC

The main findings of these studies are summarized in Table **5** [120, 133, 134, 144 - 150].

In EAC cell lines, increased concentrations of CQ (an inhibitor of AP) resulted in an increase of LC3B and p62 [145]. APT-competent (chemosensitive) EAC cells did not exhibit an increase in AP in response to treatment with chemotherapeutic agents (5-FU and/or Cisplatin) [134, 146 - 148, 150]. AP inducers (lithium and rapamycin) enhanced their sensitivity alone or in combination with chemotherapeutics [148, 149]. Moreover, in contrast to APT-incompetent (chemoresistant) counterparts in these cell lines (see below), the inhibition of anti-apoptotic Bcl-2 family members with BH3 mimetic HA14-1 resulted in more APT after treatment with 5-FU [147]. In the same cells, immunohistochemistry revealed that before and after treatment with 5-FU, the expression of LC3B was mild [134]. This finding indicates that AP is not implicated in the response to therapy in chemosensitive EAC cells. Nonetheless, in chemoresistant cells, AP increased after the treatment of 5-FU and/or Cisplatin [134, 146 - 148, 150]. The specific inhibition of Beclin-1 and ATG7 with siRNA considerably enhanced the efficacy of 5-FU and reduced the recuperation of drug-treated cells [146]. Although the inhibitors of AP did not increase the chemotherapeutic efficiency in these cells, they induced extensive vesicular accumulation [146]. Similarly, 5-FU treatment was not improved, nor was colony re-growth reduced, by HA14-1 [147]. After 5-FU treatment, these cells showed strong LC3B staining [134]. Only the drug-resistant cells showed the crescent or ring-like and globular patterns [134]. These data confirm the critical influence of AP in chemoresistance in EAC.

The role of interferon Stimulated Gene 15 (ISG15) in chemoresistance and AP has been demonstrated in many cancers, including ESCC (see below). The stimulation of these ubiquitin-like protein modifiers by IFNs allows for the transcription of multiple ISGs (reviewed in [151 - 153]). Amongst these are three enzymes: ISG15-specific E1-activating enzyme (UBE1L), ISG15/ubiquitin E2-conjugating enzyme (UBE2L6), and ISG15-specific E3 ligase (HERC5) [151 - 153]. The consecutive participation of these enzymes is necessary for the integration of ISG5 with targets [154, 155]. It has been observed that Type I IFN induces the ISGylation of Beclin-1 [156], protecting Beclin-1 from ubiquitination and inhibiting PI3KC. In a more recent study on EAC cells, ISG15 and UBE2L6 negatively modulated AP, suggesting the role of the ISG15 pathway in chemosensitivity by regulating AP [150] (Table **5**). As indicated by Falvey *et al.* [150], this pathway may constitute a choice in tumor-targeted therapy because it is not crucial in normal cells and is activated in specific conditions, including immune reactions.

Recently, Kresty *et al.* [149] studied the properties of C-PAC in two cell lines that are either sensitive or resistant to acid (Table **5**). In cells with acid sensitivity, caspase-independent cell death occurred mainly through AP and a low level of APT was observed with C-PAC induction.

It is concluded that C-PAC is a productive contributor to cell death in EAC cells. Subsequently, the same group reported that, while AP induced by rapamycin ended up with an increase in Beclin-1, providing prolonged cell survival in EAC cells, C-PAC induced significant cell death induction through AP in a Beclin--independent manner [143]. Interesting recent data showed that in EAC cells, PPIs inhibit proliferation and invasion and induce APT [144]. In the metastatic cells, it also contributes to the blockage of autophagic flux. These findings constitute important *in vitro* evidence for their potential utilization in EAC as a new drug in anti-cancer therapy [144] (Table **5**).

Table 5. Data About the Modulation of AP Obtained *In Vitro* Studies in EAC.

Ref/Year	Method	Drugs	Results
Weh, 2016 [120]	-	C-PAC	Although in EAC cells, C-PAC significantly enhances ROS it significantly decreases ROS levels in cells from BE. On the other hand, the amount of is also increased in C-PAC treated EAC cells. However. H_2O_2 levels did not change in C-PAC treated BE cells
Weh, 2015 [133]	Beclin-1 *	C-PAC, RPM	C-PAC induces Beclin-1-independent AP characterized by significant cell death induction. In EAC, Beclin-dependent AP induction is agent specific
El-Mashed, 2015 [134]	IHC	5-FU	In contrast to CS cells, CR cells show strong LC3B staining following 5-FU treatment. Untreated CS cells express diffuse cytoplasmic staining. However only CR cells show the crescent or ring-like and the globular patterns of staining
Chueca; 2016 [144]	WB, LC3B p62	PPIs	PPIs inhibit proliferation and cell invasion and induce APT. It also induces AP. On the other hand, in metastatic cells the blockade of autophagic flux is activated by PPIs
Adams, 2016 [145]	WB, LC3B p62	CQ	In EAC cell lines, LC3B and p62 are increased parallel to the increasing concentrations of the AP inhibitor CQ

(Table 5) cont.....

Ref/Year	Method	Drugs	Results
O'Donovan, 2011 [146]	INH: Beclin-1*, ATG7*, 3MA, Baf, CQ	5-FU, CPT	CS cells exhibit APT whereas CR population exhibitsSpecific inhibition of early AP significantly enhances the effect of 5-FU. 3MA, Baf or CQ did not improve chemotherapeutic effect
Nyhan, 2012 [147]	HA14-1	5-FU	CS cells exhibit more APT following 5-FU and HA14-1 treatment. However CR cells exhibit HA14-1 did not ameliorate 5-FU treatment or decrease re-growth in CR cells. The efficacity of HA14-1depends on cell line
O'Donovan, 2015 [148]	IND: Li, RPM	5-FU	In CS cells, AP inducers stimulate APT and AP. They also influence these cells through increasing their sensitivity to the 5-FU. The combination of Li or RPM with 5-FU enhances AP and APT in these cells
	INH: CQ		
Kresty, 2015 [149]	TEM	C-PAC	In cells with acid sensitivity, caspase-independent cell death occurs mainly through AP and low level of APT by C-PAC induction. However, in cells with acid resistance C-PAC results in cell necrosis
Falvey, 2017 [150]	IND: RPM	5-FU	ISG15 conjugation pathway is upregulated in CS cells. This pathway is downregulated in CR cells. In CS cells while inhibition of UBE2L6 or ISG15 promotes the induction of autophagic flux and AP respectively
	INH: CQ, ISG15*, UBE2L6/UBCH8*		

Abbreviations: **Ref**: Reference; **C-PAC**: Cranberry derived-proanthocyanidin extract; **EAC**: Esophageal adenocarcinoma; **BE**: Barrett esophagus; *Inhibited by siRNA; **RPM**: Rapamycin; **AP**: Autophagy; **IHC**: Immunohistochemistry; **5-FU**: 5-Fluorourasil; **CS**: Chemosensive; **CR**: Chemoresistant; **WB**: Western blotting; **PPIs**: Proton pump inhibitors; **APT**: Apoptosis; **INH**: Inhibition; **CQ**: Chloroquine; **3-MA**: 3-Methyladenine; **Baf**: Bafilomycin A1; **CPT**: Cisplatin; **HA14-1**: BH-3 mimetic; **IND**: Induction; **Li**: Lithium; **TEM**: Transmission electron microscopy; **ISG-15**: Interferon Stimulated Gene 15

Taken together, these data demonstrate the potential role of AP in EAC chemoresistance and necessitate further investigations of not only AP-related proteins, but also their related pathways to open up new areas for therapeutic intervention.

4.4. Autophagy in ESCC Behavior and Treatment

In ESCC, the role of AP in tumor behavior and resistance to therapy has been investigated both in *in vivo* and *in vitro* studies. The results of these investigations are outlined in Tables **6-9**. Similar to EAC, there are more *in vitro* studies than clinicopathological studies.

4.4.1. AP-Related Findings in Tumor Behavior and Progression in Patients with ESCC

In patients with ESCC, the role of AP in tumor behavior and progression has been evaluated in a limited number of reports [130, 131, 157 - 164] (Table **6**). Different research groups have assessed ULK-1, Beclin-1, and LC3 expressions with the aim of defining the role of AP in these tumors [130, 131, 157 - 164]. Although the evaluation of ULK1 expression has highlighted the role of AP in ESCC progression in two recent studies, their data was not consistent. Jiang *et al.* [131] observed that a high level of ULK1 expression is related to an advanced T status and poor prognosis. Moreover, its expression was found to be an independent prognostic factor. In contrast, in another study, low ULK1 expression was found to be significantly related with the presence of metastasis in lymph nodes and decreased survival time, and ULK-1 was not detected as an independent prognostic factor [130]. Despite the fact that ULK1 might represent a potential prognostic biomarker in ESCC, these data warrant further research to more fully understand the precise impact of ULK1 expression on predicting the prognosis in ESCC.

Similar to ULK-1 expression, the results of studies addressing Beclin-1 expression are also different [157, 158, 163]. In 54 patients with ESCC, low Beclin-1 expression was found to be related with invasion, lymph node metastasis, and the stage [157]. Similar to EAC, the prognosis of the Beclin-1-positive group was found to be better when compared to that of the Beclin-1-negative group. Interestingly, in patients with advanced-stage ESCC, Beclin-1 expression and HIF-1α expression were inversely correlated. The survival time of this group was shorter than that of the Beclin-1-positive and low-HIF-1α group. These data implicate Beclin-1 and HIF-1α proteins in the progression of ESCC [157]. It has been suggested that the inhibition of AP induced through Beclin-1 by the high expression of HIF-1α might contribute to aggressive tumor behavior [157]. In a more recent study, 150 cases with stages II–IVa ESCC who had been treated with chemoradiation Beclin-1 expression alone did not show any relation with clinicopathological parameters and treatment response [158]. However, when Beclin-1 expression and LC3 expression (see below) were evaluated together, it was found that the survival of patients with LC3 and Beclin-1-positive tumors was shorter than for those with LC3 and Beclin-1-negative expression [158]. Therefore, further investigations are necessary to clarify the effect of Beclin-1 in the progression of ESCC.

In patients with ESCC, the most studied AP marker is LC3 [158 - 164]. However, similar to other markers of AP, results on the association between LC3 and the prognosis of ESCC are controversial. In some recent studies, LC3 expression was not associated with clinicopathological factors, including survival [159]. However, in other studies, LC3 expression was correlated with clinicopathologic factors and prognosis [158, 160]. In a recent meta-analysis, Zeng *et al.* [164] demonstrated that a high LC3 level was correlated with shorter survival and might act as a promising AP-related prognostic predictor of ESCC. The opposing roles of AP and APT in the overall survival of ESCC have also been demonstrated. In conclusion, these different results on LC3 may be related to differences in the criteria used in the evaluation of IHC staining, the use of different antibodies, and the differences in overall tumor area with positive LC3 expression despite the fact that all these differences in data suggest that AP might be associated with tumor behavior in ESCC.

Table 6. Results of the Studies that Investigated AP in Patients with ESCC.

Ref/Year	Markers	CLONES	N	LGD	HGD	Expression	HP Parameters, Survival
Jiang, 2014 [130]	ULK-1	Dako	L	NI	NI	H, L	A cytoplasmic ULK1 expression is related to with LNM and survival
Jiang, 2011 [131]	ULK-1*	Cambridge	L	NI	NI	H, L	ULK1 positivity was related to T status. Tumors with higher expression of ULK-1 had a poor prognosis. ULK1 expression is an independent prognostic indicator
Chen, 2009 [157]	Beclin-1, HIF-1a	Rabbit polyclonal, Santa-Cruz	H	NI	NI	L	Positive staining with Beclin-1 correlates with depth of invasion, LNM and stage. Beclin-1 negative tumors have poor prognosis
Chen, 2013 [158]	LC3*, Beclin 1	Rabbit polyclonal, Santa-Cruz	NI	NI	NI	P, N	Any association with hp parameters. LC3 and Beclin-1-expression correlate with poor prognosis. LC3 expression is an important predictor of prognosis in patients treated with chemotherapy and radiotherapy
Yoshioka, 2008 [159]	LC3*, CAIX, Ki-67	Rabbit polyclonal custom.	0	10%	32%	L, H	The LC3 expression did not correlate with clinicopathological factors, including survival
Wang, 2013 [160]	LC3A, p53	Rabbit monoclonal, Cell Signaling Technology	NI	NI	NI	L, H	High p53 and LC3A co-expression are related to shorter survival
Sakurai, 2013 [161]	LC3	Rabbit monoclonal, Abgent	NI	NI	NI	L, M, H	LC3 expression inversely correlates with depth of invasion, LNM, LI, MVD, VEGF-A expression, and poor prognosis

(Table 6) cont.....

Ref/Year	Markers	CLONES	N	LGD	HGD	Expression	HP Parameters, Survival
Hao, 2014 [162]	LC3	Rabbit polyclonal, Novus	L	NI	NI	L, H	High level of LC3 is related to shorter survival for resectable ESCC patients and is an independent prognostic factor
Chen, 2016 [163]	LC3, Beclin-1 CASP-3	-	NA	NA	NA	NA	A decrease in CASP-3 expression and an increase in LC3B expression correlate with diminished survival time
Zheng, 2016 [164]	Meta-analysis	-	NI	NI	NI	NI	High LC3 level correlates with worse prognosis of EC

Abbreviations: **Ref**: Reference; **HP**: Histopathological; **ULK-1**: Unc-51-Like Kinase 1; **N**: Normal esophagus; **NI**: Not investigated; **H**: High; **L**: Low; **LNM**: Lymph node metastasis; *: Investigated also with immunoblotting **T**: Level of invasion; **HIF-1a**: Hypoxia inducible factor1a; **LC3**: Microtubule-associated protein 1 light chain; **P**: Positive; **N**: Negative; **CAIX**: Carbonic anhydrase IX; **Ki-67**: A marker of proliferating cells; **LC3A**: Microtubule-associated protein 1 light chain 3A; **M**: Moderate; **LI**: Lymphatic invasion; **MVD:** Microvessel density; **VEGF-A**: Vascular endothelial growth factor-A; **CASP-3**: Caspase-3

In ESCC, the co-expression of LC3 with p53 and its relation with angiogenesis have also been investigated recently [161]. The data indicated that there is an inverse correlation between their high co-expression and prognosis. Therefore, this parameter is stated to be an independent predictor of survival. It has been hypothesized that in patients with ESCC, the survival of tumor cells is promoted by a decrease in APT and an increase in AP by means of the inactivating mutations in p53 [161]. On the other hand, LC3 expression was inversely correlated with microvessel density and VEGF-A expression, supporting that tumors with LC3 expression induce AP and suppress angiogenesis in ESCC [161]. Because the proliferative capacity of tumor cells is higher than neoangiogenesis, tumor cells have to survive in an avascular milieu [165]. This milieu is suitable for the induction of AP. A supporting finding is the co-expression of LC3 together with carbonic anhydrase IX, a hypoxia marker [159]. Therefore, it is possible to suggest that in the early hypoxic phase of ESSC, AP is necessary for tumor growth. These findings suggest that tumors with LC3-positive expression induce AP in the early stage of ESCC.

Alterations in AP and CD44 expression are related to shorter survival in many cancer types. Because CD44 expression has a critical influence on the epithelial-mesenchymal transition (EMT), the role of AP (defined as the LC3 expression) in this process has been studied recently in ESCC [166]. It has been demonstrated that AP facilitates the EMT-mediated generation of high CD44-expressing ESCC cells via mitochondrial clearance, emerging as a potential novel therapeutic target in ESCC [166].

4.4.2. In Vitro Investigation of AP in ESCC

4.4.2.1. Inhibition of AP in ESCC

4.4.2.1.1. siRNAs against Beclin-1, Atg5, Atg7, Bafilomycin A1, CQ, and 3−methyladenine (3-MA):

Studies concerning the specific inhibition of AP by these agents are presented in Table **7** [146, 167 - 176]. The early inhibition of AP through the blockage of Beclin-1, Atg5, and Atg7 with siRNAs significantly enhances chemosensitization and reduces the recovery of drug-treated cells, supporting that the inhibition of AP has the potential to improve chemotherapy. On the other hand, the pharmacological inhibition of AP with either Bafilomycin A1 or CQ through the interruption of lysosomal activity did not exert this effect. These results suggest that not only the blockade of AP, but also its inhibition step are important in the cell response to chemotherapeutic agents.

4.4.2.1.2. Ro and Gypenoside L (Gyp-L)

The long-term effect of some inhibitors has also been observed. Ro (a ginsenoid extracted from *Panax ginseng*) inhibits AP, allowing the sensitization of cells resistant to chemotherapy with 5-FU [173] (Table **7**). It delays the degradation of checkpoint kinase 1 (CHK1) and DNA repair through the downregulation of DNA replication potentiation of the cytotoxic effect of 5-FU. Additionally, RAD51 (a recombinase) negatively modulates AP by stabilizing CHK1, suggesting that RAD51-targeted therapy can be individually used to cure RAD51-overexpressed ESCC. The anti-cancer activity of a saponin, Gyp-L, has been demonstrated in ESCC cell lines [175]. Gyp-L inhibits AP by blocking the fusion between autophagosomes and lysosomes. This agent showed its activity through increasing the levels of ROS, leading to protein ubiquitination and ER stress response, and has been suggested as a novel therapeutic option in ESCC [175].

Table 7. Data about the Inhibition of AP Acquired *In Vitro* Studies in ESCC. Many Results Point out that AP Might have a Role in Resistance to Therapy and its Inhibition Might Improve the Cytotoxycity.

Ref/Year	AP Inhibition	Treatment	Results
O'Donovan, 2011 [146]	Beclin-1*, ATG7*, 3-MA, Baf, CQ	5-FU, CPT	Inhibition of early AP significantly enhances the efficacy of 5- FU. But 3-MA, Baf or CQ does not increase the influence of 5-FU
Liu, 2011 [167]	3-MA	CPT	AP is a self-protective mechanism in drug treated cells

(Table 7) cont.....

Ref/Year	AP Inhibition	Treatment	Results
Tang, 2013 [168]	Beclin-1*, ATG7*, 3-MA, and CQ	RVS	Inhibition of AP enhances Resveratrol-induced APT
Zhu, 2013 [169]	ATG7*	CPT	Inhibition of AP potentiates the cytotoxicity
Yu, 2014 [170]	Beclin-1*, ATG7*, 3-MA, Baf, CQ	CPT	AP is a crucial mechanism of acquired drug resistance
Yang, 2014 [171]	Insulin (induces PI3K/Akt/mTOR)	CPT	Insulin could enhance cisplatin-induced APT by inhibition of AP
Chen, 2015 [172]	3-MA	RT	Blockade of AP with 3-MA enhances cytotoxicity of RT
Zheng, 2016 [173]	Beclin 1*, ATG5*, ATG7*, LC3B *, Ginsenoside Ro	5-FU	Ro potentiates cytotoxicity via delaying CHK1
Zhu, 2016 [174]	3-MA and CQ	-	RAD51 interacts with CHK1 and stabilize its level by inhibiting AP, thus leading to the promotion of cell growth
Liao, 2016 [175]	ATG5*, ATG7*, LC3*, 3-MA, CQ	Gyp-L	Gyp-L triggers the generation of ROS and UPR response leading to its induction. Autophagic flux is prevented by Gyp-L. It also stimulates non-apoptotic cell death. Cells are protected from Gyp-L cytotoxicity through silencing of LC3, ATG7, and ATG5. While CQ enhances the cytotoxicity of Gyp-L, 3-MA does not exert such an effect
Lu, 2016 [176]	3-MA	RT	In resistance to RT, radiation induces AP through LKB1 to favor cell survival

Abbreviations: **Ref**: Reference; **AP**: Autophagy; * Inhibited by siRNA; **3-MA:** 3-Methyladenine**; Baf:** Bafilomycin **A1; CQ**: Chloroquine; **5-FU**: 5-Fluorourasil; **CPT**: Cisplatin; **APT**: Apoptosis; **RVS**: Resveratrol; **RT**: Radiotherapy; **CHK-1**: Check point kinase 1; **Gyp L**: Gypenoside L; **ROS**: Reactive oxygen species; **UPR**: Unfolded protein response**; LKB1**: Liver kinase B1

4.4.2.1.3. Insulin

The function of insulin in the modulation of metabolic events, DNA synthesis, and modulation of transcription is well documented because insulin also has an impact on the cellular uptake of various nutritional substances by facilitating diffusion. Many years ago, its use as an adjunct in the management of cancer was proposed. It was hypothesized that insulin-induced cellular stress might allow the selective endocytosis of metabolic agents even in low doses. *In vitro* studies found that the activity of various chemotherapeutic agents, such as paclitaxel, 5-FU, cisplatin, or methotrexate, can be considerably enhanced in the presence of insulin. Although the influence of insulin in cancer therapy is not defined, studies are reporting its novel application. Regarding ESCC, an investigation has been focused on the effects of insulin on the activity of cisplatin and the underlying mechanisms in the ESCC cell line [171] (Table **7**). The protein expression levels of AKT, mTOR, PI3K, PTEN, and AP indicators LC3-II and Beclin-1 during the course of treatment were evaluated. In cells treated with cisplatin alone, a large number of autophagosomes were detected. However, in co-treatment with insulin, the expression levels of LC3-II, Beclin-1, and PTEN were significantly downregulated, but AKT, mTOR, and PI3K expressions were considerably upregulated. These results suggest that insulin can enhance cisplatin-induced APT in ESCC cells through the inhibition of AP. Moreover, the induction of PI3K/AKT/mTOR signaling induced through insulin resulted in the suppression of AP in these cells, which may be attributed to the anticancer effects of cisplatin [171].

4.4.2.1.4. Protein Kinase Cι (PKCι)

PKCι is an oncoprotein that is observed in many organ tumors [177 - 179]. Recently, ESCC data indicating an effect of PKCι in cell motility and tumor behavior have been obtained [180]. Indeed, the migration capacity of ESCC cells and their resistance to anoikis decrease with PKCι consumption [181]. Furthermore, in different ESCC cell lines, the depletion of PKCι induces APT [181]. In this process, AP plays a critical role in the downregulation of β-catenin, suggesting the participation of AP in PKCι-related oncogenic signals. The examination of fresh tissues of ESCC by immunohistochemistry has revealed similar findings. Although these data indicate the role of PKCPι as an activator of AP, its knockdown may influence esophageal cancer cell death, and other studies should confirm these results.

4.4.2.2. Induction of AP in ESCC

Although it seems contradictory, the results of many recent works promote the induction of AP as a possible alternative modality for the treatment of cancer.

4.4.2.2.1. Rapamycin, Lithium, Dichloroacetate (DCA), and BEZ235 in ESCC Cells

More recently, in APT-resistant ESCC cells, the role of AP activators, such as rapamycin and lithium, and their influence on drug sensitivity have been studied [148]. It was observed that in lithium-treated cells, the processing of the autophagosome was not efficient; in other words, autophagic flux was compromised. However, rapamycin did not show this effect, and autophagic flux was maintained. That is why its combination with rapamycin provided cellular protection, which contrasted with the effect of lithium, which enhanced non-apoptotic cell death (PCD II). It was concluded that the stimulation of disrupted AP may contribute to cytotoxicity [148] (Table **9**). Similarly, the inhibition of

DCA-induced AP with 3-MA significantly enhanced DCA-induced APT and improved the drug sensitivity of ESCC cells to DCA and 5-FU [182] (Table **9**). In ESCC cells, the combination of tunicamycin (which induces ER stress) developed the sensitivity to cisplatin by mediating the PI3K/AKT/mTOR pathway and PI3K inhibitor BEZ235 enhanced AP and APT and increased cell sensitivity to cisplatin [182] (Table **9**). Similar results have been obtained in radiosensitivity (see below).

4.4.2.2.2. UPS Inhibitors and Dihydroartemisinin (DHA)

Previously, it was reported that the inhibition of UPS resulted in the upregulation of AP [183], demonstrating that both might act as equilibrating systems in the cellular degradation of proteins [184]. Proteasome inhibitor-induced AP is capable of manipulating ER stress and decreasing cell death in cancer cells. Thus, the inhibition of UPS by proteasome inhibitors has emerged as a new target for chemotherapy [183, 184]. In ESCC, the co-administration of proteasome inhibitors with 3-MA and Bafilomycin A1 results in the enhancement of cell death, supporting the effect of proteasome inhibitors as potential novel anticancer agents for the adjuvant treatment of ESCC [185, 186] (Table **9**). Similarly, DHA reduces the viability of ESCC cells by inducing both APT and AP [187] (Table **8**).

4.4.2.2.3. Bardoxolone Methyl

The anticancer effects of Bardoxolone methyl (CDDO-Me, a synthetic tripenoid) on human ESCC cells have been described [188, 189]. Besides its role in the inhibition of ROS, cell invasion, EMT, and stemness, CDDO-Me induces APT and AP (by inhibiting the PI3K/AKT/mTOR pathway) in ESCC cells. Although further mechanistic studies are needed, CDDO-Me has been proposed as a potentially powerful and promising agent in the treatment of ESCC [188, 189] (Table **8**).

4.4.2.2.4. BH3 Mimetics

Although in many organ tumors, the strategy to manipulate APT is designed to engage the APT pathways, it is clear that two anti-apoptotic proteins, Bcl-xL and Bcl-2, are involved in AP [190 - 192]. The BH3 domain in Beclin-1 constitutes a connection site for both proteins. ABT-737, a BH3 mimetic, induces AP through the disruption of the binding of these proteins [190]. Moreover, the BH3-only proteins (Bid, Bad, and BNIP3) stimulate AP in cancer cells [190, 191]. In an earlier study with Ethyl-3, 4-Dihydroxybenzoate (EDBH), a prolyl-hydroxylase inhibitor in ESCC lines, the inductions of both APT and early AP via the up-regulation of BNIP3 were observed [193] (Table **8**). Moreover, it has been demonstrated that ESCC cells with AKR1C1 and AKR1C2 (the aldo-keto reductase superfamily of enzymes that is critical for the detoxification of drugs and toxins) expressions are more sensitive to EDBH and these enzymes may facilitate EDBH-induced AP-inhibition through co-treatment with 3-MA, providing potential guidance for chemotherapy [194] (Table **9**). Recently, in ESCC cells, the influence of HA14-1 (BH3 mimetic) was investigated in cell lines including APT-sensitive and APT-resistant cells [147]. The anti-apoptotic proteins Mcl-1, Bcl-2, and Bcl-xL and pro-apoptotic protein Bax were present in all cells. In APT-sensitive cell lines, while the expression of Bcl-2 and Bcl-xL was marginally decreased, Bax was higher. It is suggested that these different expressions may be important in sensitivity to APT [147] (Table **5** and Table **8**). Moreover, the levels and expression of NOXA have been analyzed in these cells [147].

To date, NOXA is a BH3-only protein involved in stress response and an inducer of APT [195]. Although APT-resistant cells had lower basal NOXA expression, after 5-FU, its expression was under the normal concentrations observed in APT-sensitive cells. It is suggested that there is a deficiency in BH3-only signaling in APT-sensitive cells. The combined administration of 5-FU and HA14-1 in APT-sensitive cells promoted early APT and reduced clonogenic survival compared with 5-FU alone [147]. On the other hand, while the combined administration of HA14-1 with 5-FU resulted in enhanced AP and PCD II in some of the APT-resistant cells, not all chemoresistant cells were affected by this type of administration [147]. These data demonstrate that the efficacy of HA14-1 depends on the cell line and the real benefit of this mimetic may be enhancing PCD II in APT-resistant cells. Although the combined administration of HA14-1 and 5-FU could be an effective therapy for ESCC, the poor solubility and stability of HA14-1 is another problem to be resolved. In this regard, the development of new analogs is already promising. Similar observations were detected with ABT-263 (Navitoclax) [196] (Table **8**). This is a Bcl-2 family inhibitor that is suitable for peroral use and shows its effect via BH-3 [196]. The effect of Navitoclax in cancer therapy is still under investigation in clinical trials [196]. On the other hand, Obatoclax, which inhibits the anti-apoptotic proteins, is trapped in lysosome in both chemosensitive and chemoresistant ESCC cells and induces cytotoxicity through impairing the lysosomal function in AP flux and cell viability [197, 198] (Table **9**). Furthermore, the combined administration of Obatoclax with proteasome inhibitor MG-132 exhibits a synergistic effect in the aggregation of polyubiquitinated proteins, implying its contribution to the blockade of autophagic degradation [198]. These findings suggest a possible option for further investigations of Obatoclax, especially in chemoresistant tumors in ESCC.

4.4.2.2.5. Phytoalexins

The anti-tumor activities of phytoalexins and their derivatives (such as paclitaxel and vinorelbine) have been demonstrated in previous studies [199 - 202]. Resveratrol is one of these phytoalexins and is frequently found in grapes, red wine, and peanuts, etc. Due to its cytotoxic effect in the cancer cells of different organs, it has been found as an active natural compound with sizeable therapeutic potential [199 - 202]. It has been evidenced that resveratrol prevents tumor progression through different steps depending on cell type [203, 204]. It stimulates APT in various cancer cells and induces AP in some cancers [201, 205 - 207]. Moreover, the role of AMPK and p62/SQSTM1-related AP has been demonstrated in resveratrol-induced cell death [208]. However, AP induced by resveratrol has been found to conduce cells toward resistance to death and provides cell viability in some cancers [209]. Currently, although some phytoalexins and their derivatives have been utilized in the treatment of esophageal cancers [210, 211], the effect of resveratrol in ESCC treatment has been investigated in few studies. Experimental studies have indicated that resveratrol serves a significant function in EC cell death [212 - 214]. Tang et al. [168] investigated the anti-cancer effect of resveratrol in ESCC, focusing on its impact both in AP and APT. It has been observed that resveratrol stimulates APT and consequently inhibits ESCC cell growth in a dose-dependent manner. It also induced AP through a mechanism independent from the AMPK/mTOR pathway in the ESCC cells (Table 7). Furthermore, the inhibition of AP with genetic and pharmacological agents increases the cytotoxicity of resveratrol in ESCC cells, providing a new approach to potentiating the efficacy of resveratrol in ESCC cancer treatment.

4.4.2.2.6. Metformin

Recent evidence has indicated that an antidiabetic, metformin, acts with an either chemopreventive or antineoplastic influence in numerous organ tumors [215 - 218]. However, epidemiological and preclinical investigations have pointed out that metformin exhibits a wide variety of effects through different mechanisms in various tumors [215, 216, 218]. Although the effect of metformin has been investigated in patients with varying types of cancer, it has not yet been clinically studied in ESCC. A recent *in vitro* study indicated that metformin prevents the proliferation of ESCC cells, and this effect was found to be related to AP [219] (Table **9**). In ESCC cell lines, metformin induces APT and inhibits cell proliferation. More importantly, the blockade of AP, which is stimulated by metformin, renders ESCC cells more sensitive to metformin-induced APT [219]. In ESCC cells in inoculated nude mice, metformin treatment resulted in a decrease in tumor size and weight [219], indicating that metformin decreases tumor growth in animals. These data contrast with the view on the effect of metformin-mediated AP as an alternative survival pathway to an APT inducer. However, similar results have been observed in other organ tumors [220, 221].

Although the role of metformin-induced AP in cancer necessitates further studies, it is suggested that in malignant cells with preserved apoptotic mechanisms, the blockade of AP results in APT [222]. However, in ESCC, the exact function of AP stimulated by metformin as well as the pathways involved in this process remain to be elucidated.

4.4.2.2.7. Anti-EGFR Monoclonal Antibodies

In ESCC, although chemotherapy and radiotherapy are essential in the treatment, especially in recurrence and metastasis, the toxic effects of therapy are the most critical challenge to overcome. In ESCC, the treatment efficiency of nimotuzumab (anti-EGFR monoclonal antibody) combined with chemoradiotherapy has been investigated in cells with a high and low amount of EGFR [223] (Table 8). The effect of cytotoxic drugs (paclitaxel and cisplatin) and radiotherapy was found to be increased in cells with high EGFR expression through nimotuzumab administration. Additionally, a significant association was observed between cytotoxicity and increased AP. In contrast, in cells with low EGFR expression, the chemosensitivity and radiosensitivity did not improve with the combination of nimotuzumab. However, the combination with an AP inducer (rapamycin) increased the sensitivity of these cells. It is concluded that nimotuzumab, through activating AP, leading to cell death, generates an additive therapeutic impact against tumor cells [223].

4.4.2.2.8. Eustradiol and its Analogs

The new *in silico*-designed estradiol analog 2-ethyl-3-*O*-sulfamoyl-estra-1, 3,5(10) 16-tetraene (ESE-16) has been investigated from the point of its inhibitor activities in the proliferation of the ESCC cell line [224] (Table 8). In ESE-16-treated cells, cell density was found to be decreased, metaphase was arrested, and apoptotic bodies had become evident. These cells also showed an increase in AP. In addition, the mitochondrial membrane potential was found to be diminished, suggesting that in ESCC cells, ESE-16 promotes cell death through its effects on both AP and APT. These data warrant further studies about the influence of ESE-16 in ESCC as a possible anticancer agent [224].

4.4.2.3. MicroRNA in the Regulation of AP in ESCC

MicroRNAs (miRNAs) are involved in the regulation of the proliferation, migration, angiogenesis, and metastatic processes in many tumors. However, the findings of the effect of miRNAs in APT and AP have been discovered more recently.

It has been revealed that miRNAs have various effects on the different steps of

AP [225 - 228]. For instance, mir-101, miR-30a, miR-181a, mir-34a, and miR-17/20/93/106 complexes individually contribute to induction, vesicle formation, elongation/completion, fusion, and degradation, respectively [225 - 228]. Through switching the intracellular number of proteins that play a crucial role in AP, such as SQSTM1, Atgs, Beclin-1, and ULK1/2, these miRNAs might influence autophagic events [229 - 239]. Recently, three miRNAs (miR20b, miR498, and miR196) were found to be involved in both the APT and AP processes in ESCC. Therefore, in these tumors, a connective role of miRNAs between these two cell death mechanisms has been indicated [239]. miR-193b, which has been accepted as a tumor suppressor, is another miR whose expression differs according to the chemotherapeutic sensitivity of ESCC cells. It was observed that cells with miR-193b overexpression were more sensitive to 5-FU and this sensitization was related to its negative regulation of Stathmin 1 (a potential AP regulator). Although the overexpression of miR-193b together with 5-FU administration do not activate APT, this affects autophagic flux, leading to chemosensitivity, suggesting that miR-193b has a potential application in ESCC [239]. Recently, miR-638 was determined as a crucial regulator of starvation and rapamycin-induced AP by targeting the tumor suppressor DACT in ESCC [135]. The influence of this regulation has been found to be significant in the promotion of malignant phenotypes in cancer cells [135]. It is hypothesized that the AP-related miR-638-DACT3 axis may be an attractive target for ESCC therapy [135].

4.4.2.4. AP and Radioresistance in ESCC

The current findings demonstrate that the effect of AP on sensitivity to radiation is more significant than its protective effect against radiation. The inducer role of radiation in the stimulation of AP-related genes has been proposed as a novel mechanism of cell death and has emerged as a novel target for cancer treatment [240, 241]. The use of radiation in the treatment of ESCC has limitations related to the heterogeneity in radiosensitivity even in tumors within the same grade [158]. Solutions for increasing radiotherapy sensitivity in esophageal cancer remain to be investigated. In an earlier study, the inhibition of AP through 3-MA increased the cytotoxic effect of radiation in ESCC cells [172] (Table **7**). It is suggested that the blockade of AP as an adjuvant therapy could be a promising approach in the treatment of esophageal SCC [172]. Moreover, the combination of radiation and AP inhibition has been found to end with a significant decrease in tumor size and angiogenesis [172]. In another study investigating the influence of ER stress and the molecular pathways activated after radiotherapy, tunicamycin was administered to the ESCC cell line [242] (Table **9**). A significant increase in cell death was found in cells treated with the combination of radiation with tunicamycin, indicating that tunicamycin could sensitize ESCC cells to radiation. Moreover, with this combined treatment, a significant increase in G2/M arrest and

APT was observed. Tunicamycin treatment also led to an increase in LC3 and ATG5 levels, which were further increased after combination with radiation, supporting the role of ER stress-related AP in the sensitization to radiation. 3-MA inhibited this AP response. While the cell survival after radiation treatment was not changed substantially in cells treated with 3-MA, it reduced considerably after combined treatment with tunicamycin. Similarly, in chemosensitivity (see above), it was observed that the PI3K/AKT/mTOR pathway was implicated in the increase of radiosensitivity stimulated by tunicamycin. The assessment of tumor growth in nude mice also demonstrated that the growth of tumor xenografts in tunicamycin-treated animals was significantly decreased when compared to animals that were not treated with tunicamycin [241] (Table 9). Recently, the influence of Gambogic acid (GA) on radiosensitivity was studied in ESCC cell lines [243, 244] (Table 8). In one study, it was observed that the sensitivity to radiation stimulated via GA included AP and APT, which were modulated through ROS hypergeneration and AKT/mTOR inhibition [244]. In contrast, Liu *et al.* [243] did not observe this influence of GA on AP in the ESCC cell line. It is crucial to state that the role of GA in AP appears complicated, warranting further studies to clarify how GA influences AP.

LKB1, which is assumed to be a tumor suppressor, is vital in the radiation therapy of many tumors. In ESCC cells, the potential role of LKB1 in radiotherapy has been investigated in *in vitro* studies [176, 245] (Table 7 and Table 9). In ESCC cell lines with LKB1 overexpression, LKB1 induced radioresistance through the inhibition of APT and stimulation of AP, and these functions were mediated by AMP-Activated Protein Kinase. These data revealed that LKB1 might function as a new target to enhance the efficacy of radiation therapy in esophageal cancer [176].

Although the mechanism underlying radiosensitivity and AP remains to be elucidated, all of these findings indicate that the manipulation of AP might be useful in the treatment of ESCC with radiotherapy.

Table 8. Data about the Induction of AP Obtained *In Vitro* Studies in ESCC. Results Demonstrate that AP Might have a Role in Resistance to Therapy as a Survival Mechanism of ESCC Cells.

Ref/Year	AP Induction	Results
Nyhan, 2012 [147]	HA14-1	A combination with 5-FU augments of APT CS cells. However, CR cells did not show such an effect. The efficacity of HA14-1 is cell line dependent
Du, 2013 [187]	DHA	DHA induces APT, cell cycle arrest and AP
Wang, 2015 [188]	CDDO-Me	CDDO-Me induces AP via inhibition of Pi3K/ mTOR pathway
Wang, 2016 [189]	CDDO-Me	CaMKIIα mediates AP-induced by CDDO-Me

(Table 8) cont.....

Ref/Year	AP Induction	Results
Han, 2014 [193]	EDHB	EDHB treatment induce AP by up-regulation of BNIP3 and Beclin-1 and the down-regulation of bcl-2
Lin, 2017 [196]	ABT-263	Navitoclax induces APT and prosurvival-AP
Song, 2014 [223]	NM, RPM	In CS cells with high EGFR expression nimotuzumab increases their sensitivity to therapy (RT, PXT, CPT) by AP
		In CR cells with low-EGFR expression only the combination of NM with RPM increases their sensitivity to therapy (RT, PXT, CPT) via AP
Wolmarans, 2014 [224]	ESE-16	ESE-16 promotes cell death through both AP and APT
Liu, 2016 [243]	GA	GA does not induce AP. In contrast, it induces APT via suppression of the Nuclear Factor-κB pathway
Yang, 2016 [244]	GA	AP and APT that are regulated through hypergeneration of ROS and inhibition of AKT/mTOR contribute to radiosensitivity stimulated by GA

Abbreviations: **Ref**: Reference; **AP**: Autophagy; **HA14-1**: A BH-3 mimetic; **5-FU**: 5-Fluorourasil; **APT**: Apoptosis; **CS**: Chemosensitive; **CR**: Chemoresistant; **DHA**: Dihydroartemisinin; **CDDO-Me**: 2-Cyano-3 ,12-dioxoolean-1,9- dien-28-oic acid methyl ester (Bardoxolone methyl); **EDHB**: Ethyl-3,4-dihy-r-oxybenzoate; **BNIP3**: AMP-Activated Protein Kinase; **Navtioclax**: ABT-263, a pan-inhibitor of anti-apoptotic members.**NM**: Nimotuzumab; **RPM**: Rapamycin; **EGFR**: Epidermal growth factor receptor; **RT**: Radiotherapy; **PXT**: Paclitaxel; **CPT**; Cisplatin; **ESE-16**: Estradiol analogue; **GA**: Gambogic acid

Table 9. data about the Modulation of AP Obtained *In Vitro* Studies in ESCC. Although Results are Promising, Further Studies are Required to Better Define AP as a Promising Target to Therapy.

Ref/Year	AP Modulation	Treatment	Results
O'Donovan, 2015 [148]	IND:Li, RPM	5-FU	Combination of 5-FU with RPM is protective against cytotoxicity. In contrast, Li shows strong enhancement of cell death
	INH: CQ		
Jia, 2017 [182]	IND: DCA	5-FU	The inhibition of DCA-induced AP facilitates cell APT and improves the cytotoxicity to DCA and 5-FU
	INH: 3-MA		
Liu, 2015 [185]	IND: MG-132	MG-132	MG-132 induces AP in cells, and also increases cell death
	INH: 3-MA		
Wang, 2014 [186]	IND: MG-132	-	Inhibition of PKCi induces APT through autophagic degradation of β-Catenin
	INH: Baf		
Li, 2016 [194]	IND: EDHB	EDHB	AKR1C1/C2 promotes EDHB-induced early AP
	INH: 3-MA		
Pan, 2010 [197]	OBX	5-FU, CDBCA	OBX and 5-FU/ CDBCA may provoke stronger stimuli inducing APT. Inhibition of AP potentiates the cytotoxic effect of OBX
	INH: 3-MA and CQ		

(Table 9) cont.....

Ref/Year	AP Modulation	Treatment	Results
Yu, 2016 [198]	OBX	CPT	OBX disrupts the function of lysosomes consequently blocks AP flux. It is the sole agent with the capability to stimulate the loss of cell viability in CS and CR cells equivalently
	INH: ATG5*, ATG7*		
Feng, 2014 [219]	IND: Metformin	-	The sensitization of ESCC cells to metformin stimulated APT is augmented through either pharmacological or genetic inhibition of AP
	INH:Beclin-1*, Atg5*, 3-MA, CQ		
Pang, 2013 [241]	IND: TM	RT	Through its influence both in APT and AP, TM enhances the sensitization of cells to radiation
	INH: 3-MA, Beclin-1*		
Zhou, 2017 [242]	IND: TM, BEZ235	CPT	TM and BEZ235 improve CPT-induced cytotoxicity via modulation of AP
	INH: 3-MA, CQ		
He, 2017 [245]	LKB1	RT	LKB1 suppresses APT and induces AP through AMPK signalling during the stimulation of radioresistance in cancer cells

Abbreviations: **Ref**: Reference; **AP**: Autophagy; **IND**: Induction; **Li**: Lithium; **RPM**: Rapamycin; **INH**: Inhibition; **CQ**: Chloroquine; **5-FU**: 5-Fluorourasil; **DCA**: Dichloroacetate; **3-MA**: 3-Methyladenine; **APT**: Apoptosis; **MG-132**: Proteasome inhibitor; **Baf**: Bafilomycin A1; **PKCi**: Protein kinase Cι; **EDHB**: Ethyl-3,4-dihydroxybenzoate; **AKR1C1/C2**: Aldo-keto reductase superfamily; **OBX**: Obatoclax (GX15-070), a pan-inhibitor of anti-apoptotic Bcl-2 proteins (BH-3 mimetic); **CBDCA**: Carboplatin; ***: İnhibition with siRNA; **CPT**: Cisplatin; **CS**: Chemosensitive; **CR**: Chemoresistant; **TM**: Tunicamycin; **RT**: Radiotherapy; **BEZ235**: A PI3K inhibitor; **LKB1**: Liver kinase B1

CONCLUSION

AP has crucial functions in oncogenesis, tumor behavior, and response to treatment in EC. Therefore, the modulation of AP can be relevant in these tumors. The first problem to be resolved is defining whether AP should be stimulated or inhibited in EC. From the data presented in this chapter, it seems that both strategies are encouraging. However, several parameters, such as the composition of the tumor microenvironment, might influence treatment efficacy. The identification of patients who will benefit from this therapy is another critical parameter necessitating further large-scale clinical studies. Another problem is reassigning existing drugs in AP modulation, which does not specifically modulate AP and may have off-target effects, warranting the development of specific AP-modulating compounds suitable for use in patients suffering from EC.

CURRENT & FUTURE DEVELOPMENTS

In vitro evidence indicates the contribution of AP to esophageal carcinogenesis. However, the relation of AP with other risk factors for esophageal carcinoma, such as tobacco, alcohol consumption, and dietary factors, remains to be investigated.

Clinical studies support that autophagy markers might be useful in the prognosis evaluation of patients with esophageal carcinoma. In particular, LC3 expression is a promising AP-related prognostic marker in ESCC. On the other hand, the immunohistochemical evaluation of these markers needs to be standardized.

The modulation of AP improves therapeutic efficacy in preclinical esophageal carcinoma models. Nevertheless, the mechanistic contribution of AP to therapeutic response remains elusive.

CONSENT FOR PUBLICATION

Not applicable.

CONFLICT OF INTEREST

The authors confirm that this chapter content has no conflict of interest.

ACKNOWLEDGEMENTS

Erdem Ayik and his supervisor Gulsum O. Elpek have worked together in this chapter's texting, design and analysis.

LIST OF ABBREVIATIONS

3-MA	3-Methyladenine
5-FU	5-Fluorourasil
AP	Autophagy
APT	Apoptosis
ATF	Activating Transcription Factor
ATGs	Autophagy -related Genes
Bcl-2	B-cell lymphoma 2
BNIP3	Bcl-2 19kDa İnteracting Protein
BE	Barrett Esophagus
CHK1	Checkpoint Kinase 1
C-PAC	Cranberry Proanthocyanidin Rich Extract
CQ	Chloroquine
DCA	Dichloroacetate
DHA	Dihydroartemisinin
EAC	Esophageal Adenocarcinoma
EC	Esophageal Cancer
EDBH	Ethyl-3,4-Dihydroxybenzoate

EMT	Epithelial- Mesenchymal Transition
ESCC	Esophageal Squamous Cell Carcinoma
ESE-16	2-Ethyl-3-*O*-Sulfamoyl-Estra-1 3,5(10)16-Tetraene
FIP200	Focal Adhesion Kinase Family İnteracting Protein of 200 kD
GA	Gambogic Acid
GSK3	Glycogen Synthase Kinase-3
Gyp-L	Gypenoside L
HIF-1	Hypoxia-İnducible Factor 1
IHC	Immunohistochemical
ISG	Interferon Stimulated Gene
LKB1	Liver Kinase B1
miRNAs	MicroRNAs
mTOR	mechanistic Target of Rapamycin
PE	Phosphatidylethanolamine
PI3K	Phosphoinositide3-Kinase
PI3P	Phosphatidylinositol 3-Phosphate
PKCι	Protein Kinase Cι
PPIs	Proton Pump İnhibitors
PTEN	Phosphatase and Tensin Homolog Deleted on Chromosome10
ROS	Reactive Oxygen Species
SQSTM1	Sequestosome Cytoplasm 1
STAT	Signal Transducers and Activators of Transcription
TNF	Tumor Necrosis Factor
UBE2L6	ISG15/Ubiquitin E2 Conjugating Enzyme
ULK	UNC-51-Like Kinase Complex
UPR	Unfolded Protein Response
UPS	Ubiquitin-Proteasome System
WIPI	WD-repeat protein interacting with phosphoinositides

REFERENCES

[1]   de Reuck AVS, Cameron MP. Lysosomes. London: Ciba Found. Symp., J&A; 1963.

[2]   Ozpolat B, Benbrook DM. Targeting autophagy in cancer management - strategies and developments. Cancer Manag Res 2015; 7: 291-9.
[http://dx.doi.org/10.2147/CMAR.S34859] [PMID: 26392787]

[3]   Russell RC, Yuan H-X, Guan K-L. Autophagy regulation by nutrient signaling. Cell Res 2014; 24(1): 42-57.
[http://dx.doi.org/10.1038/cr.2013.166] [PMID: 24343578]

[4]   Rebecca VW, Massaro RR, Fedorenko IV, *et al.* Inhibition of autophagy enhances the effects of the AKT inhibitor MK-2206 when combined with paclitaxel and carboplatin in BRAF wild-type melanoma. Pigment Cell Melanoma Res 2014; 27(3): 465-78.
[http://dx.doi.org/10.1111/pcmr.12227] [PMID: 24490764]

[5]   Nagelkerke A, Sweep FC, Geurts-Moespot A, Bussink J, Span PN. Therapeutic targeting of autophagy in cancer. Part I: Molecular pathways controlling autophagy. Semin Cancer Biol 2015; 31: 89-98.
[http://dx.doi.org/10.1016/j.semcancer.2014.05.004] [PMID: 24879905]

[6]   Amaravadi R, Kimmelman AC, White E. Recent insights into the function of autophagy in cancer. Genes Dev 2016; 30(17): 1913-30.
[http://dx.doi.org/10.1101/gad.287524.116] [PMID: 27664235]

[7]   Fuertes G, Martín De Llano JJ, Villarroya A, Rivett AJ, Knecht E. Changes in the proteolytic activities of proteasomes and lysosomes in human fibroblasts produced by serum withdrawal, amino-acid deprivation and confluent conditions. Biochem J 2003; 375(Pt 1): 75-86.
[http://dx.doi.org/10.1042/bj20030282] [PMID: 12841850]

[8]   Rubinsztein DC, Codogno P, Levine B. Autophagy modulation as a potential therapeutic target for diverse diseases. Nat Rev Drug Discov 2012; 11(9): 709-30.
[http://dx.doi.org/10.1038/nrd3802] [PMID: 22935804]

[9]   Mizushima N, Komatsu M. Autophagy: Renovation of cells and tissues. Cell 2011; 147(4): 728-41.
[http://dx.doi.org/10.1016/j.cell.2011.10.026] [PMID: 22078875]

[10]   Wirawan E, Vanden Berghe T, Lippens S, Agostinis P, Vandenabeele P. Autophagy: For better or for worse. Cell Res 2012; 22(1): 43-61.
[http://dx.doi.org/10.1038/cr.2011.152] [PMID: 21912435]

[11]   Mijaljica D, Prescott M, Devenish RJ. V-ATPase engagement in autophagic processes. Autophagy 2011; 7(6): 666-8.
[http://dx.doi.org/10.4161/auto.7.6.15812] [PMID: 21494095]

[12]   Sahu R, Kaushik S, Clement CC, *et al.* Microautophagy of cytosolic proteins by late endosomes. Dev Cell 2011; 20(1): 131-9.
[http://dx.doi.org/10.1016/j.devcel.2010.12.003] [PMID: 21238931]

[13]   Uttenweiler A, Mayer A. Microautophagy in the yeast *Saccharomyces cerevisiae*. Methods Mol Biol 2008; 445: 245-59.
[http://dx.doi.org/10.1007/978-1-59745-157-4_16] [PMID: 18425455]

[14]   Li W, Yang Q, Mao Z. Chaperone-mediated autophagy: Machinery, regulation and biological consequences. Cell Mol Life Sci 2011; 68(5): 749-63.
[http://dx.doi.org/10.1007/s00018-010-0565-6] [PMID: 20976518]

[15]   Dice JF. Peptide sequences that target cytosolic proteins for lysosomal proteolysis. Trends Biochem Sci 1990; 15(8): 305-9.
[http://dx.doi.org/10.1016/0968-0004(90)90019-8] [PMID: 2204156]

[16]   Mizushima N. The pleiotropic role of autophagy: From protein metabolism to bactericide. Cell Death Differ 2005; 12 (Suppl. 2): 1535-41.
[http://dx.doi.org/10.1038/sj.cdd.4401728] [PMID: 16247501]

[17]   Feng Y, He D, Yao Z, Klionsky DJ. The machinery of macroautophagy. Cell Res 2014; 24(1): 24-41.
[http://dx.doi.org/10.1038/cr.2013.168] [PMID: 24366339]

[18]   Choi AM, Ryter SW, Levine B. Autophagy in human health and disease. N Engl J Med 2013; 368(7): 651-62.
[http://dx.doi.org/10.1056/NEJMra1205406] [PMID: 23406030]

[19]   Lapaquette P, Guzzo J, Bretillon L, Bringer M-A. Cellular and molecular connections between autophagy and inflammation. Mediators Inflamm 2015; 2015.

[http://dx.doi.org/10.1155/2015/398483]

[20] Klionsky DJ, Cregg JM, Dunn WA Jr, *et al.* A unified nomenclature for yeast autophagy-related genes. Dev Cell 2003; 5(4): 539-45.
[http://dx.doi.org/10.1016/S1534-5807(03)00296-X] [PMID: 14536056]

[21] Thumm M, Egner R, Koch B, *et al.* Isolation of autophagocytosis mutants of *Saccharomyces cerevisiae.* FEBS Lett 1994; 349(2): 275-80.
[http://dx.doi.org/10.1016/0014-5793(94)00672-5] [PMID: 8050581]

[22] Boya P, Reggiori F, Codogno P. Emerging regulation and functions of autophagy. Nat Cell Biol 2013; 15(7): 713-20.
[http://dx.doi.org/10.1038/ncb2788] [PMID: 23817233]

[23] Bento CF, Renna M, Ghislat G, *et al.* Mammalian autophagy: How does it work? Annu Rev Biochem 2016; 85: 685-713.
[http://dx.doi.org/10.1146/annurev-biochem-060815-014556] [PMID: 26865532]

[24] McAlpine F, Williamson LE, Tooze SA, Chan EY. Regulation of nutrient-sensitive autophagy by uncoordinated 51-like kinases 1 and 2. Autophagy 2013; 9(3): 361-73.
[http://dx.doi.org/10.4161/auto.23066] [PMID: 23291478]

[25] Green DR, Levine B. To be or not to be? How selective autophagy and cell death govern cell fate. Cell 2014; 157(1): 65-75.
[http://dx.doi.org/10.1016/j.cell.2014.02.049] [PMID: 24679527]

[26] Nguyen TN, Padman BS, Usher J, Oorschot V, Ramm G, Lazarou M. Atg8 family LC3/GABARAP proteins are crucial for autophagosome-lysosome fusion but not autophagosome formation during PINK1/Parkin mitophagy and starvation. J Cell Biol 2016; 215(6): 857-74.
[PMID: 27864321]

[27] Lebovitz CB, Bortnik SB, Gorski SM. Here, there be dragons: Charting autophagy-related alterations in human tumors. Clin Cancer Res 2012; 18(5): 1214-26.
[http://dx.doi.org/10.1158/1078-0432.CCR-11-2465] [PMID: 22253413]

[28] Geng J, Klionsky DJ. The Atg8 and Atg12 ubiquitin-like conjugation systems in macroautophagy. 'Protein modifications: Beyond the usual suspects' review series. EMBO Rep 2008; 9(9): 859-64.
[http://dx.doi.org/10.1038/embor.2008.163] [PMID: 18704115]

[29] Hanada T, Noda NN, Satomi Y, *et al.* The Atg12-Atg5 conjugate has a novel E3-like activity for protein lipidation in autophagy. J Biol Chem 2007; 282(52): 37298-302.
[http://dx.doi.org/10.1074/jbc.C700195200] [PMID: 17986448]

[30] Weidberg H, Shvets E, Shpilka T, Shimron F, Shinder V, Elazar Z. LC3 and GATE-16/GABARAP subfamilies are both essential yet act differently in autophagosome biogenesis. EMBO J 2010; 29(11): 1792-802.
[http://dx.doi.org/10.1038/emboj.2010.74] [PMID: 20418806]

[31] Fujita N, Itoh T, Omori H, Fukuda M, Noda T, Yoshimori T. The Atg16L complex specifies the site of LC3 lipidation for membrane biogenesis in autophagy. Mol Biol Cell 2008; 19(5): 2092-100.
[http://dx.doi.org/10.1091/mbc.e07-12-1257] [PMID: 18321988]

[32] Zhang L, Li J, Ouyang L, Liu B, Cheng Y. Unraveling the roles of Atg4 proteases from autophagy modulation to targeted cancer therapy. Cancer Lett 2016; 373(1): 19-26.
[http://dx.doi.org/10.1016/j.canlet.2016.01.022] [PMID: 26805760]

[33] Tanida I, Sou YS, Ezaki J, Minematsu-Ikeguchi N, Ueno T, Kominami E. HsAtg4B/HsApg4B/autophagin-1 cleaves the carboxyl termini of three human Atg8 homologues and delipidates microtubule-associated protein light chain 3- and GABAA receptor-associated protein-phospholipid conjugates. J Biol Chem 2004; 279(35): 36268-76.
[http://dx.doi.org/10.1074/jbc.M401461200] [PMID: 15187094]

[34] Satoo K, Noda NN, Kumeta H, *et al.* The structure of Atg4B-LC3 complex reveals the mechanism of

LC3 processing and delipidation during autophagy. EMBO J 2009; 28(9): 1341-50.
[http://dx.doi.org/10.1038/emboj.2009.80] [PMID: 19322194]

[35]   Klionsky DJ, Abdelmohsen K, Abe A, Abedin MJ, Abeliovich H, Acevedo Arozena A, *et al.*
       Guidelines for the use and interpretation of assays for monitoring autophagy. Autophagy 2016; 12(1):
       1-222.

[36]   Rebecca VW, Amaravadi RK. Emerging strategies to effectively target autophagy in cancer.
       Oncogene 2016; 35(1): 1-11.
       [http://dx.doi.org/10.1038/onc.2015.99] [PMID: 25893285]

[37]   Thorburn A, Thamm DH, Gustafson DL. Autophagy and cancer therapy. Mol Pharmacol 2014; 85(6):
       830-8.
       [http://dx.doi.org/10.1124/mol.114.091850] [PMID: 24574520]

[38]   Lippai M, Szatmári Z. Autophagy-from molecular mechanisms to clinical relevance. Cell Biol Toxicol
       2017; 33(2): 145-68.
       [http://dx.doi.org/10.1007/s10565-016-9374-5] [PMID: 27957648]

[39]   DeMartino GN. Introduction to the thematic minireview series: Autophagy. J Biol Chem 2018;
       293(15): 5384-5.
       [http://dx.doi.org/10.1074/jbc.TM118.002429] [PMID: 29467224]

[40]   Zhang J, Wang G, Zhou Y, Chen Y, Ouyang L, Liu B. Mechanisms of autophagy and relevant small-
       molecule compounds for targeted cancer therapy. Cell Mol Life Sci 2018; 75(10): 1803-26.
       [http://dx.doi.org/10.1007/s00018-018-2759-2] [PMID: 29417176]

[41]   Smith M, Wilkinson S. ER homeostasis and autophagy. Essays Biochem 2017; 61(6): 625-35.
       [http://dx.doi.org/10.1042/EBC20170092] [PMID: 29233873]

[42]   Zheng HC. The molecular mechanisms of chemoresistance in cancers. Oncotarget 2017; 8(35): 59950-
       64.
       [http://dx.doi.org/10.18632/oncotarget.19048] [PMID: 28938696]

[43]   Bortnik S, Gorski SM. Clinical applications of autophagy proteins in cancer: From potential targets to
       biomarkers. Int J Mol Sci 2017; 18(7): E1496.
       [http://dx.doi.org/10.3390/ijms18071496] [PMID: 28696368]

[44]   New M, Van Acker T, Long JS, Sakamaki JI, Ryan KM, Tooze SA. Molecular pathways controlling
       autophagy in pancreatic cancer. Front Oncol 2017; 7: 28.
       [http://dx.doi.org/10.3389/fonc.2017.00028] [PMID: 28316954]

[45]   Mazure NM, Pouysségur J. Hypoxia-induced autophagy: Cell death or cell survival? Curr Opin Cell
       Biol 2010; 22(2): 177-80.
       [http://dx.doi.org/10.1016/j.ceb.2009.11.015] [PMID: 20022734]

[46]   Swart C, Du Toit A, Loos B. Autophagy and the invisible line between life and death. Eur J Cell Biol
       2016; 95(12): 598-610.
       [http://dx.doi.org/10.1016/j.ejcb.2016.10.005] [PMID: 28340912]

[47]   Li M, Gao P, Zhang J. Crosstalk between autophagy and apoptosis: Potential and emerging therapeutic
       targets for cardiac diseases. Int J Mol Sci 2016; 17(3): 332.
       [http://dx.doi.org/10.3390/ijms17030332] [PMID: 26950124]

[48]   Lee J-S, Li Q, Lee J-Y, *et al.* FLIP-mediated autophagy regulation in cell death control. Nat Cell Biol
       2009; 11(11): 1355-62.
       [http://dx.doi.org/10.1038/ncb1980] [PMID: 19838173]

[49]   Betin VM, Lane JD. Atg4D at the interface between autophagy and apoptosis. Autophagy 2009; 5(7):
       1057-9.
       [http://dx.doi.org/10.4161/auto.5.7.9684] [PMID: 19713737]

[50]   Radoshevich L, Murrow L, Chen N, *et al.* ATG12 conjugation to ATG3 regulates mitochondrial

homeostasis and cell death. Cell 2010; 142(4): 590-600.
[http://dx.doi.org/10.1016/j.cell.2010.07.018] [PMID: 20723759]

[51] Wu H, Che X, Zheng Q, *et al.* Caspases: A molecular switch node in the crosstalk between autophagy and apoptosis. Int J Biol Sci 2014; 10(9): 1072-83.
[http://dx.doi.org/10.7150/ijbs.9719] [PMID: 25285039]

[52] Wirawan E, Vande Walle L, Kersse K, *et al.* Caspase-mediated cleavage of Beclin-1 inactivates Beclin-1-induced autophagy and enhances apoptosis by promoting the release of proapoptotic factors from mitochondria. Cell Death Dis 2010; 1(1): e18.
[http://dx.doi.org/10.1038/cddis.2009.16] [PMID: 21364619]

[53] Vousden KH, Lane DP. p53 in health and disease. Nat Rev Mol Cell Biol 2007; 8(4): 275-83.
[http://dx.doi.org/10.1038/nrm2147] [PMID: 17380161]

[54] Crighton D, Wilkinson S, O'Prey J, *et al.* DRAM, a p53-induced modulator of autophagy, is critical for apoptosis. Cell 2006; 126(1): 121-34.
[http://dx.doi.org/10.1016/j.cell.2006.05.034] [PMID: 16839881]

[55] Zeng X, Kinsella TJ. A novel role for DNA mismatch repair and the autophagic processing of chemotherapy drugs in human tumor cells. Autophagy 2007; 3(4): 368-70.
[http://dx.doi.org/10.4161/auto.4205] [PMID: 17426439]

[56] Zeng X, Yan T, Schupp JE, Seo Y, Kinsella TJ. DNA mismatch repair initiates 6-thioguanine--induced autophagy through p53 activation in human tumor cells. Clin Cancer Res 2007; 13(4): 1315-21.
[http://dx.doi.org/10.1158/1078-0432.CCR-06-1517] [PMID: 17317843]

[57] Rizzuto R, Pozzan T. Microdomains of intracellular Ca^{2+}: Molecular determinants and functional consequences. Physiol Rev 2006; 86(1): 369-408.
[http://dx.doi.org/10.1152/physrev.00004.2005] [PMID: 16371601]

[58] Lavieu G, Scarlatti F, Sala G, *et al.* Regulation of autophagy by sphingosine kinase 1 and its role in cell survival during nutrient starvation. J Biol Chem 2006; 281(13): 8518-27.
[http://dx.doi.org/10.1074/jbc.M506182200] [PMID: 16415355]

[59] Scherz-Shouval R, Shvets E, Fass E, Shorer H, Gil L, Elazar Z. Reactive oxygen species are essential for autophagy and specifically regulate the activity of Atg4. EMBO J 2007; 26(7): 1749-60.
[http://dx.doi.org/10.1038/sj.emboj.7601623] [PMID: 17347651]

[60] Corcelle EA, Puustinen P, Jäättelä M. Apoptosis and autophagy: Targeting autophagy signalling in cancer cells -'trick or treats'? FEBS J 2009; 276(21): 6084-96.
[http://dx.doi.org/10.1111/j.1742-4658.2009.07332.x] [PMID: 19788415]

[61] Levine B, Kroemer G. Autophagy in the pathogenesis of disease. Cell 2008; 132(1): 27-42.
[http://dx.doi.org/10.1016/j.cell.2007.12.018] [PMID: 18191218]

[62] Mathew R, Karantza-Wadsworth V, White E. Role of autophagy in cancer. Nat Rev Cancer 2007; 7(12): 961-7.
[http://dx.doi.org/10.1038/nrc2254] [PMID: 17972889]

[63] Hewitt G, Korolchuk VI. Repair, reuse, recycle: The expanding role of autophagy in genome maintenance. Trends Cell Biol 2017; 27(5): 340-51.
[http://dx.doi.org/10.1016/j.tcb.2016.11.011] [PMID: 28011061]

[64] Xie Z, Klionsky DJ. Autophagosome formation: Core machinery and adaptations. Nat Cell Biol 2007; 9(10): 1102-9.
[http://dx.doi.org/10.1038/ncb1007-1102] [PMID: 17909521]

[65] Mathew R, Karantza-Wadsworth V, White E. Assessing metabolic stress and autophagy status in epithelial tumors. Methods Enzymol 2009; 453: 53-81.
[http://dx.doi.org/10.1016/S0076-6879(08)04004-4] [PMID: 19216902]

[66]   Koneri K, Goi T, Hirono Y, Katayama K, Yamaguchi A. Beclin 1 gene inhibits tumor growth in colon cancer cell lines. Anticancer Res 2007; 27(3B): 1453-7.
[PMID: 17595761]

[67]   Maiuri MC, Tasdemir E, Criollo A, *et al.* Control of autophagy by oncogenes and tumor suppressor genes. Cell Death Differ 2009; 16(1): 87-93.
[http://dx.doi.org/10.1038/cdd.2008.131] [PMID: 18806760]

[68]   Miracco C, Cosci E, Oliveri G, *et al.* Protein and mRNA expression of autophagy gene Beclin 1 in human brain tumours. Int J Oncol 2007; 30(2): 429-36.
[PMID: 17203225]

[69]   Qu X, Yu J, Bhagat G, *et al.* Promotion of tumorigenesis by heterozygous disruption of the beclin 1 autophagy gene. J Clin Invest 2003; 112(12): 1809-20.
[http://dx.doi.org/10.1172/JCI20039] [PMID: 14638851]

[70]   Lee S-J, Kim H-P, Jin Y, Choi AM, Ryter SW. Beclin 1 deficiency is associated with increased hypoxia-induced angiogenesis. Autophagy 2011; 7(8): 829-39.
[http://dx.doi.org/10.4161/auto.7.8.15598] [PMID: 21685724]

[71]   White EJ, Martin V, Liu J-L, *et al.* Autophagy regulation in cancer development and therapy. Am J Cancer Res 2011; 1(3): 362-72.
[PMID: 21969237]

[72]   Galluzzi L, Pietrocola F, Bravo-San Pedro JM, *et al.* Autophagy in malignant transformation and cancer progression. EMBO J 2015; 34(7): 856-80.
[http://dx.doi.org/10.15252/embj.201490784] [PMID: 25712477]

[73]   Lambert AJ, Brand MD. Reactive oxygen species production by mitochondria. Mitochondrial DNA: Methods and Protocols 2009; 165-81.
[http://dx.doi.org/10.1007/978-1-59745-521-3_11]

[74]   Payne CM, Waltmire CN, Crowley C, *et al.* Caspase-6 mediated cleavage of guanylate cyclase alpha 1 during deoxycholate-induced apoptosis: Protective role of the nitric oxide signaling module. Cell Biol Toxicol 2003; 19(6): 373-92.
[http://dx.doi.org/10.1023/B:CBTO.0000013331.70391.0e] [PMID: 15015762]

[75]   Takamura A, Komatsu M, Hara T, *et al.* Autophagy-deficient mice develop multiple liver tumors. Genes Dev 2011; 25(8): 795-800.
[http://dx.doi.org/10.1101/gad.2016211] [PMID: 21498569]

[76]   Zhang Y, Goldman S, Baerga R, Zhao Y, Komatsu M, Jin S. Adipose-specific deletion of autophagy-related gene 7 (ATG7) in mice reveals a role in adipogenesis. Proc Natl Acad Sci USA 2009; 106(47): 19860-5.
[http://dx.doi.org/10.1073/pnas.0906048106] [PMID: 19910529]

[77]   Poillet-Perez L, Despouy G, Delage-Mourroux R, Boyer-Guittaut M. Interplay between ROS and autophagy in cancer cells, from tumor initiation to cancer therapy. Redox Biol 2015; 4: 184-92.
[http://dx.doi.org/10.1016/j.redox.2014.12.003] [PMID: 25590798]

[78]   Kong J, Whelan KA, Laczkó D, *et al.* Autophagy levels are elevated in Barrett's esophagus and promote cell survival from acid and oxidative stress. Mol Carcinog 2016; 55(11): 1526-41.
[http://dx.doi.org/10.1002/mc.22406] [PMID: 26373456]

[79]   White E, Karp C, Strohecker AM, Guo Y, Mathew R. Role of autophagy in suppression of inflammation and cancer. Curr Opin Cell Biol 2010; 22(2): 212-7.
[http://dx.doi.org/10.1016/j.ceb.2009.12.008] [PMID: 20056400]

[80]   Stroikin Y, Dalen H, Lööf S, Terman A. Inhibition of autophagy with 3-methyladenine results in impaired turnover of lysosomes and accumulation of lipofuscin-like material. Eur J Cell Biol 2004; 83(10): 583-90.
[http://dx.doi.org/10.1078/0171-9335-00433] [PMID: 15679103]

[81]   Chen H-Y, White E. Role of autophagy in cancer prevention. Cancer Prev Res (Phila) 2011; 4(7): 973-83.
[http://dx.doi.org/10.1158/1940-6207.CAPR-10-0387] [PMID: 21733821]

[82]   Sharifi MN, Mowers EE, Drake LE, *et al.* Autophagy promotes focal adhesion disassembly and cell motility of metastatic tumor cells through the direct interaction of paxillin with LC3. Cell Reports 2016; 15(8): 1660-72.
[http://dx.doi.org/10.1016/j.celrep.2016.04.065] [PMID: 27184837]

[83]   Macintosh RL, Timpson P, Thorburn J, Anderson KI, Thorburn A, Ryan KM. Inhibition of autophagy impairs tumor cell invasion in an organotypic model. Cell Cycle 2012; 11(10): 2022-9.
[http://dx.doi.org/10.4161/cc.20424] [PMID: 22580450]

[84]   Lock R, Kenific CM, Leidal AM, Salas E, Debnath J. Autophagy-dependent production of secreted factors facilitates oncogenic RAS-driven invasion. Cancer Discov 2014; 4(4): 466-79.
[http://dx.doi.org/10.1158/2159-8290.CD-13-0841] [PMID: 24513958]

[85]   Qiang L, Zhao B, Ming M, *et al.* Regulation of cell proliferation and migration by p62 through stabilization of Twist1. Proc Natl Acad Sci USA 2014; 111(25): 9241-6.
[http://dx.doi.org/10.1073/pnas.1322913111] [PMID: 24927592]

[86]   Kenific CM, Stehbens SJ, Goldsmith J, *et al.* NBR1 enables autophagy-dependent focal adhesion turnover. J Cell Biol 2016; 212(5): 577-90.
[http://dx.doi.org/10.1083/jcb.201503075] [PMID: 26903539]

[87]   Sousa CM, Biancur DE, Wang X, *et al.* Pancreatic stellate cells support tumour metabolism through autophagic alanine secretion. Nature 2016; 536(7617): 479-83.
[http://dx.doi.org/10.1038/nature19084] [PMID: 27509858]

[88]   Kraya AA, Piao S, Xu X, *et al.* Identification of secreted proteins that reflect autophagy dynamics within tumor cells. Autophagy 2015; 11(1): 60-74.
[http://dx.doi.org/10.4161/15548627.2014.984273] [PMID: 25484078]

[89]   Sun W-L, Chen J, Wang Y-P, Zheng H. Autophagy protects breast cancer cells from epirubicin-induced apoptosis and facilitates epirubicin-resistance development. Autophagy 2011; 7(9): 1035-44.
[http://dx.doi.org/10.4161/auto.7.9.16521] [PMID: 21646864]

[90]   Sun WL, Lan D, Gan TQ, Cai ZW. Autophagy facilitates multidrug resistance development through inhibition of apoptosis in breast cancer cells. Neoplasma 2015; 62(2): 199-208.
[http://dx.doi.org/10.4149/neo_2015_025] [PMID: 25591585]

[91]   Chittaranjan S, Bortnik S, Dragowska WH, *et al.* Autophagy inhibition augments the anticancer effects of epirubicin treatment in anthracycline-sensitive and -resistant triple-negative breast cancer. Clin Cancer Res 2014; 20(12): 3159-73.
[http://dx.doi.org/10.1158/1078-0432.CCR-13-2060] [PMID: 24721646]

[92]   Samaddar JS, Gaddy VT, Duplantier J, *et al.* A role for macroautophagy in protection against 4-hydroxytamoxifen-induced cell death and the development of antiestrogen resistance. Mol Cancer Ther 2008; 7(9): 2977-87.
[http://dx.doi.org/10.1158/1535-7163.MCT-08-0447] [PMID: 18790778]

[93]   Vazquez-Martin A, Oliveras-Ferraros C, Menendez JA. Autophagy facilitates the development of breast cancer resistance to the anti-HER2 monoclonal antibody trastuzumab. PLoS One 2009; 4(7): e6251.
[http://dx.doi.org/10.1371/journal.pone.0006251] [PMID: 19606230]

[94]   Ajabnoor GM, Crook T, Coley HM. Paclitaxel resistance is associated with switch from apoptotic to autophagic cell death in MCF-7 breast cancer cells. Cell Death Dis 2012; 3(1): e260.
[http://dx.doi.org/10.1038/cddis.2011.139] [PMID: 22278287]

[95]   Sui X, Chen R, Wang Z, *et al.* Autophagy and chemotherapy resistance: A promising therapeutic target for cancer treatment. Cell Death Dis 2013; 4(10): e838.

[http://dx.doi.org/10.1038/cddis.2013.350] [PMID: 24113172]

[96]   Sun WL. Ambra1 in autophagy and apoptosis: Implications for cell survival and chemotherapy resistance. Oncol Lett 2016; 12(1): 367-74.
[http://dx.doi.org/10.3892/ol.2016.4644] [PMID: 27347152]

[97]   Chengyu J, Rao S, Liu H, Guo F, Wang H, Sun Y, *et al.* Use of cell autophagy (type ii cell apoptosis) inhibitors. WO2010124618, 2010.

[98]   Matsui M, Yarosh D. Small molecule inhibitors of p-type atpases. WO2013130407, 2013.

[99]   Korur S, Beaufils F, Wymann M. Combination of lysosomotropic or autophagy modulating agents and a gsk-3 inhibitor for treatment of cancer. WO2013182519, 2013.

[100]   Levy N, Cau P, De Sandre-Giovannoli A, Harhori K, Perrin S, Navarro C, *et al.* Proteasome inhibitors for treating a disorder related to an accumulation of non-degraded abnormal protein or a cancer. WO2016113357, 2016.

[101]   Zaupa C, Hortelano J, Silvestre N, Spindler A. Combination product with autophagy modulator. WO2016131945, 2016.

[102]   Amaravadi RK, Winkler J. Dimeric quinacrine derivatives as autophagy inhibitors for cancer therapy. WO2016168721, 2016.

[103]   Deckwerth T, Kleinman E, Ruan F, Baker W, Klinghoffer R. Autophagy-inhibiting compounds and uses thereof. WO2016196393, 2016.

[104]   Spada AP. Caspase inhibitors for use in the treatment of liver cancer. WO2017079566, 2017.

[105]   FaraciI WS, Fendrock BC, Herrera R. Particle delivery of rapamycin to the liver. WO2017139212, 2017.

[106]   Siegelin MD, Altieri DC. Combination therapies with mitochondrial-targeted anti-tumor agents. US20110268722, 2011.

[107]   Cho M-L, Lee S-Y, Park M-J. Composition using metformin for preventing or treating immune diseases including lupus. US20150238445, 2015.

[108]   Desai SD. Therapeutic and diagnostic method for ataxia-telangiectasia. US20170196871, 2017.

[109]   Espina V, Liotta L. Methods of treating pre-malignant ductal cancer with autophagy inhibitors. US9096833, 2015.

[110]   McKenna S, O'Sullivan GC, O'Donovan T. Method for the treatment of cancer. US9155761, 2015.

[111]   Huijun Z, Xiuhua W, Li J, Jiali Z, Weixin H, Zhancheng X. Application of dihydroartemisinin to preparation of tumor cell autophagy induction medicament. CN102038678, 2011.

[112]   Zhenghong Q, Rui S, Bo G. Application of tunicamycin in preparing medicament for treating ischemic cerebral apoplexy. CN102119935, 2012.

[113]   Zhang S, Cui S, Zhi D, Zhao Y, Meng Y. 20(R)-ginsenoside Rg3/cationic lipid/cholesterol/folic acid liposome medicine as well as preparation method and application thereof. CN105534911, 2016.

[114]   Yu D, Su L, Wei J, Ding Y. Application of diisopropylamine dichloroacetate in treating tumors. CN105748455, 2016.

[115]   Peng Y, Liu T, Li X. Tumor-targeting gambogic acid compound, and preparation method and application thereof. CN106083898, 2016.

[116]   Zhang Y. Epidemiology of esophageal cancer. World J Gastroenterol 2013; 19(34): 5598-606.
[http://dx.doi.org/10.3748/wjg.v19.i34.5598] [PMID: 24039351]

[117]   Jain S, Dhingra S. Pathology of esophageal cancer and Barrett's esophagus. Ann Cardiothorac Surg 2017; 6(2): 99-109.
[http://dx.doi.org/10.21037/acs.2017.03.06] [PMID: 28446998]

[118] Glickman JN, Odze RD. Epithelial Neoplasms of the Esophagus. In: Odze RD, Goldblum JR, Eds. Odze and Goldblum Pathology of the Gastrointestinal Tract, Liver, Biliary-tract and Pancreas. 3rd ed.; Philadelphia, Elsevier; 2015, pp: 680-701.

[119] Roesly HB, Khan MR, Chen HDR, *et al.* The decreased expression of Beclin-1 correlates with progression to esophageal adenocarcinoma: The role of deoxycholic acid. Am J Physiol Gastrointest Liver Physiol 2012; 302(8): G864-72.
[http://dx.doi.org/10.1152/ajpgi.00340.2011] [PMID: 22301112]

[120] Weh KM, Aiyer HS, Howell AB, Kresty LA. Cranberry proanthocyanidins modulate reactive oxygen species in Barrett's and esophageal adenocarcinoma cell lines. J Berry Res 2016; 6(2): 125-36.
[http://dx.doi.org/10.3233/JBR-160122] [PMID: 27583064]

[121] Dvorak K, Payne CM, Chavarria M, *et al.* Bile acids in combination with low pH induce oxidative stress and oxidative DNA damage: Relevance to the pathogenesis of Barrett's oesophagus. Gut 2007; 56(6): 763-71.
[http://dx.doi.org/10.1136/gut.2006.103697] [PMID: 17145738]

[122] McQuaid KR, Laine L, Fennerty MB, Souza R, Spechler SJ. Systematic review: The role of bile acids in the pathogenesis of gastro-oesophageal reflux disease and related neoplasia. Aliment Pharmacol Ther 2011; 34(2): 146-65.
[http://dx.doi.org/10.1111/j.1365-2036.2011.04709.x] [PMID: 21615439]

[123] Federico A, Morgillo F, Tuccillo C, Ciardiello F, Loguercio C. Chronic inflammation and oxidative stress in human carcinogenesis. Int J Cancer 2007; 121(11): 2381-6.
[http://dx.doi.org/10.1002/ijc.23192] [PMID: 17893868]

[124] Chen X, Ding YW, Yang G-y, Bondoc F, Lee M-J, Yang CS. Oxidative damage in an esophageal adenocarcinoma model with rats. Carcinogenesis 2000; 21(2): 257-63.
[http://dx.doi.org/10.1093/carcin/21.2.257] [PMID: 10657966]

[125] Inayama M, Hashimoto N, Tokoro T, Shiozaki H. Involvement of oxidative stress in experimentally induced reflux esophagitis and esophageal cancer. Hepatogastroenterology 2007; 54(75): 761-5.
[PMID: 17591057]

[126] Valko M, Leibfritz D, Moncol J, Cronin MT, Mazur M, Telser J. Free radicals and antioxidants in normal physiological functions and human disease. Int J Biochem Cell Biol 2007; 39(1): 44-84.
[http://dx.doi.org/10.1016/j.biocel.2006.07.001] [PMID: 16978905]

[127] Clements DM, Oleesky DA, Smith SC, *et al.* A study to determine plasma antioxidant concentrations in patients with Barrett's oesophagus. J Clin Pathol 2005; 58(5): 490-2.
[http://dx.doi.org/10.1136/jcp.2004.023721] [PMID: 15858119]

[128] Guo JY, Xia B, White E. Autophagy-mediated tumor promotion. Cell 2013; 155(6): 1216-9.
[http://dx.doi.org/10.1016/j.cell.2013.11.019] [PMID: 24315093]

[129] Lorin S, Hamaï A, Mehrpour M, Codogno P, Eds. Autophagy regulation and its role in cancer Seminars in cancer biology. Elsevier 2013.

[130] Jiang L, Duan B-S, Huang J-X, *et al.* Association of the expression of unc-51-Like kinase 1 with lymph node metastasis and survival in patients with esophageal squamous cell carcinoma. Int J Clin Exp Med 2014; 7(5): 1349-54.
[PMID: 24995094]

[131] Jiang S, Li Y, Zhu YH, *et al.* Intensive expression of UNC-51-like kinase 1 is a novel biomarker of poor prognosis in patients with esophageal squamous cell carcinoma. Cancer Sci 2011; 102(8): 1568-75.
[http://dx.doi.org/10.1111/j.1349-7006.2011.01964.x] [PMID: 21518141]

[132] Huang N, Liu Z, Zhu J, *et al.* Sirtuin 6 plays an oncogenic role and induces cell autophagy in esophageal cancer cells. Tumour Biol 2017; 39(6): 1010428317708532.
[http://dx.doi.org/10.1177/1010428317708532] [PMID: 28653878]

[133] Weh KM, Howell AB, Kresty LA. Expression, modulation, and clinical correlates of the autophagy protein Beclin-1 in esophageal adenocarcinoma. Mol Carcinog 2016; 55(11): 1876-85.
[http://dx.doi.org/10.1002/mc.22432] [PMID: 27696537]

[134] El-Mashed S, O'Donovan TR, Kay EW, *et al.* LC3B globular structures correlate with survival in esophageal adenocarcinoma. BMC Cancer 2015; 15(1): 582.
[http://dx.doi.org/10.1186/s12885-015-1574-5] [PMID: 26265176]

[135] Ren Y, Chen Y, Liang X, Lu Y, Pan W, Yang M. MiRNA-638 promotes autophagy and malignant phenotypes of cancer cells via directly suppressing DACT3. Cancer Lett 2017; 390: 126-36.
[http://dx.doi.org/10.1016/j.canlet.2017.01.009] [PMID: 28108314]

[136] Hwang JW, Chung S, Sundar IK, *et al.* Cigarette smoke-induced autophagy is regulated by SIRT1-PARP-1-dependent mechanism: Implication in pathogenesis of COPD. Arch Biochem Biophys 2010; 500(2): 203-9.
[http://dx.doi.org/10.1016/j.abb.2010.05.013] [PMID: 20493163]

[137] Lin M-H, Hsieh W-F, Chiang W-F, *et al.* Autophagy induction by the 30-100kDa fraction of areca nut in both normal and malignant cells through reactive oxygen species. Oral Oncol 2010; 46(11): 822-8.
[http://dx.doi.org/10.1016/j.oraloncology.2010.08.002] [PMID: 20920876]

[138] Chen Z-H, Lam HC, Jin Y, *et al.* Autophagy protein microtubule-associated protein 1 light chain-3B (LC3B) activates extrinsic apoptosis during cigarette smoke-induced emphysema. Proc Natl Acad Sci USA 2010; 107(44): 18880-5.
[http://dx.doi.org/10.1073/pnas.1005574107] [PMID: 20956295]

[139] Was H, Dulak J, Jozkowicz A. Heme oxygenase-1 in tumor biology and therapy. Curr Drug Targets 2010; 11(12): 1551-70.
[http://dx.doi.org/10.2174/138945011109011551] [PMID: 20704546]

[140] Kim HP, Wang X, Chen ZH, *et al.* Autophagic proteins regulate cigarette smoke-induced apoptosis: Protective role of heme oxygenase-1. Autophagy 2008; 4(7): 887-95.
[http://dx.doi.org/10.4161/auto.6767] [PMID: 18769149]

[141] Li X, Xu HL, Liu YX, An N, Zhao S, Bao JK. Autophagy modulation as a target for anticancer drug discovery. Acta Pharmacol Sin 2013; 34(5): 612-24.
[http://dx.doi.org/10.1038/aps.2013.23] [PMID: 23564085]

[142] Janku F, McConkey DJ, Hong DS, Kurzrock R. Autophagy as a target for anticancer therapy. Nat Rev Clin Oncol 2011; 8(9): 528-39.
[http://dx.doi.org/10.1038/nrclinonc.2011.71] [PMID: 21587219]

[143] Kresty L, Howell A, Baird M. A cranberry proanthocyanidin rich extract induces both apoptosis and autophagy in human SEG-1 esophageal adenocarcinoma cells. AACR 2008.

[144] Chueca E, Apostolova N, Esplugues JV, García-González MA, Lanas Á, Piazuelo E. Proton pump inhibitors display antitumor effects in Barrett's adenocarcinoma cells. Front Pharmacol 2016; 7: 452.
[http://dx.doi.org/10.3389/fphar.2016.00452] [PMID: 27932981]

[145] Adams O, Dislich B, Berezowska S, *et al.* Prognostic relevance of autophagy markers LC3B and p62 in esophageal adenocarcinomas. Oncotarget 2016; 7(26): 39241-55.
[http://dx.doi.org/10.18632/oncotarget.9649] [PMID: 27250034]

[146] O'Donovan TR, O'Sullivan GC, McKenna SL. Induction of autophagy by drug-resistant esophageal cancer cells promotes their survival and recovery following treatment with chemotherapeutics. Autophagy 2011; 7(5): 509-24.
[http://dx.doi.org/10.4161/auto.7.5.15066] [PMID: 21325880]

[147] Nyhan MJ, O'Donovan TR, Elzinga B, Crowley LC, O'Sullivan GC, McKenna SL. The BH3 mimetic HA14-1 enhances 5-fluorouracil-induced autophagy and type II cell death in oesophageal cancer cells. Br J Cancer 2012; 106(4): 711-8.
[http://dx.doi.org/10.1038/bjc.2011.604] [PMID: 22240779]

[148] O'Donovan TR, Rajendran S, O'Reilly S, O'Sullivan GC, McKenna SL. Lithium modulates autophagy in esophageal and colorectal cancer cells and enhances the efficacy of therapeutic agents *in vitro* and *in vivo*. PLoS One 2015; 10(8): e0134676.
[http://dx.doi.org/10.1371/journal.pone.0134676] [PMID: 26248051]

[149] Kresty LA, Weh KM, Zeyzus-Johns B, Perez LN, Howell AB. Cranberry proanthocyanidins inhibit esophageal adenocarcinoma *in vitro* and *in vivo* through pleiotropic cell death induction and PI3K/AKT/mTOR inactivation. Oncotarget 2015; 6(32): 33438-55.
[http://dx.doi.org/10.18632/oncotarget.5586] [PMID: 26378019]

[150] Falvey CM, O'Donovan TR, El-Mashed S, Nyhan MJ, O'Reilly S, McKenna SL. UBE2L6/UBCH8 and ISG15 attenuate autophagy in esophageal cancer cells. Oncotarget 2017; 8(14): 23479-91.
[http://dx.doi.org/10.18632/oncotarget.15182] [PMID: 28186990]

[151] Jeon YJ, Yoo HM, Chung CH. ISG15 and immune diseases. BBA-MOL BASIS DIS 2010; 1802(5): 485-96.
[http://dx.doi.org/10.1016/j.bbadis.2010.02.006]

[152] Pitha-Rowe IF, Pitha PM. Viral defense, carcinogenesis and ISG15: Novel roles for an old ISG. Cytokine Growth Factor Rev 2007; 18(5-6): 409-17.
[http://dx.doi.org/10.1016/j.cytogfr.2007.06.017] [PMID: 17689132]

[153] Sgorbissa A, Brancolini C. IFNs, ISGylation and cancer: Cui prodest? Cytokine Growth Factor Rev 2012; 23(6): 307-14.
[http://dx.doi.org/10.1016/j.cytogfr.2012.07.003] [PMID: 22906767]

[154] Kim KI, Zhang D-E. ISG15, not just another ubiquitin-like protein. Biochem Biophys Res Commun 2003; 307(3): 431-4.
[http://dx.doi.org/10.1016/S0006-291X(03)01216-6] [PMID: 12893238]

[155] Serniwka SA, Shaw GS. The structure of the UbcH8-ubiquitin complex shows a unique ubiquitin interaction site. Biochemistry 2009; 48(51): 12169-79.
[http://dx.doi.org/10.1021/bi901686j] [PMID: 19928833]

[156] Xu D, Zhang T, Xiao J, *et al*. Modification of BECN1 by ISG15 plays a crucial role in autophagy regulation by type I IFN/interferon. Autophagy 2015; 11(4): 617-28.
[http://dx.doi.org/10.1080/15548627.2015.1023982] [PMID: 25906440]

[157] Chen Y, Lu Y, Lu C, Zhang L. Beclin-1 expression is a predictor of clinical outcome in patients with esophageal squamous cell carcinoma and correlated to hypoxia-inducible factor (HIF)-1α expression. Pathol Oncol Res 2009; 15(3): 487-93.
[http://dx.doi.org/10.1007/s12253-008-9143-8] [PMID: 19130303]

[158] Chen Y, Li X, Wu X, *et al*. Autophagy-related proteins LC3 and Beclin-1 impact the efficacy of chemoradiation on esophageal squamous cell carcinoma. Pathol Res Pract 2013; 209(9): 562-7.
[http://dx.doi.org/10.1016/j.prp.2013.06.006] [PMID: 23880165]

[159] Yoshioka A, Miyata H, Doki Y, *et al*. LC3, an autophagosome marker, is highly expressed in gastrointestinal cancers. Int J Oncol 2008; 33(3): 461-8.
[PMID: 18695874]

[160] Wang ZB, Peng XZ, Chen SS, *et al*. High p53 and MAP1 light chain 3A co-expression predicts poor prognosis in patients with esophageal squamous cell carcinoma. Mol Med Rep 2013; 8(1): 41-6.
[http://dx.doi.org/10.3892/mmr.2013.1451] [PMID: 23632916]

[161] Sakurai T, Okumura H, Matsumoto M, *et al*. The expression of LC-3 is related to tumor suppression through angiogenesis in esophageal cancer. Med Oncol 2013; 30(4): 701.
[http://dx.doi.org/10.1007/s12032-013-0701-x] [PMID: 24122254]

[162] Hao C-L, Li Y, Yang H-X, *et al*. High level of microtubule-associated protein light chain 3 predicts poor prognosis in resectable esophageal squamous cell carcinoma. Int J Clin Exp Pathol 2014; 7(7): 4213-21.

[PMID: 25120801]

[163] Chen H-I, Tsai H-P, Chen Y-T, Tsao S-C, Chai C-Y. Autophagy and apoptosis play opposing roles in overall survival of esophageal squamous cell carcinoma. Pathol Oncol Res 2016; 22(4): 699-705. [http://dx.doi.org/10.1007/s12253-016-0051-z] [PMID: 26980476]

[164] Zheng T, Li D, Zhang K, Guo H, Cui G, Zhao S. Prognostic value of autophagy marker LC3 in esophageal cancer: A meta-analysis. Int J Clin Exp Med 2016; 9(11): 21535-41.

[165] Brahimi-Horn MC, Chiche J, Pouysségur J. Hypoxia and cancer. J Mol Med (Berl) 2007; 85(12): 1301-7. [http://dx.doi.org/10.1007/s00109-007-0281-3] [PMID: 18026916]

[166] Whelan KA, Chandramouleeswaran PM, Tanaka K, *et al.* Autophagy supports generation of cells with high CD44 expression via modulation of oxidative stress and Parkin-mediated mitochondrial clearance. Oncogene 2017; 36(34): 4843-58. [http://dx.doi.org/10.1038/onc.2017.102] [PMID: 28414310]

[167] Liu D, Yang Y, Liu Q, Wang J. Inhibition of autophagy by 3-MA potentiates cisplatin-induced apoptosis in esophageal squamous cell carcinoma cells. Med Oncol 2011; 28(1): 105-11. [http://dx.doi.org/10.1007/s12032-009-9397-3] [PMID: 20041317]

[168] Tang Q, Li G, Wei X, *et al.* Resveratrol-induced apoptosis is enhanced by inhibition of autophagy in esophageal squamous cell carcinoma. Cancer Lett 2013; 336(2): 325-37. [http://dx.doi.org/10.1016/j.canlet.2013.03.023] [PMID: 23541682]

[169] Zhu L, Du H, Shi M, Chen Z, Hang J. ATG7 deficiency promote apoptotic death induced by cisplatin in human esophageal squamous cell carcinoma cells. Bull Cancer 2013; 100(7-8): 15-21. [PMID: 23823853]

[170] Yu L, Gu C, Zhong D, *et al.* Induction of autophagy counteracts the anticancer effect of cisplatin in human esophageal cancer cells with acquired drug resistance. Cancer Lett 2014; 355(1): 34-45. [http://dx.doi.org/10.1016/j.canlet.2014.09.020] [PMID: 25236911]

[171] Yang Y, Wen F, Dang L, *et al.* Insulin enhances apoptosis induced by cisplatin in human esophageal squamous cell carcinoma EC9706 cells related to inhibition of autophagy. Chin Med J (Engl) 2014; 127(2): 353-8. [PMID: 24438628]

[172] Chen Y, Li X, Guo L, *et al.* Combining radiation with autophagy inhibition enhances suppression of tumor growth and angiogenesis in esophageal cancer. Mol Med Rep 2015; 12(2): 1645-52. [http://dx.doi.org/10.3892/mmr.2015.3623] [PMID: 25891159]

[173] Zheng K, Li Y, Wang S, *et al.* Inhibition of autophagosome-lysosome fusion by ginsenoside Ro via the ESR2-NCF1-ROS pathway sensitizes esophageal cancer cells to 5-fluorouracil-induced cell death via the CHEK1-mediated DNA damage checkpoint. Autophagy 2016; 12(9): 1593-613. [http://dx.doi.org/10.1080/15548627.2016.1192751] [PMID: 27310928]

[174] Zhu X, Pan Q, Huang N, *et al.* RAD51 regulates CHK1 stability via autophagy to promote cell growth in esophageal squamous carcinoma cells. Tumour Biol 2016; 37(12): 16151-61. [http://dx.doi.org/10.1007/s13277-016-5455-6] [PMID: 27743378]

[175] Liao C, Zheng K, Li Y, *et al.* Gypenoside L inhibits autophagic flux and induces cell death in human esophageal cancer cells through endoplasm reticulum stress-mediated Ca^{2+} release. Oncotarget 2016; 7(30): 47387-402. [http://dx.doi.org/10.18632/oncotarget.10159] [PMID: 27329722]

[176] Lu C, Xie C. Radiation-induced autophagy promotes esophageal squamous cell carcinoma cell survival via the LKB1 pathway. Oncol Rep 2016; 35(6): 3559-65. [http://dx.doi.org/10.3892/or.2016.4753] [PMID: 27109915]

[177] Regala RP, Weems C, Jamieson L, *et al.* Atypical protein kinase Cι is an oncogene in human non-small cell lung cancer. Cancer Res 2005; 65(19): 8905-11.

[http://dx.doi.org/10.1158/0008-5472.CAN-05-2372] [PMID: 16204062]

[178] Eder AM, Sui X, Rosen DG, *et al.* Atypical PKCiota contributes to poor prognosis through loss of apical-basal polarity and cyclin E overexpression in ovarian cancer. Proc Natl Acad Sci USA 2005; 102(35): 12519-24.
[http://dx.doi.org/10.1073/pnas.0505641102] [PMID: 16116079]

[179] Takagawa R, Akimoto K, Ichikawa Y, *et al.* High expression of atypical protein kinase C λ/ι in gastric cancer as a prognostic factor for recurrence. Ann Surg Oncol 2010; 17(1): 81-8.
[http://dx.doi.org/10.1245/s10434-009-0708-x] [PMID: 19774416]

[180] Yang YL, Chu JY, Luo ML, *et al.* Amplification of PRKCI, located in 3q26, is associated with lymph node metastasis in esophageal squamous cell carcinoma. Genes Chromosomes Cancer 2008; 47(2): 127-36.
[http://dx.doi.org/10.1002/gcc.20514] [PMID: 17990328]

[181] Liu S-G, Wang B-S, Jiang Y-Y, *et al.* Atypical protein kinase Cι (PKCι) promotes metastasis of esophageal squamous cell carcinoma by enhancing resistance to Anoikis via PKCι-SKP2-AKT pathway. Mol Cancer Res 2011; 9(4): 390-402.
[http://dx.doi.org/10.1158/1541-7786.MCR-10-0359] [PMID: 21310827]

[182] Jia HY, Wang HN, Xia FY, *et al.* Dichloroacetate induces protective autophagy in esophageal squamous carcinoma cells. Oncol Lett 2017; 14(3): 2765-70.
[http://dx.doi.org/10.3892/ol.2017.6562] [PMID: 28928817]

[183] Wu WK, Sakamoto KM, Milani M, *et al.* Macroautophagy modulates cellular response to proteasome inhibitors in cancer therapy. Drug Resist Updat 2010; 13(3): 87-92.
[http://dx.doi.org/10.1016/j.drup.2010.04.003] [PMID: 20462785]

[184] Wojcik S. Crosstalk between autophagy and proteasome protein degradation systems: Possible implications for cancer therapy. Folia Histochem Cytobiol 2013; 51(4): 249-64.
[http://dx.doi.org/10.5603/FHC.2013.0036] [PMID: 24497130]

[185] Liu D, Gao M, Yang Y, Qi YU, Wu K, Zhao S. Inhibition of autophagy promotes cell apoptosis induced by the proteasome inhibitor MG-132 in human esophageal squamous cell carcinoma EC9706 cells. Oncol Lett 2015; 9(5): 2278-82.
[http://dx.doi.org/10.3892/ol.2015.3047] [PMID: 26137056]

[186] Wang BS, Yang Y, Lu HZ, *et al.* Inhibition of atypical protein kinase Cι induces apoptosis through autophagic degradation of β-catenin in esophageal cancer cells. Mol Carcinog 2014; 53(7): 514-25.
[http://dx.doi.org/10.1002/mc.22003] [PMID: 23359356]

[187] Du X-X, Li Y-J, Wu C-L, *et al.* Initiation of apoptosis, cell cycle arrest and autophagy of esophageal cancer cells by dihydroartemisinin. Biomed Pharmacother 2013; 67(5): 417-24.
[http://dx.doi.org/10.1016/j.biopha.2013.01.013] [PMID: 23582790]

[188] Wang Y-Y, Yang Y-X, Zhao R, *et al.* Bardoxolone methyl induces apoptosis and autophagy and inhibits epithelial-to-mesenchymal transition and stemness in esophageal squamous cancer cells. Drug Des Devel Ther 2015; 9: 993-1026.
[PMID: 25733817]

[189] Wang Y-Y, Zhou S, Zhao R, Hai P, Zhe H. The therapeutic response of CDDO-Me in the esophageal squamous cell carcinoma (ESCC) cells is mediated by CaMKIIα. Am J Transl Res 2016; 8(4): 1695-707.
[PMID: 27186293]

[190] Maiuri MC, Le Toumelin G, Criollo A, *et al.* Functional and physical interaction between Bcl-X(L) and a BH3-like domain in Beclin-1. EMBO J 2007; 26(10): 2527-39.
[http://dx.doi.org/10.1038/sj.emboj.7601689] [PMID: 17446862]

[191] Lamparska-Przybysz M, Gajkowska B, Motyl T. Cathepsins and BID are involved in the molecular switch between apoptosis and autophagy in breast cancer MCF-7 cells exposed to camptothecin. J

Physiol Pharmacol 2005; 56 (Suppl. 3): 159-79.
[PMID: 16077201]

[192] Hamacher-Brady A, Brady NR, Logue SE, *et al.* Response to myocardial ischemia/reperfusion injury involves Bnip3 and autophagy. Cell Death Differ 2007; 14(1): 146-57.
[http://dx.doi.org/10.1038/sj.cdd.4401936] [PMID: 16645637]

[193] Han B, Li W, Sun Y, Zhou L, Xu Y, Zhao X. A prolyl-hydroxylase inhibitor, ethyl-3,--dihydroxybenzoate, induces cell autophagy and apoptosis in esophageal squamous cell carcinoma cells via up-regulation of BNIP3 and N-myc downstream-regulated gene-1. PLoS One 2014; 9(9): e107204.
[http://dx.doi.org/10.1371/journal.pone.0107204] [PMID: 25232961]

[194] Li W, Hou G, Zhou D, *et al.* The roles of AKR1C1 and AKR1C2 in ethyl-3,4-dihydroxybenzoate induced esophageal squamous cell carcinoma cell death. Oncotarget 2016; 7(16): 21542-55.
[http://dx.doi.org/10.18632/oncotarget.7775] [PMID: 26934124]

[195] Ploner C, Kofler R, Villunger A. Noxa: At the tip of the balance between life and death. Oncogene 2008; 27 (Suppl. 1): S84-92.
[http://dx.doi.org/10.1038/onc.2009.46] [PMID: 19641509]

[196] Lin QH, Que FC, Gu CP, Zhong DS, Zhou D, Kong Y, *et al.* ABT-263 induces G 1/G 0-phase arrest, apoptosis and autophagy in human esophageal cancer cells *in vitro.* Acta Pharmacol Sin 2017; aps201778.

[197] Pan J, Cheng C, Verstovsek S, Chen Q, Jin Y, Cao Q. The BH3-mimetic GX15-070 induces autophagy, potentiates the cytotoxicity of carboplatin and 5-fluorouracil in esophageal carcinoma cells. Cancer Lett 2010; 293(2): 167-74.
[http://dx.doi.org/10.1016/j.canlet.2010.01.006] [PMID: 20153924]

[198] Yu L, Wu WK, Gu C, *et al.* Obatoclax impairs lysosomal function to block autophagy in cisplatin-sensitive and -resistant esophageal cancer cells. Oncotarget 2016; 7(12): 14693-707.
[http://dx.doi.org/10.18632/oncotarget.7492] [PMID: 26910910]

[199] Fuggetta MP, D'Atri S, Lanzilli G, *et al. In vitro* antitumour activity of resveratrol in human melanoma cells sensitive or resistant to temozolomide. Melanoma Res 2004; 14(3): 189-96.
[http://dx.doi.org/10.1097/01.cmr.0000130007.54508.b2] [PMID: 15179187]

[200] Osman A-MM, Bayoumi HM, Al-Harthi SE, Damanhouri ZA, Elshal MF. Modulation of doxorubicin cytotoxicity by resveratrol in a human breast cancer cell line. Cancer Cell Int 2012; 12(1): 47.
[http://dx.doi.org/10.1186/1475-2867-12-47] [PMID: 23153194]

[201] Delmas D, Rébé C, Lacour S, *et al.* Resveratrol-induced apoptosis is associated with Fas redistribution in the rafts and the formation of a death-inducing signaling complex in colon cancer cells. J Biol Chem 2003; 278(42): 41482-90.
[http://dx.doi.org/10.1074/jbc.M304896200] [PMID: 12902349]

[202] Shi WF, Leong M, Cho E, *et al.* Repressive effects of resveratrol on androgen receptor transcriptional activity. PLoS One 2009; 4(10): e7398.
[http://dx.doi.org/10.1371/journal.pone.0007398] [PMID: 19816598]

[203] Cheson B. Resveratrol and cancer prevention. Clin Adv Hematol Oncol: H&O 2009; 7(3): 142.

[204] Bishayee A. Cancer prevention and treatment with resveratrol: From rodent studies to clinical trials. Cancer Prev Res (Phila) 2009; 2(5): 409-18.
[http://dx.doi.org/10.1158/1940-6207.CAPR-08-0160] [PMID: 19401532]

[205] Pozo-Guisado E, Merino JM, Mulero-Navarro S, *et al.* Resveratrol-induced apoptosis in MCF-7 human breast cancer cells involves a caspase-independent mechanism with downregulation of Bcl-2 and NF-kappaB. Int J Cancer 2005; 115(1): 74-84.
[http://dx.doi.org/10.1002/ijc.20856] [PMID: 15688415]

[206] Scarlatti F, Maffei R, Beau I, Codogno P, Ghidoni R. Role of non-canonical Beclin 1-independent

autophagy in cell death induced by resveratrol in human breast cancer cells. Cell Death Differ 2008; 15(8): 1318-29.
[http://dx.doi.org/10.1038/cdd.2008.51] [PMID: 18421301]

[207] Hsu K-F, Wu C-L, Huang S-C, *et al.* Cathepsin L mediates resveratrol-induced autophagy and apoptotic cell death in cervical cancer cells. Autophagy 2009; 5(4): 451-60.
[http://dx.doi.org/10.4161/auto.5.4.7666] [PMID: 19164894]

[208] Estrov Z, Shishodia S, Faderl S, *et al.* Resveratrol blocks interleukin-1β-induced activation of the nuclear transcription factor NF-kappaB, inhibits proliferation, causes S-phase arrest, and induces apoptosis of acute myeloid leukemia cells. Blood 2003; 102(3): 987-95.
[http://dx.doi.org/10.1182/blood-2002-11-3550] [PMID: 12689943]

[209] Li J, Qin Z, Liang Z. The prosurvival role of autophagy in Resveratrol-induced cytotoxicity in human U251 glioma cells. BMC Cancer 2009; 9(1): 215.
[http://dx.doi.org/10.1186/1471-2407-9-215] [PMID: 19566920]

[210] Cho S-H, Chung I-J, Song S-Y, *et al.* Bi-weekly chemotherapy of paclitaxel and cisplatin in patients with metastatic or recurrent esophageal cancer. J Korean Med Sci 2005; 20(4): 618-23.
[http://dx.doi.org/10.3346/jkms.2005.20.4.618] [PMID: 16100454]

[211] Conroy T, Etienne P-L, Adenis A, *et al.* Vinorelbine and cisplatin in metastatic squamous cell carcinoma of the oesophagus: Response, toxicity, quality of life and survival. Ann Oncol 2002; 13(5): 721-9.
[http://dx.doi.org/10.1093/annonc/mdf063] [PMID: 12075740]

[212] Li ZG, Hong T, Shimada Y, *et al.* Suppression of N-nitrosomethylbenzylamine (NMBA)-induced esophageal tumorigenesis in F344 rats by resveratrol. Carcinogenesis 2002; 23(9): 1531-6.
[http://dx.doi.org/10.1093/carcin/23.9.1531] [PMID: 12189197]

[213] Zhou H-B, Yan Y, Sun Y-N, Zhu J-R. Resveratrol induces apoptosis in human esophageal carcinoma cells. World J Gastroenterol 2003; 9(3): 408-11.
[http://dx.doi.org/10.3748/wjg.v9.i3.408] [PMID: 12632486]

[214] Fan Y, Chiu JF, Liu J, *et al.* Resveratrol induces autophagy-dependent apoptosis in HL-60 cells. BMC Cancer 2018; 18(1): 581.
[http://dx.doi.org/10.1186/s12885-018-4504-5] [PMID: 29788929]

[215] Pollak MN. Investigating metformin for cancer prevention and treatment: The end of the beginning. Cancer Discov 2012; 2(9): 778-90.
[http://dx.doi.org/10.1158/2159-8290.CD-12-0263] [PMID: 22926251]

[216] Taubes G. Cancer research. Cancer prevention with a diabetes pill? Science 2012; 335(6064): 29.
[http://dx.doi.org/10.1126/science.335.6064.29] [PMID: 22223788]

[217] Goodwin PJ, Stambolic V, Lemieux J, *et al.* Evaluation of metformin in early breast cancer: A modification of the traditional paradigm for clinical testing of anti-cancer agents. Breast Cancer Res Treat 2011; 126(1): 215-20.
[http://dx.doi.org/10.1007/s10549-010-1224-1] [PMID: 20976543]

[218] Hadad S, Iwamoto T, Jordan L, *et al.* Evidence for biological effects of metformin in operable breast cancer: A pre-operative, window-of-opportunity, randomized trial. Breast Cancer Res Treat 2011; 128(3): 783-94.
[http://dx.doi.org/10.1007/s10549-011-1612-1] [PMID: 21655990]

[219] Feng Y, Ke C, Tang Q, *et al.* Metformin promotes autophagy and apoptosis in esophageal squamous cell carcinoma by downregulating Stat3 signaling. Cell Death Dis 2014; 5(2): e1088.
[http://dx.doi.org/10.1038/cddis.2014.59] [PMID: 24577086]

[220] Tomic T, Botton T, Cerezo M, *et al.* Metformin inhibits melanoma development through autophagy and apoptosis mechanisms. Cell Death Dis 2011; 2(9): e199.
[http://dx.doi.org/10.1038/cddis.2011.86] [PMID: 21881601]

[221] Shi WY, Xiao D, Wang L, *et al.* Therapeutic metformin/AMPK activation blocked lymphoma cell growth via inhibition of mTOR pathway and induction of autophagy. Cell Death Dis 2012; 3(3): e275. [http://dx.doi.org/10.1038/cddis.2012.13] [PMID: 22378068]

[222] Ben Sahra I, Laurent K, Giuliano S, *et al.* Targeting cancer cell metabolism: The combination of metformin and 2-deoxyglucose induces p53-dependent apoptosis in prostate cancer cells. Cancer Res 2010; 70(6): 2465-75. [http://dx.doi.org/10.1158/0008-5472.CAN-09-2782] [PMID: 20215500]

[223] Song H, Pan B, Yi J, Chen L. Featured article: Autophagic activation with nimotuzumab enhanced chemosensitivity and radiosensitivity of esophageal squamous cell carcinoma. Exp Biol Med (Maywood) 2014; 239(5): 529-41. [http://dx.doi.org/10.1177/1535370214525315] [PMID: 24625442]

[224] Wolmarans E, Mqoco TV, Stander A, *et al.* Novel estradiol analogue induces apoptosis and autophagy in esophageal carcinoma cells. Cell Mol Biol Lett 2014; 19(1): 98-115. [http://dx.doi.org/10.2478/s11658-014-0183-7] [PMID: 24563014]

[225] Chen Y, Fu LL, Wen X, *et al.* Oncogenic and tumor suppressive roles of microRNAs in apoptosis and autophagy. Apoptosis 2014; 19(8): 1177-89. [http://dx.doi.org/10.1007/s10495-014-0999-7] [PMID: 24850099]

[226] Frankel LB, Lund AH. MicroRNA regulation of autophagy. Carcinogenesis 2012; 33(11): 2018-25. [http://dx.doi.org/10.1093/carcin/bgs266] [PMID: 22902544]

[227] Fu LL, Wen X, Bao JK, Liu B. MicroRNA-modulated autophagic signaling networks in cancer. Int J Biochem Cell Biol 2012; 44(5): 733-6. [http://dx.doi.org/10.1016/j.biocel.2012.02.004] [PMID: 22342941]

[228] Zhai H, Fesler A, Ju J. MicroRNA: A third dimension in autophagy. Cell Cycle 2013; 12(2): 246-50. [http://dx.doi.org/10.4161/cc.23273] [PMID: 23255136]

[229] Jing Z, Han W, Sui X, Xie J, Pan H. Interaction of autophagy with microRNAs and their potential therapeutic implications in human cancers. Cancer Lett 2015; 356(2 Pt B): 332-8. [http://dx.doi.org/10.1016/j.canlet.2014.09.039] [PMID: 25304373]

[230] Zhu H, Wu H, Liu X, *et al.* Regulation of autophagy by a beclin 1-targeted microRNA, miR-30a, in cancer cells. Autophagy 2009; 5(6): 816-23. [http://dx.doi.org/10.4161/auto.9064] [PMID: 19535919]

[231] Tang B, Li N, Gu J, *et al.* Compromised autophagy by MIR30B benefits the intracellular survival of Helicobacter pylori. Autophagy 2012; 8(7): 1045-57. [http://dx.doi.org/10.4161/auto.20159] [PMID: 22647547]

[232] Korkmaz G, le Sage C, Tekirdag KA, Agami R, Gozuacik D. miR-376b controls starvation and mTOR inhibition-related autophagy by targeting ATG4C and BECN1. Autophagy 2012; 8(2): 165-76. [http://dx.doi.org/10.4161/auto.8.2.18351] [PMID: 22248718]

[233] Frankel LB, Wen J, Lees M, *et al.* microRNA-101 is a potent inhibitor of autophagy. EMBO J 2011; 30(22): 4628-41. [http://dx.doi.org/10.1038/emboj.2011.331] [PMID: 21915098]

[234] Chang Y, Yan W, He X, Zhang L, Li C, Huang H, *et al.* miR-375 inhibits autophagy and reduces viability of hepatocellular carcinoma cells under hypoxic conditions. Gastroenterology 2012; 143(1): 177-87.

[235] Mikhaylova O, Stratton Y, Hall D, *et al.* VHL-regulated MiR-204 suppresses tumor growth through inhibition of LC3B-mediated autophagy in renal clear cell carcinoma. Cancer Cell 2012; 21(4): 532-46. [http://dx.doi.org/10.1016/j.ccr.2012.02.019] [PMID: 22516261]

[236] Lu C, Chen J, Xu HG, *et al.* MIR106B and MIR93 prevent removal of bacteria from epithelial cells by

disrupting ATG16L1-mediated autophagy. Gastroenterology 2014; 146(1): 188-99.
[http://dx.doi.org/10.1053/j.gastro.2013.09.006] [PMID: 24036151]

[237]   Zhai Z, Wu F, Dong F, *et al.* Human autophagy gene ATG16L1 is post-transcriptionally regulated by MIR142-3p. Autophagy 2014; 10(3): 468-79.
[http://dx.doi.org/10.4161/auto.27553] [PMID: 24401604]

[238]   Wan G, Xie W, Liu Z, *et al.* Hypoxia-induced MIR155 is a potent autophagy inducer by targeting multiple players in the mTOR pathway. Autophagy 2014; 10(1): 70-9.
[http://dx.doi.org/10.4161/auto.26534] [PMID: 24262949]

[239]   Nyhan MJ, O'Donovan TR, Boersma AW, Wiemer EA, McKenna SL. MiR-193b promotes autophagy and non-apoptotic cell death in oesophageal cancer cells. BMC Cancer 2016; 16(1): 101.
[http://dx.doi.org/10.1186/s12885-016-2123-6] [PMID: 26878873]

[240]   Cui L, Song Z, Liang B, Jia L, Ma S, Liu X. Radiation induces autophagic cell death via the p53/DRAM signaling pathway in breast cancer cells. Oncol Rep 2016; 35(6): 3639-47.
[http://dx.doi.org/10.3892/or.2016.4752] [PMID: 27109777]

[241]   Pang X-L, He G, Liu Y-B, Wang Y, Zhang B. Endoplasmic reticulum stress sensitizes human esophageal cancer cell to radiation. World J Gastroenterol 2013; 19(11): 1736-48.
[http://dx.doi.org/10.3748/wjg.v19.i11.1736] [PMID: 23555162]

[242]   Zhou F, Li Y-H, Wang J-J, Pan J, Lu H. Endoplasmic reticulum stress could induce autophagy and apoptosis and enhance chemotherapy sensitivity in human esophageal cancer EC9706 cells by mediating PI3K/Akt/mTOR signaling pathway. Tumour Biol 2017; 39(6): 1010428317705748.
[http://dx.doi.org/10.1177/1010428317705748] [PMID: 28631572]

[243]   Liu WY, Wu XU, Liao CQ, Shen J, Li J. Apoptotic effect of gambogic acid in esophageal squamous cell carcinoma cells via suppression of the NF-κB pathway. Oncol Lett 2016; 11(6): 3681-5.
[http://dx.doi.org/10.3892/ol.2016.4437] [PMID: 27284372]

[244]   Yang Y, Sun X, Yang Y, *et al.* Gambogic acid enhances the radiosensitivity of human esophageal cancer cells by inducing reactive oxygen species via targeting Akt/mTOR pathway. Tumour Biol 2016; 37(2): 1853-62.
[http://dx.doi.org/10.1007/s13277-015-3974-1] [PMID: 26318432]

[245]   He Q, Li J, Dong F, Cai C, Zou X. LKB1 promotes radioresistance in esophageal cancer cells exposed to radiation, by suppression of apoptosis and activation of autophagy via the AMPK pathway. Mol Med Rep 2017; 16(2): 2205-10.
[http://dx.doi.org/10.3892/mmr.2017.6852] [PMID: 28656285]

CHAPTER 5

Recent Patents on Smart Nano-Formulations for Cancer Therapy

Shaheen Sultana*, **Mohammad Yusuf** and **Maria Khan**

Assistant Professor, Department of Pharmaceutics, College of Pharmacy, Taif University, P.O. Box 888, Hawiyah, Taif, Zip Code 21974, Kingdom of Saudi Arabia

Abstract: Treatment of cancer using nanoparticle-based approaches being explored extensively to overcome the drawbacks associated with conventional treatment. Progress in nanotechnology for cancer therapy has led to the development of smart nanoformulations which improve the intracellular delivery of drugs due to their augmented multi-functionality and targeting potential. Smart nanoformulations are nano range particles which release the drug in accordance with the biological stimuli pre-existing at the disease site. This chapter summarizes most of the recent patents related to smart nanopreparations for cancer therapy. Such a smart system has shown to enhance the therapeutic effect of current standard treatment modalities such as chemotherapies and radiotherapies. Several polymeric nanoparticles were patented that destroy tumors by thermal energy deposition and thus enhanced tumor therapy. Patented thermoresponsive solid lipid nanoformulations which act as smart drug delivery systems showed temperature sensitivity (39°C-45°C) and release payload at target sites of cancerous cells. The pH-sensitive polymeric drug delivery system containing adornment acidic or basic groups to accept or donate protons in response to environmental pH showed accelerated drug release at the tumor site. A novel liposome linked thermosensitive peptide was invented which showed temperature dependent peptide shrinkage and drug release. Likewise, due to unique properties of metallic nanoparticles in imaging and diagnostic field, they are gaining interest widely as stimuli-sensitive drug delivery system. Gold nanoparticles can absorb light strongly and convert photon energy into heat quickly and efficiently escalating the temperature of a tumor cell (41°C-47°C) and thus destroying cancerous cells specifically. Coupling metallic nanoparticle properties with pH-sensitive targeting, resulted in an enhanced anti-tumor effect as observed in recently granted patents.

Keywords: Cancer, carbon nanotubes, controlled release, dendrimers, gold nanoparticles, hydrogels, ligand, liposomes, magnetic nanoparticles, metallic nanoparticles, micelles, nanoformulation, nanotechnology, pH-sensitive targeting, polymeric nanoparticles, smart nanoformulation, solid lipid nanoparticles,

* **Corresponding author Shaheen Sultana:** Assistant Professor, Department of Pharmaceutics, College of Pharmacy, Taif University, P.O. Box 888, Hawiyah, Taif, Zip Code 21974, Kingdom of Saudi Arabia; Tel: +966544122485; E-mail: shaheen634@yahoo.co.uk

Atta-ur-Rahman and Khurshid Zaman (Eds.)

stimuli-sensitive, thermosensitive nanoparticles, virus-based nanoparticles.

1. INTRODUCTION

The development of cancer nanoformulations has attracted great interest in the recent decade due to their targeting potential and selective killing of cancer cells while leaving healthy cells unscathed. Nanoformulations are man-made formulations where particle size varies preferably in the range of 5-200nm size range. Nanoformulations have affectively led to a significant reduction in toxicity and an increased efficacy due to the enhanced permeation and retention (EPR) effect [1]. Nanoparticles created for cancer treatment are synthesized from various materials, including polymers (e.g., polymeric nanoparticles, micelles, vesicles, or dendrimers), lipids (liposomes, lipid nanoparticles), viruses (viral nanoparticles) and certain metals [2, 3]. Such formulations are characterized by unique physical, optical and electronic properties that are attractive for specific targeting and treatment opportunities in cancer therapy. In the past few years, smart nano-formulations have been extensively developed for cancer treatment, which improves the distribution of the chemotherapeutic agent by adapting to chemo-physical properties in accordance with the biological stimuli pre-existing at the tumor site [4]. To be a smart drug delivery system, it should have the targeting ability and release the drug only in the specific tumor environment. Such system identifies target and kills just the cancer cells leaving the healthy cells intact. In this chapter, we will focus on the recent progress in the development of smart nanoparticles as drug delivery systems with advanced properties and high sensitivity to tumor microenvironments for improved cancer treatment.

1.1. Polymer-Based Nano-Formulations

In the last decades, polymers having been widely used as biomaterials for smart drug delivery due to their favorable properties such as biocompatibility, tunable size and shape, enhance permeation, flexibility, solubility and targeting potential, specific activity at a predetermined rate and time and interesting bio-mimetic character [5]. With modification in polymeric science smart nano-preparations can be formulated. Recently, modifications in the polymeric system to achieve nanometer structures have been instituted as a strong strategy for the development of smart drug delivery system. Such modified systems can achieve desired qualities such as pre-scheduled rate, self-controlled, targeting, predetermined release time and ease of monitoring [6, 7]. The smart drug delivery system has shown to enhance the therapy regimen for cancer targeting.

1.1.1. Polymeric Nanoparticles

Polymeric nanoparticles are nanometer size range particles made up of polymers which are exploited as a carrier of therapeutic agents for invasive and non-invasive routes of delivery [8]. Such systems are designed to respond to a variety of different internal stimuli that characterize diseased tissues such as pH, reductive environment, temperature, and enzyme concentration to maximize drug delivery at the target site [9]. These nanoparticles undergo physiochemical structural changes when exposed to these stimuli and thus lose their well-defined nanoarchitecture and release the drugs directly into tumor cells [10]. Polymers used to prepare such formulations hold at least one moiety from acrylamide, acrylate, acrylic acid and other moiety from cellulose derivatives, poly(vinyl alcohol), polystyrene, polypropylene, polycaprolactone, poly(lactic acid-co-glycolic acid), polyanhydride etc. [11].

Targeting ligands for specific delivery may be incorporated in polymeric nanoparticles to target them to a specific type of cell or an intracellular region, or to specific organ/tissues. A combination of targeted delivery through ligands, imaging and therapeutics is shown in Fig. (**1**) [12]. By binding a ligand to polymeric nanoparticles, it is possible to deliver site-specific delivery and develop a more favorable therapeutic regime. Recently, Mn^{2+}-coordinated doxorubicin (DOX)-loaded polylactic-co-glycolic acid (PLGA) nanoparticles were synthesized that directly destroy tumors in a mouse model, by thermal energy deposition, and also enhance tumor therapy [13]. Resistance to chemotherapeutic drugs is a major challenge to a successful chemotherapeutic regimen acquired through a variety of mechanisms such as tumor genetic alteration, epigenetic changes, changes in the microenvironment of tumor cells, modification of the drug's cellular target, or blocking the drug's entry into the tumor cell [14, 15]. One such polymeric nanoparticle with a hydrophobic core that encapsulates curcumin and a hydrophilic shell with one or more chemotherapeutic agents (e.g., doxorubicin) associated with the shell surface is formed from N-isopropylacryl Amide (NIPAAM), Acrylic Acid (AA), and at least one vinyl monomer which effectively overcome multidrug resistance and ameliorate cardiomyopathy [16]. In one invention, PLGA nanoparticle was formulated with a nucleophilic ligand (antibody, receptor proteins, localization sequences, organic molecules) attached through the grafting of polyethylene glycol to the exterior surface of a biodegradable nanoshell. The designed formulation showed quick internalization and eradication of prostate tumors in mice without toxicity [17]. A stimulus-responsive phosphorescent hybrid system was developed comprising light-emitting transition metal complex in a wide variety of hydrogels and polymers for biological labeling, imaging, and optical sensing [18]. Winchurch and Yeoman, 2014, disclosed the chemical conjugation of polysaccharides and poloxamers to nanoparticles for controlled therapeutic drug delivery, imaging, and theragnostic applications [19]. A dual block copolymer (PCL-PEGSeSe-PCL) in response to selenium-containing double, in the aqueous solution assembled into polymeric nanoparticles, which in the oxidizing or reducing conditions, leads to diselenide bond breakage and release of drugs. *In vivo* study reveals that the polymeric system can be efficiently endocytosed into the HeLa cells, and effectively release the drug in the tumor cells loaded with concentrations of Glutathione (GSH) or ROS (reactive oxygen species) [20].

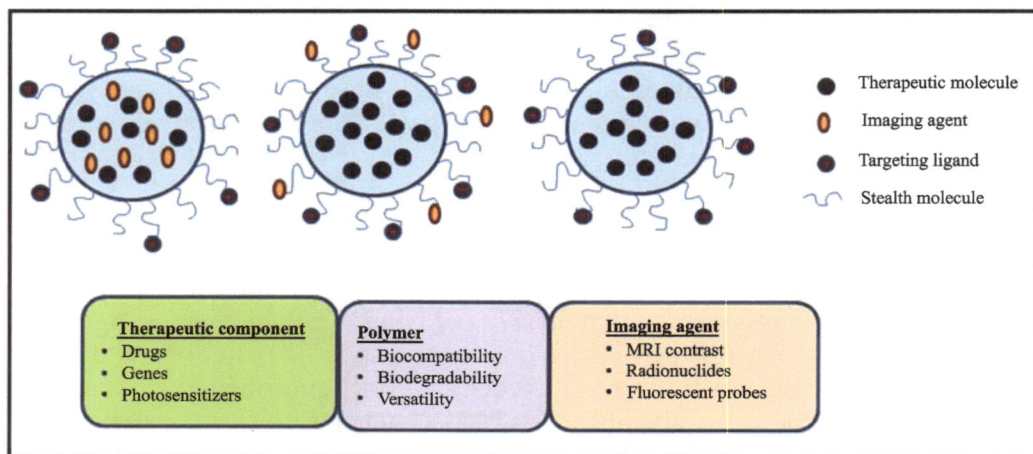

Fig. (1). Polymeric nanoparticles showing multifunctional system [12].

1.1.1.1. pH-Sensitive Polymeric Nanoparticles

pH-Sensitive polymeric nanoparticles respond to acidic pH in the tumor microenvironment (pH 6.5-7.2) to achieve accelerated drug release at the tumor site (Fig. **2**). The pH-responsive nanoparticles can be accumulated in a tumor acidic environment via the Enhanced Permeability and Retention (EPR) effect by means of surface charge conversion (from negative charge trending to neutral charge) and thus enhance the interaction with the cancer cells and permeation into a deep area of the tumor tissues [21]. Researchers developed pH-sensitive polymeric nanoparticles with gold (I) compound payloads which can synergistically induce cancer cell death through regulation of autophagy [22]. Recently, PEG-DOX-Cur prodrug nanoparticle approach has been developed through Schiff base reaction for simultaneous delivery of doxorubicin (DOX) and curcumin (Cur) into the nuclei and cytoplasma of the tumor cells resulting in enhanced tumor penetration [23]. The pH-sensitive polymers must contain adornment acidic or basic groups to accept or donate protons in response to environmental pH to achieve accelerated drug release at the tumor site.

Polymethacrylic Acid (PMAA), poly (ethylene amine), poly (L-lysine), Polymethacrylic Acid (PMAA), poly (ethylene amine), poly(L-lysine), chitosan and eudragit are the various pH sensitive polymers [11, 24]. In one patent, pH-sensitive peptide-based nanoparticles were constructed using pH-sensitive hydrophilic and hydrophobic amino acids in the backbone. As the pH of the environment changes from physiological pH level to a weakly acidic environment as found near a tumor site (pH~6.5-6.9), the peptides start to dissolve, releasing the biological substance [25]. A pH-responsive nanoparticle made of a pH-responsive polymer and a poly(lactic-co-glycolic acid) is formed by the self-assembly of polyethylene glycol derivative and an R-Histidine derivative. A surface zeta potential of the pH-responsive nanoparticle is converted from negative charge to positive charge depending upon an external environment [26]. Similar features of nanoparticles are also explored by researchers where the degradation and release are favored at low temperature and/or ROS (Reactive Oxygen Species) [27]. Recent patents on smart polymeric nanoparticles for cancer therapy are shown in Table **1**.

Table 1. Recent Patents on Smart Polymeric Nanoparticles for Cancer Treatment.

Reference	Inventors	Patent Number	Title
[16]	Maitra, A., Pramanik, D.	US20130330412	Smart polymeric nanoparticles which overcome multidrug resistance to cancer therapeutics and treatment-related systemic toxicity
[17]	Arthur, R.C.B., Jamboor, K.V.	EP2146694	Formulation of active agent loaded activated PLGA nanoparticles for targeted cancer nano-therapeutics
[18]	Omary, M.A., Hu, Z., Marpu, S.	US20120065614	Polyionic transitional metal phosphorescent complex/polymer hybrid systems for bioimaging and sensing applications
[19]	Richard A.W., Roy R.Y.	US20140199232	Targeted therapeutic nanoparticles
[20]	Peihong, N., Yue, S., Jinlin, H., Mingzu, Z.	CN107641201	Preparation method of the block copolymer with dual responsiveness of rapid oxidization/reduction and selenium bonds and application of block copolymer
[21]	Almutairi, A., Sankaranarayanan, J., Mahmoud, E., Schopf, E.	US20120070383	Polymeric nano-carriers with a linear dual response mechanism and uses thereof
[22]	Chen, W., Zhou, R.	US20160213790	pH-Sensitive nanoparticles for drug delivery
[23]	Nguyen, K.T., Rahmi, M., Kona, S., Lin, A.	US9216220	Compositions and methods for thermo-sensitive nanoparticles and magnetic nanoparticles

(Table 1) cont.....

Reference	Inventors	Patent Number	Title
[24]	Chopra, S., Karnik, R., Wang, A., Farokhzad, O., Zhang, X.Q.	WO2017062920	Nanoparticles with pH-triggered drug release
[25]	Chen, I.W., Choi, H., Zhou, R.	US9687563	pH-Sensitive peptides and their nanoparticles for drug delivery.
[26]	Chiu, H.C., Chiang, W.H., Hung, C.C., Yu, T.W.	US20160367489	Preparation of pH-responsive nanoparticles and promoted delivery of anticancer drugs into deep tumor tissues and application thereof
[27]	Almutairi, A., Sankaranarayanan, J., Mahmoud, E., Schopf, E.	US20120070383	Polymeric nano-carriers with a linear dual response mechanism and uses thereof
[28]	Nguyen, K.T., Rahimi, M., Kona, S., Lin, A.H.	US9216220	Compositions and methods for thermo-sensitive nanoparticles and magnetic nanoparticles

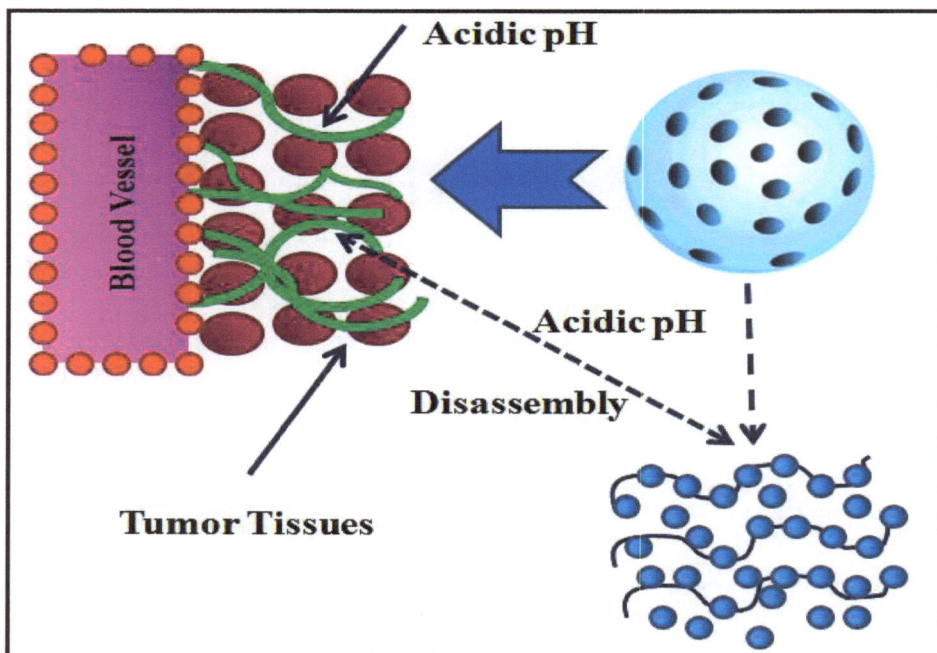

Fig. (2). Schematic representation showing the mechanism of drug release from pH-sensitive polymer.

1.1.1.2. Temperature Responsive Polymeric Nanoparticles

The temperature responsive polymeric nanoparticles comprise of polymers with thermo-responsive blocks which destabilize the particles in response to the change of temperature and undergo a sharp change of their physical properties, facilitating drug release [28, 29]. These polymers like poly (N-isopropylacrylamide), Pluronic F-127 and chitosan undergo a temperature-dependent phase transition known as the Critical Solution Temperature (CST) [30]. Wang and coworkers, covalently interact thermo-sensitive Polymeric Nanoparticles (PNPs) on functionalized Graphene Oxide (GO) nanosheets to create novel GO–PNP hybrids that have selective anti-tumor potential [31]. Recently, an enhanced drug release and cell uptake in tumor microenvironment were predicted with biodegradable, thermo and pH dual responsive oxaliplatin-loaded chitosan-graft-poly-N-isopropylacrylamide (CS-g-PNIPAAm) co-polymeric nanoparticles [32]. Similarly, chitosan-g-poly (N-vinylcaprolactam) nanoparticles showed specific toxicity to cancer cells and increased apoptosis [33].

1.1.2. Hydrogels

Hydrogel nanoparticles, also referred to as polymeric nanogels or macromolecular micelles are nanostructures made of the polymeric network with a three-dimensional configuration that absorb large quantities of water or biological fluids [34]. The system exhibit stimuli-responsive changes in the gel network and hence leading to the controlled drug release at a predetermined site [35]. Hydrogel nanoparticles were prepared by inventors using cross-linked polymer in which drug conjugated to the cross-linked polymer, pH-sensitive moiety and a redox-sensitive moiety that showed the accelerated release of antitumor agent when observed under cancer cell-mimicking conditions [36]. Recently, Gan *et al.* prepared nanogel by cross-linking of thermo-sensitive monomer with controllable radical polymerization. In normal tissues, the nanogel is in a hydrophilic swelling state that is favorable for avoiding being phagocytosed by the Reticuloendothelial System (RES) and thus long circulation capacity; while at the tumor site the state of the nanogel is reversed into a hydrophobic shrinking state and thereby releases the drugs responsively, achieving a good tumor inhibition effect [37]. In one invention nanoparticle-polymer, injectable composite hydrogel with double drug loading system was constructed, which was expected to show better penetration and adsorption of drug into tumor tissues specifically [38]. Recently, a new technology was invented in which Minjinnami cage based hydrogel drug system was synthesized which comprises of light-heat conversion gold cage, smart responsive polymer and an antitumor agent. When the system was irradiated with near-infrared light, the light energy absorbed by the gold cage converted into heat energy that increased the temperature of the system rapidly and thus killed cancer cells selectively. Simultaneously, high temperature accelerates the Brownian motion of drug molecules and ultimately releases it [39]. Recent patents on smart hydrogel-based nano-preparations for cancer therapy are shown in Table **2**.

Table 2. Recent Patents on Smart Hydrogel Based Nano-Formulations for Cancer Treatment.

Reference	Inventors	Patent Number	Title
[36]	Artzi, N., Zhang, Y., Jorge, N.O., Conde, J.	US20170333304	Hydrogel particles, compositions, and methods
[37]	Gan, Y., Wang, Q., Yang, X., Yang, W., Li, F.	CN106810636	Nanogel and nanogel drug carrier system both with smart response to the tumor microenvironment
[38]	Wang, L., Yang, W., Liang, L., Zhou, P.	CN107550921	Nano particle-polymer injectable composite hydrogel double drug loading system and preparation method thereof
[39]	Zhao, Y., Wan, J., Yang, X., Yan, H.	CN106890332	Photo-thermal and chemotherapeutic precise synergic antitumor temperature-sensitive gold nanocage hydrogel drug carrying system

1.1.3. Dendrimers

Dendrimers are highly branched, 3D macromolecules with modifiable surface functionalities and available internal cavities that make them attractive as delivery systems for drug and gene delivery applications. Targeting molecules can be attached that can recognize a cancer cell, distinguishing it from a healthy cell and applied to a variety of cancer therapies to improve the safety and effectiveness of many common therapeutics [36]. A nano-smart drug delivery system was invented in which carrier is connected to a dendrimer molecule ligand to improve the ability to induce differentiation of cancer cells as well as reduce toxicity [37]. A dendrimer conjugate comprising a dendrimer can be associated with an antitumor agent through an aromatic azo linkage that can cleave with a tissue-specific enzyme [38]. Recently, paclitaxel-loaded nano-carrier asymmetric PEGylated dendrimer drug delivery system conjugated with the tumor cell sensitive enzyme GFLG peptide was invented. The nano-conjugate enriched tumor via EPR effect, inhibiting rapid clearance and resulted in enhanced anti-cancer effect [39].

1.1.4. Micelles

Micelles are polymeric self-assemblies which can accommodate various anticancer agents within their core [40]. Polymeric micelles can be modified to confer stimuli-responsiveness and active targeting for cancer drug delivery [41]. An intelligent amphiphilic polymer nano micelle comprising of targeted peptide-polyethylene glycol-B-polyhistidine-B-polycysteine-phenylpropionic acid was synthesized by Lintao *et al.* wherein the innermost layer is a cysteine disulfide crosslinked poly segment; the intermediate layer consists of a pH sensitive polyhistidine segment and an outer layer comprising of polyethylene glycol. In an acidic environment of the tumor, poly-histidine side chains matrix imidazole protonated and release drug rapidly [42]. In one patent, cell microenvironment-sensitive, oxidized, ascorbic acid-modified tumor-targeting polymer micelle was formulated using polyethylene glycol - polylysine - polyphenylalanine (MPEG-pLys- pPhe)as a polymer and DHA glucose transporter molecule as a targeted moiety. When tested in mice, targeting micelles were found to be superior to non-targeted micelles groups resulting in significant prolongation of survival time [43]. Hydrazone bond-containing copolymer was synthesized using a hydrophilic polymer such as N-(2- hydroxypropyl) methacrylamide with folic acid as a targeting moiety. The micelles smartly released the drug at acidic pH with greatly extending the drug residence time [44]. An intelligent system was developed by Jianping *et al.* in which a "shell" which is cross-linked Hyaluronic Acid (HA), adsorbed onto the surfaces of the cationic micelles through electrostatic interaction, forming a "core-shell" nano-composition. This composition was susceptible to degradation by high-concentration HA enzyme found in tumor microenvironment and efficiently achieve a high concentration in tumor cells [45]. In one invention, micelle is formed by self-assembly of hydrophobically modified polysaccharide polymer with an endosome pH sensitive characteristic. Antitumor activity of designed micelle was expected to significantly improve via EPR-mediated passive targeting, CD44 receptor initiative targeting and pH-sensitive targeting strategies [46]. In other invention, multi-stimuli responsive shell crosslinked polymeric micelle was prepared using Polydimethylaminoethyl Methacrylate (PDMAEMA) as the hydrophilic chain and polymethacrylateferrocenylformyloxy ethyl ester (PMAFFEE) as the hydrophobic chain that can achieve controlled release through joint triggering of multiple stimuli [47] (Table **3**).

Table 3. Recent Patents on Smart Dendrimers and Miceller Based Nano-Formulations for Cancer Treatment.

Reference	Inventors	Patent Number	Title
[42]	Lintao, C., Huqiang, Y., Lijiao, L., Yifan, M., Peng, L., Gaofeng, X.	CN103690961	Intelligent amphiphilic polymer nano micelle and preparation method and application thereof
[43]	Chen, J., Yu S., Yang, Y.	CN104274834	Environment-sensitive tumor-targeting polymer micelle and preparation method thereof
[44]	Jianchao, Y., Yan, Z., Shenglan, Z., Wenbo, L., Kairun, S.	CN105061701	Hydrazone bond-containing block copolymer having targeting antitumor activity and preparation thereof, and applications of block copolymer as antitumor drug carrier
[45]	Jianping, Z., Yang, D., Qiuling, D.	CN106729737	"Shelling" type intelligent nano-drug composition and preparing method thereof

(Table 3) cont.....

Reference	Inventors	Patent Number	Title
[46]	Yanhua, L., Chengming, Z., Wenping, W., Jianhong, Y.	CN106265510	PH-Triggering-to-release multilevel targeting polymer micelle in tumor cells and preparation method of multilevel targeting polymer micelle
[47]	Zhongli, L., Kehu, Z., Hong, Y.	CN107141488	Multi-stimuli responsive shell crosslinked polymeric micelle and preparation method thereof

1.2. Virus-Based Nanoparticles

In the latest research development virus-based nanoparticles (VNP) are being highly investigated for cancer therapy [48, 49]. The VNP are empty shells from which infectious viral genes have been removed and loaded with an active agent. However, these systems typically require modification of the virus surface using chemical or genetic means to achieve tumor-specific delivery. By modifying their surfaces, smart ways can be evolved to deliver these bioactive molecules into specific cells [48]. Franzen *et al.* invented plant virus-based delivery systems, in that the targeting peptides were attached to the surface of plant viral capsid [49]. The *in vivo* study showed significant enhancement in the uptake and cytotoxicity of doxorubicin from surface attached peptide VNP, relative to free drug [50]. Papilloma-derived protein nanoparticle was invented to deliver drugs to the keratinocytes and basal membrane cells for the treatment of skin-related diseases (such as skin cancer, psoriasis). This presents an effective method for delivering small molecule nucleic acids to the epidermal cells [51]. In one invention, virion-derived nanoparticles have been designed to deliver radioactive isotopes suitable for imaging and treatment of malignant diseases. Additionally, these nanoparticles may deliver a radioisotope that enhances immune system's recognition of the tumor as well as kill tumor cells by alpha, beta or gamma radiation [52]. Moreover, these virus nanoparticles are favorable for immune cancer therapy if targeted to the immune cells and amplify immune activation via the use of stimuli-responsive or immune-stimulatory materials [53, 54].

1.3. Carbon Nanotubes

Carbon Nanotubes (CNTs), one of the unique one-dimensional nanomaterials, can be functionalized via different methods to enhance tumor therapy [54]. Mechanism of carbon nanotube for selective destructing cancer cells is shown in Fig. (3). A targeting multifunctional carbon nanotube/polyethyleneimine drug delivery carrier for prostate cancer was formulated in which amino groups on polyethyleneimine were utilized to further modify the carbon nanotube by connecting dansyl luminescent groups and human prostate stem cell antigen. The formulated drug delivery carrier showed good biocompatibility, reduce toxicity, strong drug loading capability, good luminescent properties and targeting properties [55]. Inventors synthesized immunologically modified nanotubes in which carbon nanotubes are dissolved in a solution of glycated chitosan (an immunostimulant) to deliver immunoadjuvants to tumor cells and to produce targeted, synergistic photothermal and immunological reactions for cancer treatment. These carbon nanotubes can produce spatially and temporally synchronized photothermal and immunological reactions for cancer treatment upon irradiation [56]. In one patent, carbon nanotubes were designed to target the P membrane glycoprotein and produced a high temperature that facilitated intracellular destruction of cells, in order to kill ovarian cancer cells [57]. Several inventions showed that modification of carbon nanotube surface resulted in enhancing the antitumor activity of therapeutic molecules [58 - 61]. Carboxylated multiwalled nanotubes significantly inhibited lung metastasis in tumor-bearing mice and were able to treat tumor metastases and reprogramming of tumor associated with macrophages [62]. Nevertheless, for the cancer treatment, these engineered carbon nanotubes are able to act as an excellent adjuvant Contrast Agents (CA) for many different imaging techniques [63 - 65].

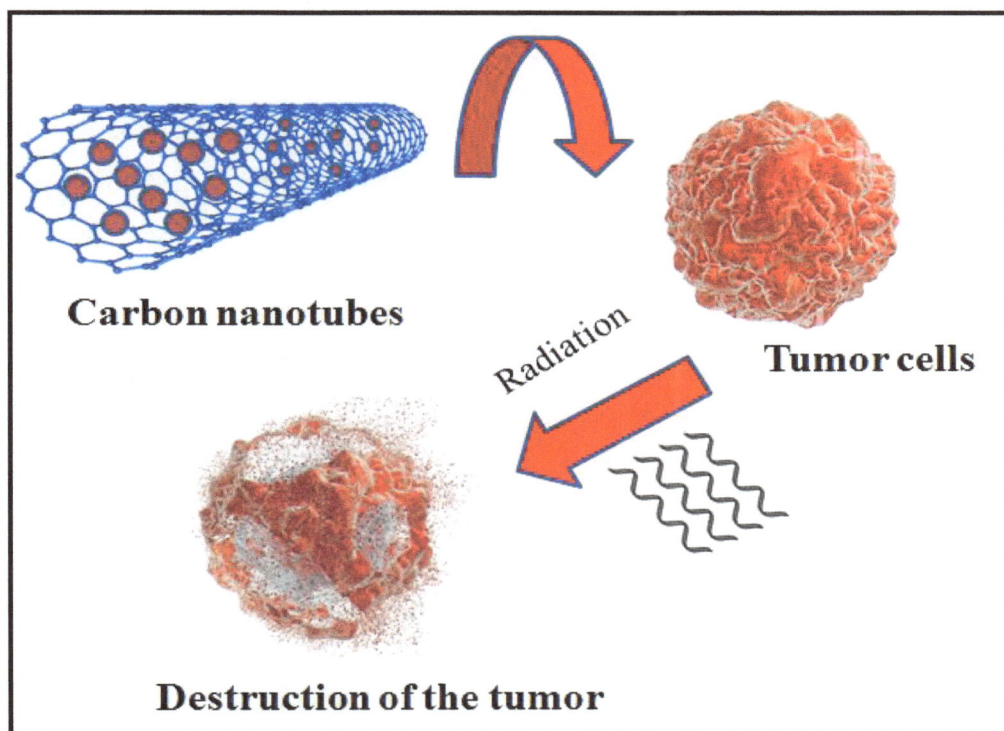

Fig. (3). Mechanism of carbon nanotubes in the selective destruction of cancer cells.

Immunologically modified nanotubes were synthesized by dissolving the nanotubes in a solution of glycated chitosan, an immunostimulant which upon laser irradiation produced spatially and temporally synchronized photothermal and immunological reactions for cancer treatment [66]. In one such patent, researchers developed fullerene nanoparticles that effectively destroyed the tumor blood vessels by the accumulation of heat, which ultimately "starves" the tumor tissue after 4h to 8h of an injection. Due to short retention period (metabolized in ~48h), the nanoparticles do not exhibit long-term retention *in vivo* toxicity [67]. In another invention, the drug molecules were adsorbed by hydrophobic interaction on the surface of chitosan modified carbon nanotube which was attached with a targeted moiety (cancer stem cells). CNT maintains high therapeutic levels, effectively repair DNA by anti-cancer stem cells and promote gastric stem cell apoptosis and necrosis [68] (Table **4**).

Table 4. Recent Patents on Virus-Based Nanoparticles (VNP) and Carbon Nanotubes (CNT) for Cancer Treatment.

Reference	Inventor	Patent Number	Title
[49]	Franzen, S., Guenther, R., Lommel, S.A., Loo, L.	US20120039799	Viral nanoparticle cell-targeted delivery platform
[50]	De Los Pinos, E.	WO2013009717	Virion derived protein nanoparticles for delivering diagnostic or therapeutic agents for the treatment of skin-related diseases
[51]	De Los Pinos, E.	US20130116408	Virion derived protein nanoparticles for delivering radioisotopes for the diagnosis and treatment of malignant and systemic disease and the monitoring of therapy
[52]	Steinmetz, N.F., Wen, A.M., Fiering, S., Lizotte, P.H.	WO2016073972	Cancer immunotherapy using virus particles
[55]	Chen, Z., Zhang, A., Wang, X., Zhu, J., Fan, Y., Yu, H., Yang, Z.	CN102626519	Targeting multifunctional carbon nanotube / polyethyleneimine drug delivery carrier, and preparation method and application thereof
[56]	Chen, W.R.	US20130172848	Immunologically modified carbon nanotubes for cancer treatment
[57]	Hongbo, W., Xiaoli, Z.	CN103191526	Thermal functionalized carbon nanotubes modified anti-ovarian tumor ablation effect
[58]	Dong, G., Kang, W., Soo, S., Jung, C., Hyun, N.T.	WO2014030975	Method for manufacturing carbon nanotube-based anti-cancer agent suppressing cancer cell resistance
[59]	Limin, Z., Lei, T.	CN103990143	Liver cancer-targeted multi-walled carbon nanotube drug-loaded composite material and preparation method thereof

(Table 4) cont.....

Reference	Inventor	Patent Number	Title
[60]	Hongjuan, Y., Yingge, Z., Yan, S., Yan, L.	WO2016023456	Carbon nanotube-drug delivery system for targeting cancer stem cells, a method for preparation of same, and use of same
[62]	Jing, Y., Lianlian, W., Xia, L., Qiqi, X., Yang, X.	CN106265735	Application of carboxylated multi-walled carbon nanotube to the preparation of anti-tumor metastasis medicine
[63]	Yingbin, L., Qinggang, T., Wei, L., Ning, W., Jian, Z., Yijian, Z., Yi, W., Zhiwei, L., Qiang, M.	CN106913886	Tumor-targeting carbon-nanotube photoacoustic contrast agent and preparation method thereof
[65]	Mohajerzadeh, S., Abdolahad, M., Sanaee, Z., Abdollahi, M.	US20130102027	Method for detecting cancer cells using vertically carbon nanotubes
[66]	Wei, R.C.	US20130172848	Immunologically modified carbon nanotubes for cancer treatment
[67]	Chunru, W., Mingming, M., Chunying, S., Taishan, W., Jie, L., Guoqiang, Z.	CN104127872	Application of metal fullerene monocrystal nanoparticles in preparation of specific tumor vascular disrupting agent
[68]	Hongjuan, Y., Yingge, Z., Yan, S., Yan, L.	WO2016023456	Carbon nanotube-drug delivery system for targeting cancer stem cells, a method for preparation of same, and use of same

1.4. Lipid-Based Nano-Formulation

Lipid-based nanoparticulate systems are a most common approach towards improved chemotherapeutic delivery through increased solubility and sustained drug release. Moreover, therapeutic efficacy can be increased by attaching the surface of these nanoparticles by tumor-specific antibodies or ligands [69].

1.4.1. Liposomes

Liposomes are a vesicular system in which phospholipid bilayers are separated by aqueous compartment. These are carriers of choice because of biocompatible and biodegradable features in addition to the flexibility of surface modifications with a suitable ligand, i.e., peptides, antibodies or their fragments, aptamers, small molecules, etc., for targeted delivery of anticancer agents. Moreover to prevent uptake by phagocytes and to make them long circulatory, their surface can be coated with a hydrophilic polymer such as polyethylene glycol which increases the repulsive forces between liposomes and serum components [69 - 71]. Stimuli-responsive smart liposomes that respond to pH, temperature, and enzymes as an internal trigger and magnetic field, ultrasound, and redox potential as external triggers have emerged as promising candidates for enhancement of drug delivery to tumors [72, 73]. pH-sensitive lipid vesicles comprised of a lipid layer, drug and an organic halogen (radiation sensitive agent) that allow controlled release of the medicament from the vesicles after exposure to ionizing radiation [74]. pH-responsive liposomes were invented, having a carboxyl group-containing polysaccharide-derived moieties and a hydrophobic moiety having at least one carboxyl group which easily destabilize in weakly acidic medium and releases the drug. These liposomes delivered antigenic protein (oval albumin) in the cytoplasm, activating the killer T cells and inhibit the growth of tumor cells through cellular immunity [75]. Robillard and coworkers synthesize liposome linked directly or indirectly, to a trigger, and an activator for the trigger that able to release the drug selectively at pH 5.5 and pH 7.4 [76]. Novel liposomes in which thermosensitive peptides were linked to the components of a phospholipid bilayer were invented. As temperature rises, the thermosensitive peptide shrinks, destroying the lipid bilayer, thus releasing the active agents entrapped inside a liposome [77]. Recently, a nanoparticle comprising of first lipid layer shell and an aqueous core comprising chemokine, which is released when the environment of the nanoparticle is in between 38°C and 43°C [78]. Rohit and coworkers invented a degradable nano-construct comprising of gold coated lipid liposome made up of phosphatidylcholine and cholesterol, where the drug is released by degradation either by the enzyme, increase in temperature or photo-thermal effect. The significant increase in cell death was observed in the group receiving the combination treatment of engineered formulation and laser technique which produced the most extensive necrotic response in tumors [79].

1.4.2. Solid Lipid Nanoparticles

SLN are sub-micron colloidal carriers ranging from 50 to 1000nm, composed of lipid dispersed in an aqueous surfactant solution, are attracting major attention as a novel colloidal drug carrier for cancer treatment due to physical stability, protection of labile drugs from degradation, ease of preparation, and low toxicity [80 - 82]. SLNs are being widely investigated as carriers for a variety of drug molecules and newer methods for production of SLNs are being patented [83]. In recent past, Resveratrol-loaded Solid Lipid Nanoparticles (Res-SLNs) prepared using emulsification and low-temperature solidification method displayed a superior ability in inhibiting the proliferation of human breast cells [84]. A new pH-sensitive phospholipid entrapped antineoplastic polyhistidine nanoparticles (Lipid Poly-L-histidine hybrid Nanoparticles, LPNs) to which iNRG ligand was attached as targeting moiety. The iNGR-LPNs showed high tumor targeting efficiency in murine 4T1 breast cancer in mice as compared to LPNs [85].

Thermo-responsive solid lipid nanoparticles which act as smart drug delivery systems are sensitive to higher temperature (39°C-45°C) and release payload at target sites, i.e., hyperthermic body tissues [86, 87]. A Solid Lipid Nanoparticle (SLN) includes an Elastin-Like Polypeptide (ELP) conjugated to a hydrophobic moiety was prepared that undergo a temperature dependent conformation change and drug release [88]. Recent patents on smart lipid nano-formulation for cancer treatment are shown in Table **5**.

Table 5. Recent Patents on Smart Lipid Nano-Formulation for Cancer Treatment.

Reference	Inventor	Patent Number	Title
[73]	Lintao, C., Pengfei, Z., Mingbin, Z., Zhenyu, L., Ping, G., Cuifang, Z., Caixia, Y.	CN103908429	Heat-sensitive liposomes and their preparation and use
[74]	Fologea, D., Henry, R., Salamo, G., Mazur, Y., Borrelli, M.J.	WO2013070872	Methods and compositions for x-ray induced release from pH-sensitive liposomes
[75]	Yuzo, E., Tajima, E.Y., Tajima, N., Kenji, K., Kono, K.	JP2012232949	pH-sensitive liposomes
[76]	Robillard, M.S., Johannes VAN D.S.M., Pouderoijen M.J., Versteegen, R.M.	WO2014081299	Activatable liposomes
[77]	Kim, H.R., Park, S.J., Kim, M.S.	US20140294932	Temperature sensitive liposome including cationic lipid and use thereof
[78]	Zhong, X., Porter, T.M., Seldine, D.C., Landesman, E., Vo, H., Chiu, J.	WO2017096139	B Cell-based cancer immunotherapy
[79]	Srivastava, R., Banerjee, R., Rengan, K.A., Pradhan, A., De, A., Bukhari, A.B.	WO2017115381	Degradable or transformable gold coated liposomal nano-construct and a process for its preparation
[85]	Osmanthus, G.W.	CN107551277	pH-Sensitive targeted LPNs (Lipid Poly-L-histidine hybrid Nanoparticles) for encapsulating anti-tumor drugs
[88]	Park, S.M., Kim, H.R., Park, J.C., Chae, S.Y.	EP2623097	Solid lipid nanoparticles including elastin-like polypeptides and use thereof

1.5. Metal-Based Nanoparticles

Metal-based nanoparticles are sub-micronic particles made up of a pure metal such as gold, platinum, silver, titanium, zinc, cerium, iron, and thallium or their compounds like oxides, hydroxides, sulfides, phosphates, fluorides, and chlorides. In particular, these nanoparticles have received increasing interest due to their widespread application in targeted drug delivery, vehicles for a gene or drug delivery and diagnostic imaging [89]. An invention described local control and prevention of spreading/diffusion of nanoparticles, thus allows full utilization of quantum physics properties of metallic nanoparticles or quantum dots to enable surgical precision of tumor removal [90]. In one patent, core-satellite nanocomposites comprise metal (such as Fe_3O_4, silicon, gold, copper) and surrounding by biocompatible coating is synthesized for treating or imaging tumors [91]. In other invention, charge-modified CdSe / ZnS nanoparticles were targeted to the tumor tissue in high concentration PEG2000 modified CdSe / ZnS nanoparticles confirming in-vivo targeting ability in liver cancer [92].

1.5.1. Gold Nanoparticles (AuNPs)

Gold nanoparticles (AuNPs) have been extensively employed for diagnostic and therapeutic purposes due to their unique physical and chemical properties together with multiple surface functionalities [93 - 95]. Gold nanoparticles can absorb light strongly and convert photon energy into heat, therefore quickly and efficiently raising the temperature of tumor cells (41°C-47°C) and destructing it [96]. Hyperthermia normally combined with other treatments, including radiotherapy and radiofrequency waves, microwaves or ultrasound is found to be more efficacious [97]. The method comprises of optically irradiating and an oscillating magnetic field applying to the nanostructure consisting of a core-shell magnetic nanosphere and a capped gold nanoparticle inducing coupled hyperthermia and oxidative stress to destroy the cell. An approach seems to be viable in guide neuroblastoma cell destruction and can be extended to treat other aggressive cancers [98]. Yanbing *et al.* invented temperature-sensitive gold nanocage hydrogel drug carrying system comprising of a light-heat conversion gold cage, smart responsive polymer and an antitumor agent which increase temperature within the tumor significantly, up to a maximum of 50°C with an increase in irradiation time [99]. Similarly, polyethylene glycol-grafted-poly-cysteine/gold composite nanoparticles with photo-thermal conversion performance were invented [100]. Siwen *et al.* developed complex intelligent nano-delivery system for treating non-small cell lung cancer in which a gold nano-shell is taken as a core, interference sequences of the ALK and the microRNA-301 are linked to the surface of the gold nano-shell by virtue of chemical bonds, and adriamycin is loaded to the outermost layer through an electrostatic adsorption action. Gold shell nano drug system has a good antitumor effect, which is stronger than the individual killing effects of hyperthermia, chemotherapy or gene therapy [101]. Similarly, a synergistic effect with an integrated approach of chemotherapy and phototherapy using pH-sensitive release medicines (10-hydroxycamptothecin) is further observed [102].

As already discussed, a tumor is accompanied with acidosis and presents a lower pH than the normal tissue surrounding it, thus, a pH-sensitive drug-delivery system can specifically target the cancer cells. In a similar type of patent, the researchers developed gold nanoparticles as an active ingredient and protein built around the particles poses sensitive behavior to different pH conditions [103]. Special pH sensitive targeting was observed by Shouju *et al.* in which nanometer gold star materials taken into tumor cells in a faintly acidic environment, and the absorbed light energy is converted into heat energy after near-infrared laser radiation, so that the local temperature is raised and significantly inhibit the growth of cervical cancer cells [104]. A similar attempt was done by Lijuan *et al.* in which gold-loaded polymer micelle systems were created using polycap-rolactone-SS-polymethacrylic acid N, N-dimethylamino ethyl methacrylate as an amphiphilic biodegradable polymer that showed significant antitumor activity on HepG2 cells [105].

1.5.2. Magnetic Nanoparticles (MNPs)

Magnetic nanoparticles are small intelligent inorganic crystals of about 5-20nm diameter used for diagnosis and treatment of cancer due to the large specific surface area, magnetic response and superparamagnetism [106, 107]. Mechanism of magnetic nanoparticles for diagnosis and treatment of cancer is shown in Fig. (**4**) [107]. The basic structure of iron oxide nanoparticles comprises of three main components: An iron oxide core serving as a Magnetic Resonance Imaging (MRI) contrast agent, a biocompatible coating on the exterior of the core, and a final therapeutic coating with specific ligands for biomarker targeting. This exclusive arrangement permits MNP accumulation at the site of interest via biomarker targeting allowing the diagnosis of diseases, evaluation of treatment efficacy, and precise, localized delivery of drugs and therapies [108, 109]. Magnetic hyperthermia which involves transferring of electromagnetic energy into heat allows the temperature increase in well- defined regions in tumor cells [110]. An intelligent multifunctional magnetic nanoparticle was invented wherein the core is a medical magnetic nanoparticle, and the shell is photodynamic drug loaded nano silica with a mesoporous structure [111]. In one invention, iron oxide nanoparticles were coated with 2 hydroxyethyl methacrylate (2-hydroxyethyl methacrylate) and dopamine methacrylamide (Dopamine methacrylamide) monomers, which lead to the formation of catechol group on the surface as a result of polymerization. pH-Dependent drug coating layer was separated in an acid environment, thus showing the controlled release of active ingredient. Thermal therapy along with pH-dependent release was found to significantly enhance the anti-tumor effect of chemotherapeutic agent [112]. Similarly, a synergistic effect of hyperthermia and chemotherapy was patented by other researchers also [113, 114]. In one invention, magnetic nanoparticles targeted, the intelligent dual-ROS system was developed in which thioketal based polymer (PPADT) drug loaded material is wrapped around Fe_3O_4 superparamagnetic magnetic core. The system showed a good dual targeting effect, entrapment efficiency, stability, and low bio-toxicity [115]. An injectable temperature-sensitive magnetic species supramolecular gel was patented recently using distearyl phosphatidyl acetamide-methoxy polyethylene glycol DSPE-mPEG2000 oil-soluble iron tetroxide nanoparticles to provide heat treatment to kill tumor cells [116].

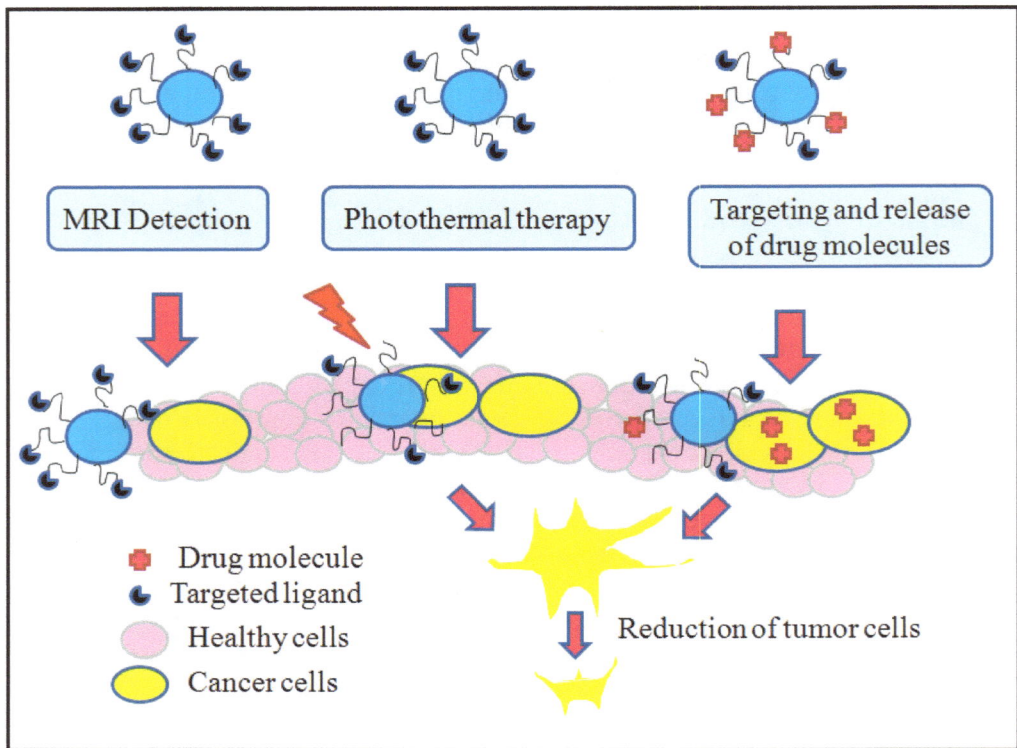

Fig. (4). Mechanism of magnetic nanoparticles for diagnosis and treatment of cancer [107].

In order to provide efficient diagnosing and targeting, micro/nano/stimuli-responsive particles conjugate to a tropic cell (stem cells or an embryoid body) that targets the pathological site well [117]. Furthermore, dextran-coated magnetic iron oxide nanoparticles loaded with Erlotinib showed significant inhibition of tumor cells by suppressing EGFR-ERK-NF-κB signaling pathway, tumor promotion associated MMP-9 and XIAP protein expression, and subsequent inhibition of migration and invasion of cancer cells [118]. In the past few decades, magnetic nanoparticles have emerged as a promising diagnostic and imaging agent due to combine complementary features of Magnetic Resonance Imaging (MRI) and optical imaging [119 - 121]. Zhang and coworker attempt to coat cross-linked copolymer comprising a chitosan and a poly(ethylene oxide) oligomer on the surface of iron oxide/metallic oxide nanoparticles for brain imaging and treatment. O^6-Benzylguanine covalently coupled to the coated surface which inhibits O^6-methylguanine-DNA methyltransferase (MGMT) and treats brain cancers [122, 123]. The nanoparticles facilitate successful BBB (blood brain barrier) permeation via receptor-mediated transcytosis through vessel endothelial cells [123]. Patents on metal-based nanoparticles for cancer treatment are given in Table **6**.

Table 6. Recent Patents on Metal-Based Nanoparticles for Cancer Treatment.

Reference	Inventor	Patent Number	Title
[90]	Greb, G., Beleke, J.P.	EP3028721	Nanoparticle formulation having reverse-thermal gelation properties for injection
[91]	Chen, H., Sun, D.	US20150065858	Core-satellite nanocomposites for MRI and photothermal therapy
[92]	Jian, Ji.,Xiangsheng, L., Qiao, J., Yangjun, C.	CN102989016	Nanoparticle material with pH sensitivity and preparation method thereof
[98]	Ghosh, S., Mitra, S.G.	US20170128573	Multimodal therapy for cancer cell destruction
[99]	Yanbing, Z., Jiangshan, W., Xiangliang, Y., Henan, Y.	CN106890332	Photo-thermal and chemotherapeutic precise synergic antitumor temperature-sensitive gold nanocage hydrogel drug carrying system
[100]	Xingjie, W., Changming, D.	CN105396134	Polyethylene glycol-grafted-polycysteine/gold composite nanoparticles, preparation thereof and applications of the nanoparticles
[101]	Siwen, L., Yueqing, G., Yuxi, L.	CN106421803	Complex intelligent nano-delivery system for treating EML4-ALK fusion mutant non-small cell lung cancer and preparation method of complex intelligent nano-delivery system
[102]	Yang, L.	CN106806900	Preparation on basis of 10-hydroxycamptothecin for pH (potential of hydrogen)-sensitive release medicines, method for preparing preparation and application thereof
[103]	Dixon, C.	KR20150007105	Biocompatible gold nanoparticle with anti-cancer efficacy, and the preparation method thereof
[104]	Shouju, W., Guangming, L., Zhaogang, T., Ying, L., Ying, T., Jing, S., Yuxia, T., Nan, L., Yuan, X., Yanzhen, Z., Xinzhi, C.	CN104083760	PH-Sensitive nanometer gold star material as well as preparation method and application thereof

(Table 6) cont.....

Reference	Inventor	Patent Number	Title
[105]	Lijuan, Z., Di, X., Xiaofang, Z., Wei, Z., Shiyuan, P.	CN106866902	Degradable double-response polymer and loading drug of the degradable double-response polymer as well as preparation method and application of gold nanoparticle micelle
[108]	Weissleder, R., Lee, H., & Yoon, T.-J.	US 8945628	Magnetic nanoparticles
[111]	Weibo, L., Xueyu, Z., Hongli, Z., Huihui, Y., Zongyan, C., Denghao, Z., Liang, T.	CN103566381	Multifunctional magnetic nanoparticle and preparation method thereof
[112]	Chul-hyeon, K., Chan-hee, P., Uni-Tan, R., Gabba, A., Amin, M., Chandra, R., Sashkala, K., Arahram, A.	KR20160145991	Magnetic nanocomposite and preparation method thereof
[113]	Xifang, Z., Yi, X.	CN105561333	Nano-drug carrier and drug with synergistic action of magnetic hyperthermia-chemotherapy and preparation method of nano-drug carrier and drug
[114]	Guangyi, W., Fang, Z., Fang, H., Wei, T., Hao, J.,Guosheng, W., Shizhao, J., Yu, S., Shi, X., Xia, C., Fan, S.	CN107551271	Magnetic-ROS dual smart targeting nanoparticles and preparation method thereof
[115]	Yu, Z., Zhengyang, J., Jun, X., Lina, S., Ning, G.	CN104258425	Preparation method and application of RGD-modified ultra-small magnetic iron oxide nanoparticles
[116]	Yuwu, Z., Ming, A.M., Ning, G.	CN108078914	Injectable types of temperature-sensitive magnetic supramolecular gel preparation and application methods
[117]	Aboody, A., Annala, A., Mooney, R., Berlin, J., Weng, Y.	US20150056144	Encapsulated diagnostics and therapeutics in nanoparticles-conjugated to tropic cells and methods for their use
[118]	Zhenyu, C., Atif, Y., Ali, Y., Feiting, H., Xushan, H.	WO2018098705	Dextran-magnetic iron oxide nanoparticle, preparation and use in treating cancer and as contrast
[119]	Josephson, L., Weissleder, R., Perez, J.M.	US8569078	Magnetic-nanoparticle conjugates and methods of use
[120]	Fu, A., Wang, S.X., Gambhir, S.S.	US8722017	Fluorescent magnetic nanoprobes, methods of making, and methods of use
[121]	Zhang, M., Gunn, J.W., Yee, C.	US20160193369	Magnetic nanoparticle and method for imaging T cells

(Table 6) cont.....

Reference	Inventor	Patent Number	Title
[122]	Zhang, M., Sun, C., Veiseh, O., Bhattarai, N.	US20150320890	Nanoparticles for brain tumor imaging
[123]	Zhang, M., Ellenbogen, R.G., Kievit, F., Silber, J.R., Stephen, Z., Veiseh, O.	US9784730	Nanoparticle for targeting brain tumors and delivery of o^6-benzylguanine

CONCLUSION

Recently, stimuli-sensitive nano preparation has grabbed attention in cancer therapy. These nanoformulations which release the drug by physical and/or chemical structural changes induced by the specific stimulus (pH, temperature or specific enzyme) showed enhanced tumor targeting and controlled drug release at the pathological sites.

CURRENT & FUTURE DEVELOPMENTS

The recent patents clearly demonstrate the potential of stimuli-sensitive nanoparticles in the selective treatment of cancer. It is clearly evident that the system paved new pathways and opened many doors for providing safer and effective treatment options. Ultimately by manipulating the surface property of smart nanoformulation, it is possible to achieve targeted therapy and controlled drug release specifically at cancer sites. But still, commercial utilization is a big challenge owing to complexity; stability and specificity of designed smart nanosystems that need further researches.

CONSENT FOR PUBLICATION

Not applicable.

CONFLICT OF INTEREST

The authors confirm that this chapter content has no conflict of interest.

ACKNOWLEDGEMENTS

Thanks to Prof. Mohammad Ali for his dedication and thoroughness in proofreading.

REFERENCES

[1] Sanchez-Moreno P, Ortega-Vinuesa JL, Peula-Garcia JM, Marchal JA, Boulaiz H. Smart drug-delivery systems for cancer nanotherapy. Curr Drug Targets 2018; 9(4): 339-59.

[2] Xin Y, Yin M, Zhao L, Meng F, Luo L. Recent progress on nanoparticle-based drug delivery systems

for cancer therapy. Cancer Biol Med 2017; 14(3): 228-41.

[3]   Swain S, Sahu PK, Beg S, Babu SM. Nanoparticles for cancer targeting: Current and future directions. Curr Drug Deliv 2016; 13(8): 1290-302.

[4]   Liu JP, Wang TT, Wang DG, Dong AJ, Li YP, Yu HJ. Smart nanoparticles improve therapy for drug-resistant tumors by overcoming pathophysiological barriers. Acta Pharmacol Sin 2017; 38(1): 1-8.
[http://dx.doi.org/10.1038/aps.2016.84] [PMID: 27569390]

[5]   Gagliardi M, Borri C. Polymer nanoparticles as smart carriers for the enhanced release of therapeutic agents to the CNS. Curr Pharm Des 2017; 23(3): 393-410.
[PMID: 27799038]

[6]   Soppimath KS, Aminabhavi TM, Kulkarni AR, Rudzinski WE. Biodegradable polymeric nanoparticles as drug delivery devices. J Control Release 2001; 70(1-2): 1-20.
[http://dx.doi.org/10.1016/S0168-3659(00)00339-4] [PMID: 11166403]

[7]   Panyam J, Labhasetwar V. Biodegradable nanoparticles for drug and gene delivery to cells and tissue. Adv Drug Deliv Rev 2003; 55(3): 329-47.
[http://dx.doi.org/10.1016/S0169-409X(02)00228-4] [PMID: 12628320]

[8]   Pandey P, Dureja H. Recent patents on polymeric nanoparticles for cancer therapy. Recent Pat Nanotechnol 2018; 12(2): 155-69.
[http://dx.doi.org/10.2174/1872210512666180327120648] [PMID: 29589551]

[9]   Mattu C, Brachi G, Ciardelli G. Smart polymeric nanoparticles in smart nanoparticles for biomedicine, micro and nano technologies. Springer 2018; 15-29.
[http://dx.doi.org/10.1016/B978-0-12-814156-4.00002-1]

[10]   Sambi M, Qorri B, Malardier-Jugroot C, Szewczuk MR. Advancements in polymer science: 'Smart' drug delivery systems for the treatment of cancer. MOJ Poly Sci 2017; 1(3): 113-8.

[11]   Yadav D, Suri S, Chaudhary AA, *et al.* Stimuli responsive polymeric nanoparticles in regulated drug delivery for cancer. Pol J Chem Technol 2012; 14(1): 57-64.
[http://dx.doi.org/10.2478/v10026-012-0060-y]

[12]   Wang Y. Smart polymeric nanoparticles: Combining targeted delivery, imaging and therapy into one nanomedicine platform. J Bioanal Biomed 2017; 9(5): 269-71.

[13]   Xi J, Da L, Yang C, *et al.* Mn^{2+}-coordinated PDA@DOX/PLGA nanoparticles as a smart theranostic agent for synergistic chemo-photothermal tumor therapy. Int J Nanomedicine 2017; 12: 3331-45.
[http://dx.doi.org/10.2147/IJN.S132270] [PMID: 28479854]

[14]   Gorre ME, Mohammed M, Ellwood K, *et al.* Clinical resistance to STI-571 cancer therapy caused by BCR-ABL gene mutation or amplification. Science 2001; 293(5531): 876-80.
[http://dx.doi.org/10.1126/science.1062538] [PMID: 11423618]

[15]   Szakács G, Paterson JK, Ludwig JA, Booth-Genthe C, Gottesman MM. Targeting multidrug resistance in cancer. Nat Rev Drug Discov 2006; 5(3): 219-34.
[http://dx.doi.org/10.1038/nrd1984] [PMID: 16518375]

[16]   Maitra A, Pramanik D. Smart polymeric nanoparticles which overcome multidrug resistance to cancer therapeutics and treatment-related systemic toxicity. US20130330412, 2013.

[17]   Arthur RCB, Jamboor KV. Formulation of active agent loaded activated PLGA nanoparticles for targeted cancer nano-therapeutics. EP2146694, 2012.

[18]   Omary MA, Hu Z, Marpu S. Polyionic transitional metal phosphorescent complex/polymer hybrid systems for bioimaging and sensing applications. US20120065614, 2012.

[19]   Richard AW, Roy RY. Targeted therapeutic nanoparticles. US20140199232, 2014.

[20]   Peihong N, Yue S, Jinlin H, Mingzu Z. Preparation method of block copolymer with dual responsiveness of rapid oxidization/reduction and selenium bonds and application of block copolymer.

CN107641201, 2018.

[21]   Almutairi A, Sankaranarayanan J, Mahmoud E, Schopf E. Polymeric nano-carriers with a linear dual response mechanism and uses thereof. US20120070383, 2012.

[22]   Chen W, Zhou R. pH-Sensitive nanoparticles for drug delivery. US20160213790, 2016.

[23]   Nguyen KT, Rahmi M, Kona S, Lin A. Compositions and methods for thermo-sensitive nanoparticles and magnetic nanoparticles. US9216220, 2015.

[24]   Chopra S, Karnik R, Wang A, Farokhzad O, Zhang XQ. Nanoparticles with pH triggered drug release. WO2017062920, 2017.

[25]   Chen IW, Choi H, Zhou R. pH-Sensitive peptides and their nanoparticles for drug delivery. US9687563, 2016.

[26]   Chiu HC, Chiang WH, Hung CC, Yu TW. Preparation of pH-responsive nanoparticles and promoted delivery of anticancer drugs into deep tumor tissues and application thereof. US20160367489, 2018.

[27]   Almutairi A, Sankaranarayanan J, Mahmoud E, Schopf E. Polymeric nano-carriers with a linear dual response mechanism and uses thereof. US20120070383, 2012.

[28]   Nguyen KT, Rahimi M, Kona S, Lin AH. Compositions and methods for thermo-sensitive nanoparticles and magnetic nanoparticles. US9216220, 2015.

[29]   Koppolu B, Bhavsar Z, Wadajkar AS, *et al.* Temperature-sensitive polymer-coated magnetic nanoparticles as a potential drug delivery system for targeted therapy of thyroid cancer. J Biomed Nanotechnol 2012; 8(6): 983-90.
        [http://dx.doi.org/10.1166/jbn.2012.1465] [PMID: 23030006]

[30]   Crucho CIC. Stimuli-responsive polymeric nanoparticles for nanomedicine. ChemMedChem 2015; 10(1): 24-38.
        [http://dx.doi.org/10.1002/cmdc.201402290] [PMID: 25319803]

[31]   Wang H, Sun D, Zhao N, *et al.* Thermo-sensitive graphene oxide-polymer nanoparticle hybrids: Synthesis, characterization, biocompatibility and drug delivery. J Mater Chem 2014.

[32]   Patil AS, Gadad AP, Hiremath RD, Josh SD. Biocompatible tumor micro-environment responsive CS-g-PNIPAAm co-polymeric nanoparticles for targeted Oxaliplatin delivery. J Polym Res 2018; 3.

[33]   Rejinold NS, Muthunarayanan M, Divyarani VV, *et al.* Curcumin-loaded biocompatible thermoresponsive polymeric nanoparticles for cancer drug delivery. J Colloid Interface Sci 2011; 360(1): 39-51.
        [http://dx.doi.org/10.1016/j.jcis.2011.04.006] [PMID: 21549390]

[34]   Gonçalves C, Pereira P, Gama M. Self-assembled hydrogel nanoparticles for drug delivery applications. Materials (Basel) 2010; 3(2): 1420-60.
        [http://dx.doi.org/10.3390/ma3021420]

[35]   Patel GC, Dalwadi CA. Recent patents on stimuli responsive hydrogel drug delivery system. Recent Pat Drug Deliv Formul 2013; 7(3): 206-15.
        [http://dx.doi.org/10.2174/1872211307666131118141600] [PMID: 24237032]

[36]   Artzi N, Zhang Y, Jorge NO, Conde J. Hydrogel particles, compositions, and methods. US20170333304, 2017.

[37]   Gan Y, Wang Q, Yang X, Yang W, Li F. Nanogel and nanogel drug carrier system both with smart response to tumor microenvironment. CN106810636, 2017.

[38]   Wang L, Yang W, Liang L, Zhou P. Nano particle-polymer injectable composite hydrogel double drug loading system and preparation method thereof. CN107550921, 2018.

[39]   Zhao Y, Wan J, Yang X, Yan H. Photo-thermal and chemotherapeutic precise synergic antitumor temperature-sensitive gold nanocage hydrogel drug carrying system. CN106890332, 2017.

[40]   Zhou Q, Zhang L, Yang T, Wu H. Stimuli-responsive polymeric micelles for drug delivery and cancer therapy. Int J Nanomedicine 2018; 13: 2921-42.
[http://dx.doi.org/10.2147/IJN.S158696] [PMID: 29849457]

[41]   Talelli M, Rijckenac CJF, Hennink WE, Lammers T. Polymeric micelles for cancer therapy: 3C's to enhance efficacy. Curr Opin Solid State Mater Sci 2012; 16(6): 302-30.
[http://dx.doi.org/10.1016/j.cossms.2012.10.003]

[42]   Lintao C, Huqiang Y, Lijiao L, Yifan M, Peng L, Gaofeng X. Intelligent amphiphilic polymer nano micelle and preparation method and application thereof. CN103690961, 2014.

[43]   Chen J, Yu S, Yang Y. Environment-sensitive tumor-targeting polymer micelle and preparation method thereof. CN104274834, 2015.

[44]   Jianchao Y, Yan Z, Shenglan Z, Wenbo L, Kairun S. Hydrazone bond-containing block copolymer having targeting antitumor activity and preparation thereof, and applications of block copolymer as antitumor drug carrier. CN105061701, 2015.

[45]   Jianping Z, Yang D, Qiuling D. Shelling" type intelligent nano-drug composition and preparing method thereof. CN106729737, 2017.

[46]   Yanhua L, Chengming Z, Wenping W, Jianhong Y. pH-Triggering-to-release multilevel targeting polymer micelle in tumor cells and preparation method of multilevel targeting polymer micelle. CN106265510, 2016.

[47]   Zhongli L, Kehu Z, Hong Y. Multi-stimuli responsive shell crosslinked polymeric micelle and preparation method thereof. CN107141488, 2017.

[48]   Hefferon KL. Repurposing plant virus nanoparticles. Vaccines (Basel) 2018; 6(1): 1-10.
[http://dx.doi.org/10.3390/vaccines6010011] [PMID: 29443902]

[49]   Franzen S, Guenther R, Lommel SA, Loo L. Viral nanoparticle cell-targeted delivery platform. US20120039799, 2012.

[50]   De Los Elisabet P. Virion derived protein nanoparticles for delivering diagnostic or therapeutic agents for the treatment of skin-related diseases. WO2013009717, 2013.

[51]   De Los Elisabet P. Virion derived protein nanoparticles for delivering radioisotopes for the diagnosis and treatment of malignant and systemic disease and the monitoring of therapy. US20130116408, 2013.

[52]   Steinmetz NF, Wen AM, Fiering S, Lizotte PH. Cancer immunotherapy using virus particles. WO2016073972, 2016.

[53]   Saleh T, Shojaosadati SA. Multifunctional nanoparticles for cancer immunotherapy. Hum Vaccin Immunother 2016; 12(7): 1863-75.
[PMID: 26901287]

[54]   Steinmetz NF, Amy M, Wen AM, Fiering S, Lizotte PH. Cancer immunotherapy using virus particles. WO2016073972, 2016.

[54]   Chen Z, Zhang A, Wang X, *et al.* The advances of carbon nanotubes in cancer diagnostics and therapeutics. J Nanomater 2017.
[http://dx.doi.org/10.1155/2017/3418932]

[55]   Haili S, Huixia W, Shiping Y, Xue W. Targeting multifunctional carbon nanotube polyethylenimine drug delivery carrier, and preparation method and application thereof. CN102626519, 2012.

[56]   Chen WR. Immunologically modified carbon nanotubes for cancer treatment. US20130172848, 2013.

[57]   Hongbo W, Xiaoli Z. Thermal functionalized carbon nanotubes modified anti-ovarian tumor ablation effect. CN103191526, 2013.

[58]   Dong G, Kang W, Soo S, Jung C, Hyun NT. Method for manufacturing carbon nanotube-based anti-

cancer agent suppressing cancer cell resistance. WO2014030975, 2014.

[59] Limin Z, Lei T. Liver cancer-targeted multi-walled carbon nanotube drug-loaded composite material and preparation method thereof. CN103990143, 2014.

[60] Hongjuan Y, Yingge Z, Yan S, Yan L. Carbon nanotube-drug delivery system for targeting cancer stem cells, method for preparation of same, and use of same. WO2016023456, 2016.

[61] Gomez S, Rendtorff NM, Aglietti EF, Sakka Y, Suárez G. Surface modification of multiwall carbon nanotubes by sulfonitric treatment. Applied Surface Sci 2016; 379: 264-9.

[62] Jing Y, Lianlian W, Xia L, Qiqi X, Yang X. Application of carboxylated multiwalled carbon nanotube to preparation of anti-tumor metastasis medicine. CN106265735, 2017.

[63] Yingbin L, Qinggang T, Wei L, *et al.* Tumor-targeting carbon-nanotube photoacoustic contrast agent and preparation method thereof. CN106913886, 2017.

[64] Sanginario A, Miccoli B, Demarchi D. Carbon nanotubes as an effective opportunity for cancer diagnosis and treatment. Biosensors (Basel) 2017; 7(1): 9.

[65] Mohajerzadeh S, Abdolahad M, Sanaee Z, Abdollahi M. Method for detecting cancer cells using vertically carbon nanotubes. US20130102027, 2013.

[66] Chen WR. Immunologically modified carbon nanotubes for cancer treatment. US9107944, 2015.

[67] Chunru W, Mingming M, Chunying S, Taishan W, Jie L, Guoqiang Z. Application of metal fullerene monocrystal nanoparticles in preparation of specific tumor vascular disrupting agent. CN104127872, 2014.

[68] Hongjuan Y, Yingge Z, Yan S, Yan L. Lipid-based nanoparticles for cancer diagnosis and therapy. Organic Materials as Smart Nanocarriers for Drug Delivery, 2018; 415-70.

[69] Palei NN, Mohanta BC, Sabapathi ML, Das MK. Lipid-Based Nanoparticles for Cancer Diagnosis and Therapy. Elsevier: Materials as Smart Nanocarriers for Drug Delivery 2018; pp. 415-70.
[http://dx.doi.org/10.1016/B978-0-12-813663-8.00010-5]

[70] Pattni BS, Chupin VV, Torchilin VP. New developments in liposomal drug delivery. Chem Rev 2015; 115(19): 10938-66.

[71] Hatakeyama H, Akita H, Harashima H. The polyethyleneglycol dilemma: Advantage and disadvantage of PEGylation of liposomes for systemic genes and nucleic acids delivery to tumors. Biol Pharm Bull 2013; 36(6): 892-9.
[http://dx.doi.org/10.1248/bpb.b13-00059] [PMID: 23727912]

[72] Jain A, Jain SK. Stimuli-responsive smart liposomes in cancer targeting. Curr Drug Targets 2018; 19(3): 259-70.
[http://dx.doi.org/10.2174/1389450117666160208144143] [PMID: 26853324]

[73] Lintao C, Pengfei Z, Mingbin Z, *et al.* A heat-sensitive liposomes and their preparation and use. CN103908429, 2014.

[74] Fologea D, Henry R, Salamo G, Mazur Y, Borrelli MJ. Methods and compositions for X-ray induced release from ph sensitive liposomes. WO2013070872, 2013.

[75] Yuzo E, Tajima EY, Tajima N, Kenji K, Kono K. pH-Sensitive liposomes. JP2012232949, 2012.

[76] Robillard MS, Johannes Van DSM, Pouderoijen MJ, Versteegen RM. Activatable liposomes. WO2014081299, 2014.

[77] Kim HR, Park SJ, Kim MS. Temperature sensitive liposome including cationic lipid and use thereof. US20140294932, 2014.

[78] Zhong X, Porter TM, Seldine DC, Landesman E, Vo H, Chiu J. B Cell-based cancer immunotherapy. WO2017096139, 2017.

[79] Srivastava R, Banerjee R, Rengan KA, Pradhan A, De A, Bukhari AB. Degradable or transformable

gold coated liposomal nano-construct and a process for its preparation. WO2017115381, 2017.

[80]   Mathur V, Satrawala Y, Rajput MS, *et al.* Solid lipid nanoparticles in cancer therapy. Int J Drug Deliv 2010; 2: 192-9.
[http://dx.doi.org/10.5138/ijdd.2010.0975.0215.02029]

[81]   Kang KW, Chun MK, Kim O, *et al.* Doxorubicin-loaded solid lipid nanoparticles to overcome multidrug resistance in cancer therapy. Nanomedicine (Lond) 2010; 6(2): 210-3.
[http://dx.doi.org/10.1016/j.nano.2009.12.006] [PMID: 20060074]

[82]   Ekambaram P, Sathali AH, Priyanka K. Solid lipid nanoparticles: A review. Sci Revs Chem Commun 2012; 2(1): 80-102.

[83]   Sawant KK, Dodiya SS. Recent advances and patents on solid lipid nanoparticles. Recent Pat Drug Deliv Formul 2008; 2(2): 120-35.
[http://dx.doi.org/10.2174/187221108784534081] [PMID: 19075903]

[84]   Wang W, Zhang L, Chen T, *et al.* Anticancer effects of resveratrol-loaded solid lipid nanoparticles on human breast cancer cells. Molecules 2017; 22(11): pii: E1814.
[http://dx.doi.org/10.3390/molecules22111814]

[85]   Osmanthus GW. pH-sensitive targeted LPNs (lipid poly-L-histidine hybrid nanoparticles) for encapsulating anti-tumor drugs. CN107551277, 2018.

[86]   Shao P, Wang B, Wang Z, Li J, Zhang Y. The application of thermosensitive nanocarriers in controlled drug delivery. J Nanomater 2011; 1-12.
[http://dx.doi.org/10.1155/2011/389640]

[87]   Rehman M, Ihsan A, Madni A, *et al.* Solid lipid nanoparticles for thermoresponsive targeting: evidence from spectrophotometry, electrochemical, and cytotoxicity studies. Int J Nanomedicine 2017; 12: 8325-36.
[http://dx.doi.org/10.2147/IJN.S147506] [PMID: 29200845]

[88]   Park SM, Kim HR, Park JC, Chae SY. Solid lipid nanoparticles including elastin-like polypeptides and use thereof. EP2623097, 2013.

[89]   Mody VV, Siwale R, Singh A, Mody HR. Introduction to metallic nanoparticles. J Pharm Bioallied Sci 2010; 2(4): 282-9.
[http://dx.doi.org/10.4103/0975-7406.72127] [PMID: 21180459]

[90]   Greb G, Beleke JP. Nanoparticle formulation having reverse-thermal gelation properties for injection. EP3028721, 2015.

[91]   Chen H, Sun D. Core-satellite nanocomposites for MRI and photothermal therapy. US20150065858, 2015.

[92]   Ji J. Nanoparticle material with pH sensitivity and preparation method thereof. CN102989016, 2013.

[93]   Yeh YC, Creran B, Rotello VM. Gold nanoparticles: preparation, properties, and applications in bionanotechnology. Nanoscale 2012; 4(6): 1871-80.
[http://dx.doi.org/10.1039/C1NR11188D] [PMID: 22076024]

[94]   Joseph MM, Sreelekha TT. Gold nanoparticles-synthesis and applications in cancer management. Recent Pat Mater Sci 2014; 1(7): 8-25.
[http://dx.doi.org/10.2174/1874464806666131220232647]

[95]   Thambiraj S, Hema S, Shankaran DR. An overview on applications of gold nanoparticle for early diagnosis and targeted drug delivery to prostate cancer. Recent Pat Nanotechnol 2018; 12(2): 110-31.
[http://dx.doi.org/10.2174/1872210511666171101120157] [PMID: 29090672]

[96]   Huang X, El-Sayed MA. Plasmonic photo-thermal therapy (PPTT). Alexandria Med J 2011; 47(1): 1-9.
[http://dx.doi.org/10.1016/j.ajme.2011.01.001]

[97]   Jain S, Hirst DG, O'Sullivan JM, O'Sullivan JM. Gold nanoparticles as novel agents for cancer therapy. Br J Radiol 2012; 85(1010): 101-13.
[http://dx.doi.org/10.1259/bjr/59448833] [PMID: 22010024]

[98]   Ghosh S, Mitra SG. Multimodal therapy for cancer cell destruction. US20170128573, 2017.

[99]   Yanbing Z, Jiangshan W, Xiangliang Y, Henan Y. Photo-thermal and chemotherapeutic precise synergic antitumor temperature-sensitive gold nanocage hydrogel drug carrying system. CN106890332, 2017.

[100]   Xingjie W, Changming D. Polyethylene glycol-grafted-polycysteine/gold composite nanoparticles, preparation thereof and applications of the nanoparticles. CN105396134, 2016.

[101]   Siwen L, Yueqing G, Yuxi L. Complex intelligent nano delivery system for treating EML4-ALK fusion mutant non-small cell lung cancer and preparation method of complex intelligent nano delivery system. CN106421803, 2017.

[102]   Yang L. Preparation on basis of 10-hydroxycamptothecin for pH (potential of hydrogen)-sensitive release medicines, method for preparing preparation and application thereof. CN106806900, 2017.

[103]   Dixon C. Biocompatible gold nanoparticle with anti-cancer efficacy, and the preparation method thereof. KR20150007105, 2015.

[104]   Shouju W, Guangming L, Zhaogang T, *et al.* pH-Sensitive nanometer gold star material as well as preparation method and application thereof. CN104083760, 2014.

[105]   Lijuan Z, Di X, Xiaofang Z, Wei Z, Shiyuan P. Degradable double-response polymer and loading drug of degradable double-response polymer as well as preparation method and application of gold nanoparticle micelle. CN106866902, 2017.

[106]   Wu M, Huang S. Magnetic nanoparticles in cancer diagnosis, drug delivery and treatment. Mol Clin Oncol 2017; 7(5): 738-46.
[PMID: 29075487]

[107]   Gobbo OL, Sjaastad K, Radomski MW, Volkov Y, Prina-Mello A. Magnetic nanoparticles in cancer theranostics. Theranostics 2015; 5(11): 1249-63.
[http://dx.doi.org/10.7150/thno.11544] [PMID: 26379790]

[108]   Weissleder R, Lee H, Yoon T. Magnetic nanoparticles. US8945628, 2015.

[109]   Zhang M, Kohler N, Gunn J W. Magnetic nanoparticle compositions and methods. US7462446, 2008.

[110]   Bañobre-López M, Teijeiro A, Rivas J. Magnetic nanoparticle-based hyperthermia for cancer treatment. Rep Pract Oncol Radiother 2013; 18(6): 397-400.
[http://dx.doi.org/10.1016/j.rpor.2013.09.011] [PMID: 24416585]

[111]   Weibo L, Xueyu Z, Hongli Z, *et al.* Multifunctional magnetic nano particle and preparation method thereof. CN103566381A, 2014.

[112]   Chul-hyeon K, Chan-hee P, Uni-Tan R, *et al.* Magnetic nano composite and preparation method thereof. KR20160145991, 2016.

[113]   Xifang Z, Yi X. Nano-drug carrier and drug with synergistic action of magnetic hyperthermia-chemotherapy and preparation method of nano-drug carrier and drug. CN105561333, 2016.

[114]   Guangyi W, Fang Z, Fang H, *et al.* Magnetic-ROS dual smart targeting nanoparticles and preparation method thereof. CN107551271, 2018.

[115]   Yu Z, Zhengyang J, Jun X, Lina S, Ning G. Preparation method and application of RGD-modified ultra-small magnetic iron oxide nanoparticles. CN104258425, 2015.

[116]   Yuwu Z, Ming AM, Ning G. Injectable types of temperature-sensitive magnetic supramolecular gel preparation and application methods. CN108078914, 2018.

[117]   Aboody A, Annala A, Mooney R, Berlin J, Weng Y. Encapsulated diagnostics and therapeutics in

nanoparticles-conjugated to tropic cells and methods for their use. US20150056144, 2015.

[118] Zhenyu C, Atif Y, Ali Y, Feiting H, Xushan H. Dextran-magnetic iron oxide nanoparticle, preparation and use in treating cancer and as contrast. WO2018098705, 2018.

[119] Josephson L, Weissleder R, Perez JM. Magnetic-nanoparticle conjugates and methods of use. US8569078, 2013.

[120] Fu A, Wang SX, Gambhir SS. Fluorescent magnetic nanoprobes, methods of making, and methods of use. US8722017, 2015.

[121] Zhang M, Gunn JW, Yee C. Magnetic nanoparticle and method for imaging T cells. US20160193369, 2016.

[122] Zhang M, Sun C, Veiseh O, Bhattarai N. Nanoparticles for brain tumor imaging. US20150320890, 2015.

[123] Zhang M, Ellenbogen RG, Kievit F, Silber JR, Stephen Z, Veiseh O. Nanoparticle for targeting brain tumors and delivery of o^6-benzylguanine. US9784730, 2017.

CHAPTER 6

Potential Inflammatory Mechanisms Underlying Chemotherapy-Induced Peripheral Neuropathy and Skeletal Muscle Effects

Claire E. Feather[1,2,4], **John B. Kwok**[4,5], **Gila Moalem-Taylor**[3,4] and **Patsie Polly**[1,2,4,*]

[1] *Mechanisms of Disease and Translational Research Group, School of Medical Sciences, University of New South Wales, NSW 2052, Sydney, Australia*

[2] *Department of Pathology, University of New South Wales, NSW 2052, Sydney, Australia*

[3] *Neuropathic Pain Research Group, Translational Neuroscience Facility, University of Sydney, NSW 2050, Sydney, Australia*

[4] *School of Medical Sciences, UNSW Sydney, NSW 2052, Sydney, Australia*

[5] *Brain & Mind Centre, The University of Sydney, NSW 2050, Sydney, Australia*

Abstract: Cancer patients receiving chemotherapy treatment frequently experience adverse side effects, including the development of chemotherapy-induced peripheral neuropathy (CIPN) and muscle wasting. Investigation into the pathophysiological mechanisms responsible for these neuromuscular effects is crucial since associated symptoms including pain and muscle fatigue can lead to chemotherapy dose reduction or discontinuation, as well as long-term effects on patient mobility and quality of life. While patient symptoms may vary depending on the chemotherapy drug type and dosage regime, inflammation has been implicated as a common mediator responsible for the peripheral tissue effects associated with chemotherapy use. Although mitochondrial dysfunction has been recently investigated as a key underlying mechanism of CIPN and chemotherapy-induced muscle atrophy, there is a close association between mitochondrial dysfunction, oxidative stress and inflammation in biological systems. Host genetic factors have also been implicated in CIPN, and further genetic studies are therefore essential for identifying biomarkers of patient susceptibility, as well as assisting in the elucidation of candidate molecular pathways. Finally, another important consideration is the relationship between cancer-induced and chemotherapy-induced effects, given that chemotherapy can exacerbate cancer cachexia-related muscle wasting. Since cancer cachexia results from excessive systemic inflammation due to the host-tumour interaction, these findings suggest that inflammation-associated molecular alterations due to chemotherapy administration

* **Corresponding author Patsie Polly:** Mechanisms of Disease and Translational Research Group Department of Pathology School of Medical Sciences University of New South Wales Sydney, NSW 2052, Sydney, Australia; Tel; +61 2 9385 2924: Fax: +61 2 9385 1389; E-mail: patsie.polly@unsw.edu.au

Atta-ur-Rahman and Khurshid Zaman (Eds.)

could contribute to muscle wasting in the treatment setting. Therefore, the purpose of this chapter is to provide evidence for a role of inflammation in chemotherapy-induced neuromuscular effects, and to summarise recent patented developments aimed at targeting these side effects.

Keywords: Cancer cachexia, cancer treatment, chemotherapy-induced peripheral neuropathy, inflammation, inflammatory cytokines, mitochondrial dysfunction, muscle wasting, reactive oxygen species, skeletal muscle atrophy.

1. INTRODUCTION

The worldwide burden of cancer is steadily increasing, with global cancer incidence expected to rise to 22 million new cases annually within the next two decades [1]. Meanwhile, advances in cancer diagnosis and treatment have contributed to a significant reduction in mortality rates, therefore raising concerns for the long-term outcomes associated with cancer survivorship [1, 2]. In particular, chemotherapy-induced peripheral neuropathy (CIPN) is a common and debilitating side effect of several frequently administered antineoplastic agents, including platinum compounds, taxanes, vinca alkaloids, bortezomib and thalidomide [3, 4]. Clinically, CIPN features the progressive onset of sensory symptoms such as burning, numbness and tingling, as well as neuropathic pain, typically in a bilateral 'stocking and glove' distribution [4]. Neuropathic pain is defined as pathological pain resulting from disease or damage to the somatosensory system [5]. These symptoms can be highly disabling, leading to impaired mobility and reduced quality of life in both the short- and long-term [3, 4].

1.1. Chemotherapy, Neuropathic Pain and Skeletal Muscle Effects

The overall prevalence of CIPN is exceptionally high, affecting as many as 68% of cancer patients within the first month following chemotherapy completion [3]. Additionally, although neuropathy may resolve over time, approximately 30% of patients continue to suffer from CIPN six months after the cessation of treatment, and symptoms may persist for years, potentially due to permanent peripheral nervous system (PNS) damage [3, 6 - 8]. The incidence and severity of CIPN are highly variable and depend on a number of factors: the specific drug used, the frequency and duration of therapy, the cumulative dose, the presence of pre-existing neuropathy and whether the drug is used in isolation or in combination [4]. Unfortunately, although the implementation of dose-dense combination chemotherapy regimes has resulted in improved patient survival, these multimodal therapeutic approaches have also contributed to increased CIPN incidence [4, 9].

Another problematic side effect of chemotherapy, which can further impair patient mobility, is the negative impact of antineoplastic agents on muscle mass and function. While patients with CIPN sometimes experience muscle pain (myalgia), which may eventually lead to disuse muscle atrophy, studies have confirmed that chemotherapy can directly induce skeletal muscle loss and contribute to muscle weakness and fatigue [2, 10 - 16]. This is particularly significant as many cancer patients already suffer from muscle wasting due to cancer cachexia, a hypercatabolic/hypermetabolic paraneoplastic syndrome in which the host-tumour interaction leads to chronic systemic inflammation and loss of lean body mass and fat [17, 18]. Importantly, experimental studies have indicated that chemotherapy may actually exacerbate cancer cachexia, irrespective of tumour burden reduction [10, 12]. Additionally, cancer patients with muscle wasting are much more susceptible to developing drug-related toxicities, including severe CIPN, and also have a poorer prognosis [19 - 21].

1.2. Clinical Insights

The clinical significance of CIPN and chemotherapy-induced muscle wasting and fatigue relates not only to the long-term effects on patient mobility and quality of life, but the efficacy and success of treatment. Development of CIPN often leads to chemotherapy dose reduction, which is highly problematic, as potentially curative treatments may not successfully eliminate the tumour burden [4, 22]. In some instances, there may be complete discontinuation of chemotherapy, potentially contributing to increased mortality and reduced long-term survival [4]. Based on these observations, the mechanisms behind CIPN and chemotherapy-induced muscle wasting warrant further investigation.

Unfortunately, the pathophysiological mechanisms responsible for CIPN development are still not well understood, while relatively few studies have investigated chemotherapy-induced effects on skeletal muscle [2]. Additionally, elucidation of the mechanisms underlying these neuromuscular effects is complicated by the fact that different classes of chemotherapy may elicit cellular changes through distinct molecular pathways [2]. Furthermore, although current treatment options for CIPN (e.g. topical agents, antidepressant and antiepileptic medications) can provide some symptomatic relief, no effective targeted treatment options currently exist [3, 23]. Therefore, there is a critical need to develop specific preventative and treatment strategies, which will stem from an improved understanding of the molecular mechanisms underlying these effects. Interestingly, studies indicate some degree of overlap in the key potential mechanisms of interest, suggesting that mitochondrial dysfunction and oxidative stress may be major contributors to PNS and skeletal muscle tissue effects elicited by various chemotherapy drugs, including platinum compounds and taxanes [10,

11, 24 - 26]. Since mitochondrial damage and oxidative stress are closely associated with inflammation, and studies report that chemotherapy contributes to increased cytokine and reactive oxygen species (ROS) production, this chapter will discuss evidence for inflammation as a potential mediator of chemotherapy-induced neuromuscular effects [27]. Finally, since the development of effective treatment options is a rapidly growing area of interest where extensive investigation is being undertaken, some recent patents related to the prevention and treatment of chemotherapy-associated effects will also be reviewed.

2. AN OVERVIEW OF CHEMOTHERAPY-INDUCED NEUROMUSCULAR EFFECTS

2.1. Chemotherapy-Induced Peripheral Neuropathy (CIPN)

Although clinical studies, primarily observational, have been useful in delineating the incidence, prevalence, clinical features and predictors of CIPN, they have not allowed for the investigation of the pathophysiological basis of neuropathic pain at the cellular and molecular levels. Consequently, most of the current understanding regarding CIPN and its development has been derived from animal models (Table **1**) [2, 4, 28 - 30].

Table 1. Chemotherapy Drugs Implicated in CIPN.

Drug Class	Chemotherapy Drug	Anti-Cancer Mechanism	Neuropathy Features (Sensory, Motor)	References
Platinum Compound	Cisplatin	DNA cross-linking, defective DNA repair	Primarily sensory	[2, 4]
	Oxaliplatin	DNA cross-linking, defective DNA repair	Primarily sensory (acute and chronic neuropathy) Muscle cramps	
Taxane	Paclitaxel	Microtubule stabilisation, defective mitosis	Primarily sensory Myalgia at higher doses	[2, 28]
	Docetaxel	Microtubule stabilisation, defective mitosis	Primarily sensory Myalgia at higher doses	
Vinca Alkaloid	Vincristine	Microtubule destabilisation, defective mitosis	Primarily sensory Muscle cramps and distal weakness	[2, 29]

(Table 1) cont.....

Drug Class	Chemotherapy Drug	Anti-Cancer Mechanism	Neuropathy Features (Sensory, Motor)	References
Other	Bortezomib	Proteasome inhibition, apoptosis	Painful sensory neuropathy	[2, 30]
	Thalidomide	Immunomodulation, inhibition of angiogenesis	Sensory neuropathy Mild distal weakness and cramps	[2]

2.1.1. Animal Models

Investigation into the impact of chemotherapy drugs on neuronal tissues at both the cellular and molecular level has been facilitated primarily through the development of CIPN rodent models involving chemotherapy administration in non-tumour-bearing rats or mice. It is now recognised that many chemotherapy agents are able to penetrate the Blood-Nerve-Barrier (BNB) and infiltrate PNS tissues, including the Dorsal Root Ganglion (DRG) and peripheral sensory nerve axons [31]. As a result, chemotherapy may produce neurotoxic effects in multiple components of the PNS. The DRG, a cluster of sensory neuron cell bodies at the posterior root of spinal nerves, is commonly affected in CIPN, potentially explaining the prevalence of sensory over motor symptoms [32, 33]. Interestingly, despite the different mechanisms of action of chemotherapy drugs including platinum compounds, taxanes and vinca alkaloids, these agents can induce similar morphological changes in peripheral nerves, and are also associated with comparable neuropathy profiles [3] (Table **1**).

Numerous cellular targets (e.g. sensory neurons, Schwann cells and Satellite glial cells) and underlying mechanisms have been implicated in the development of CIPN. Some of the mechanisms responsible for chemotherapy-induced neurotoxicity are DNA damage, alterations in cellular system repair, mitochondrial dysfunction, increased intracellular reactive oxygen species, alterations in neurotransmitter signalling and ectopic firing in primary afferents [34]. In addition, a common mechanism appears to be changes in ion channel expression and function. Several studies have demonstrated modulation of the Na^+, K^+, Ca^{2+} as well as the Transient Receptor Potential (TRP) channels by different chemotherapeutic drugs contributing to neuronal excitation [35]. Such mechanisms of chemotherapy-induced neurotoxicity can lead to peripheral nerve degeneration and loss of intraepidermal nerve fibers (IENFs), which has been characterised for multiple chemotherapeutic agents, including paclitaxel, oxaliplatin and bortezomib [24, 36 - 38]. Nerve degeneration in CIPN is mostly attributed to distal axonopathy, the disruption of normal axonal function and transport in a retrograde manner, which correlates closely with commonly reported peripheral sensory symptoms [38]. In instances where nerve damage is limited, axons may be able to repair or regenerate, explaining why many patients eventually recover from sensory symptoms following treatment completion or cessation [2]. However, aside from axonopathy, neuronopathy can also result from direct toxicity of chemotherapy drugs to DRG neuronal cell bodies, potentially leading to permanent axonal damage and long-term CIPN symptoms [2]. Axonal dysfunction is supported by electrophysiological studies, which have detected decreased nerve conduction velocity in experimental models [38 - 40]. However, although decreased conduction velocity is typical in CIPN, one study found increased afferent nerve conduction, suggesting that these measures may not necessarily be accurate indicators of neuropathy [41].

Interestingly, in some cases of chronic neuropathy induced by oxaliplatin or paclitaxel, severe mitochondrial dysfunction, observed as atypical vacuolated mitochondria in primary afferent neurons, has been demonstrated in the absence of evidence of axonal degeneration or apoptosis [24, 25, 42]. Sensory symptoms including pain and loss of sensation might therefore be explained by axonal transport disturbances resulting from mitochondrial dysfunction in DRG neurons. Mitochondrial dysfunction is closely associated with oxidative stress, a process that promotes the production of pro-inflammatory mediators [43]. Interestingly, patients receiving chemotherapy, particularly oxaliplatin, often report a phase of acute pain immediately following treatment, which may transition into a chronic pain state, although distinct mitochondrial abnormalities in animal models are not detectable until a week following treatment [3, 42]. Together, these findings suggest that other mechanisms of pain induction may be of interest, and given the association between mitochondrial dysfunction and inflammation, peripheral neuro-inflammatory processes may be significant in CIPN development.

2.2. Effects of Chemotherapy on Muscle

There is a high incidence of skeletal muscle wasting in cancer patients receiving chemotherapy treatment, and CIPN patients often experience muscle weakness and fatigue that coexists with their neurological symptoms [4, 19 - 21, 44, 45]. Although chemotherapy agents have been associated with numerous side effects including nausea and anorexia, these symptoms cannot fully account for the changes in muscle mass characterised following treatment [12, 16, 46]. Interestingly, a few novel clinical studies have supported the physical benefits of exercise for skeletal muscle fatigue and weakness following chemotherapy treatment [47, 48]. One study found that biomarkers of muscle degradation were upregulated in cancer patients after chemotherapy treatment [47], while another investigation found that chemotherapy alters mitochondrial gene expression, a potential mechanism which will be discussed further in relation to chemotherapy-induced inflammation [48]. However, similar to CIPN, the current understanding of the effects of chemotherapy on skeletal muscle is predominantly attributable to the development of pre-clinical experimental animal models.

2.2.1. Animal Models

Animal models have confirmed that chemotherapy can directly induce muscle atrophy in healthy, non-tumour-bearing hosts [10 - 16]. Antineoplastic agents also elicit muscle weakness and fatigue in mice, indicated by overall reduced contractile force of hindlimb muscles [49]. A study by Damrauer *et al.* [12] verified that substantial muscle atrophy, denoted by decreased myofiber size and overall weight loss, could be induced within 5-10 days of cisplatin administration. Interestingly, this effect was not limited to cisplatin, and was also evident after treatment with the topoisomerase inhibitors doxorubicin, irinotecan and etoposide, suggesting that similar processes of muscle loss might occur across multiple drug classes [12]. Importantly, chemotherapy has been demonstrated to promote catabolic downstream effects, with administration in healthy and tumour-bearing rats disrupting protein metabolism and up-regulating pro-atrophic gene expression [15, 50].

As mentioned, cancer cachexia, a progressive paraneoplastic wasting syndrome characterised by loss of lean body mass and fat, may actually be exacerbated by chemotherapy use [12, 13]. Cancer cachexia is hypothesised to result from systemic inflammation characterised by the excessive production of pro-inflammatory cytokines due to the host-tumour interaction [51]. Although patient studies reveal correlations between chemotherapy use and cachexia, they are ultimately quite limited as no direct causality can be inferred due to complex interactions between the host, tumour and treatment factors; the contribution of chemotherapy alone has not been clearly delineated in this setting [19, 21, 44, 45]. Therefore, although the relationship between chemotherapy and cancer cachexia remains unclear based on clinical data, animal studies have indicated that chemotherapy does contribute to muscle wasting in tumour-bearing hosts, irrespective of tumour burden reduction [12, 13]. In a model investigating docetaxel use in tumour-bearing mice, the overall tumour weight decreased significantly, but muscle loss persisted, particularly with higher drug dosages, and was even more extensive than in the untreated tumour-bearing mice [13]. Although the mechanisms by which chemotherapy might contribute to, or even have an additive effect on muscle wasting in this context remain unknown, there may be some similarities between chemotherapy-induced and cancer-induced cachexia. In fact, this is a concept that has recently been validated by a proteomics-based study which compared differential protein expression in two separate experimental mouse models: the colon-26 (C26) carcinoma model of cancer cachexia and a model of combination chemotherapy-induced muscle wasting using Folfiri (5-fluorouracil, leucovorin and CPT-11), a colorectal cancer treatment [10]. Interestingly, 240 proteins were differentially expressed in skeletal muscle across both of these models, and mitochondrial dysfunction was also common to both experimental conditions. Therefore, as in CIPN, evidence from this study and others supports a role of mitochondrial dysfunction and inflammation in chemotherapy-induced muscle atrophy [10, 11, 52].

3. CHEMOTHERAPY AND INFLAMMATION

Inflammation is a significant contributor to pain in peripheral nerve injury, diabetic neuropathy and inflammatory neuropathy, and may also play a role in CIPN pathogenesis and downstream functional effects [53 - 55]. Most recently, studies suggest that chemotherapy induces neurotoxicity through oxidative stress and impairment of mitochondrial function, processes that have also been implicated in chemotherapy-induced muscle atrophy, and can lead to the production of pro-inflammatory mediators such as cytokines and reactive oxygen species [11, 24 - 26, 52, 56]. The following discussion will draw upon relevant clinical and experimental animal studies.

3.1. Cytokines

Chemotherapy administration can contribute to systemic inflammation, including increased serum levels of the pro-inflammatory cytokines tumour necrosis factor-alpha (TNF-α), interleukin-1-beta (IL-1β) and interleukin-6 (IL-6) [57 - 61]. An investigation into chemotherapy-associated cognitive impairment revealed upregulation of these same pro-inflammatory cytokines in breast cancer patients following chemotherapy, suggesting involvement in other chemotherapy-related side effects [57]. Furthermore, given that many cancer patients already have higher pre-chemotherapy serum levels of pro-inflammatory cytokines such as TNF-α, when compared to healthy controls, these findings strongly support a role of chemotherapy in modulating systemic markers of inflammation [62, 63].

In relation to CIPN, studies have found increased levels of pro-inflammatory cytokines in the DRG and spinal cord of chemotherapy-treated rodents [25, 32]. Meanwhile, although the role of cytokines in peripheral neuropathic pain after nerve injury is well characterised, few studies have focused exclusively on CIPN [5]. Importantly, cytokines can cause neuropathic pain (e.g. hyperalgesia) through direct receptor-mediated activity or indirectly, via downstream mediators such as prostaglandins [64, 65]. Following chemotherapy administration, alterations in cellular neuro-immune responses could therefore explain the induction of an acute pain state. Most significantly, studies of paclitaxel-induced peripheral neuropathy have revealed an increase in the number of activated macrophages in the DRG, peripheral nerves and Schwann cells following paclitaxel administration, along with upregulated activating transcription factor 3 (ATF3), a marker of nerve injury [66, 67]. Macrophage infiltration may lead to the subsequent production and secretion of cytokines, chemokines and other inflammatory mediators including prostaglandins and nitric oxide [27]. The importance of this cellular response in pain development is supported by a study in which inhibition of macrophage function by clodronate leads to decreased TNF-α expression, inhibition of neuronal apoptosis and reduced mechanical hypersensitivity [33]. Furthermore, anti-TNF-α antibody treatment was protective against neuropathy induced by bortezomib, while IL-6 neutralising antibodies attenuated pain and IL-6 knockout mice were more resistant to neuropathy caused by the vinca alkaloid vincristine [68, 69]. Together, these findings demonstrate that cytokines may potentially play a major role in CIPN-related pain and hypernociception.

Contrastingly, some studies have suggested that cytokines may instead play a role in nerve repair and regeneration following chemotherapy administration. Interestingly, IL-6 has been associated with nerve fiber repair and had a neuroprotective effect in a comparative study across three CIPN models using the drugs paclitaxel, oxaliplatin or vincristine [29]. However, since IL-6 can have pro-inflammatory and anti-inflammatory effects through interactions with membrane receptors, including the gp130/IL-6 receptor complex, its role in CIPN requires further investigation. Aside from macrophages, Schwann cells can also act as a potential source of cytokines, but instead may produce anti-inflammatory interleukin-10 (IL-10) in an attempt to protect nerve axons from additional damage [27]. In fact, intravenous injection of IL-10 attenuated paclitaxel-induced peripheral neuropathy by suppressing the expression of TNF-α and IL-1β in the DRG [32]. Based on this evidence, a conceivable hypothesis is that chemotherapy can offset the balance between pro-inflammatory and anti-inflammatory mediators, leading to the characteristic features of CIPN and associated neuropathic pain.

Furthermore, increased gene and protein expression of pro-inflammatory cytokines have also been detected in skeletal muscle tissues following the administration of various chemotherapy agents. Docetaxel, a microtubule-targeting taxane drug, induced muscle atrophy and a three-fold increase in IL-6 protein expression relative to TNF-α in the gastrocnemius muscles of healthy mice [13]. While IL-6 is a chief mediator of muscle wasting in cancer cachexia, these findings also support a role of IL-6 in chemotherapy-induced muscle atrophy [17, 18, 70]. Furthermore, one study using the combination chemotherapy CAF (cyclophosphamide, doxorubicin, 5-fluorouracil) in non-tumour-bearing mice identified glucocorticoid signaling as a critical intermediary in chemotherapy-induced muscle atrophy, and detected upregulation of both systemic and local cytokine-associated inflammation [14]. Additionally, cisplatin-induced skeletal muscle atrophy was associated with increased nuclear factor-kappa B (NF-kB) activation, which is another crucial molecular pathway that has been characterized in cancer-induced cachexia, regulating the production and elaboration of cytokines [12]. It is therefore possible that chemotherapy modulates cytokine levels in both PNS and skeletal muscle tissues, although the role of cytokines in eliciting these neuromuscular effects remains unclear.

3.2. Reactive Oxygen Species

Reactive oxygen species (ROS) are generated primarily from mitochondria during normal cellular respiration and energy metabolism [56]. However, studies have revealed that chemotherapy can modulate ROS production in peripheral tissues, leading to oxidative stress and inflammation, processes that potentially play an important role in the development of chemotherapy-associated neuromuscular effects. Although oxidative stress is a crucial mechanism through which anti-cancer compounds induce cell death, it may also be involved in the collateral effects evident in PNS and skeletal muscle tissues [26]. In relation to CIPN, studies reveal that platinum agents can induce the production of ROS in sensory neurons, which occurs in a dose-dependent manner [71, 72]. Meanwhile, resulting ROS can directly sensitise primary afferent neurons to pain, which is partially attenuated by the addition of antioxidants in models of taxane and platinum-induced neuropathy [43, 56]. However, lack of complete pain reduction by antioxidants in experimental and clinical settings supports the involvement of other mediators, including pro-inflammatory cytokines [43, 56, 73]. Interestingly, in culture, superoxide species oxidise proteins and induce macrophage production of TNF-α, supporting the hypothesis that cytokines and ROS may act synergistically to cause inflammation and downstream molecular alterations in neuropathy [74].

Furthermore, oxidative stress has been closely associated with skeletal muscle fatigue and atrophy attributed to chemotherapy administration [52, 75]. In fact, mitochondrial depletion in association with muscle loss has been characterised in response to the combination chemotherapy treatments Folfox (5-fluorouracil, leucovorin, oxaliplatin) and Folfiri (5-fluorouracil, leucovorin, irinotecan) in non-tumour-bearing mice, and may result from oxidative stress [11]. Indeed, since skeletal muscle is a highly metabolic tissue that relies heavily upon mitochondrial function, disruption of normal cellular respiration may lead to fatigue and atrophy [76]. Doxorubicin treatment is known to increase ROS production, and in addition to a direct association with mitochondrial damage and dysfunction, ROS can also act as signaling molecules to activate various proteolytic pathways in skeletal muscle, including calpain and caspase-3 pathways [52]. Again, these characteristic responses are not necessarily specific to one drug class, as oxaliplatin also increases mitochondrial ROS production, and was shown to reduce both cell and mitochondrial viability in a C2C12 myotube cell culture model [76]. Finally, since skeletal muscle involvement has been characterised across multiple drug classes, increased ROS production and inflammation may not be dependent on any particular mode of drug action.

4. INFLAMMATION-ASSOCIATED MOLECULAR PATHWAYS OF INTEREST

There is the possibility of some reciprocal interplay between mitochondrial dysfunction and inflammation. In fact, although mitochondrial dysfunction may result directly from the damaging effects of pro-inflammatory cytokines and ROS, it is equally possible that mitochondrial dysfunction contributes to progressive inflammation [27]. Importantly, while proinflammatory cytokines and ROS may play a pertinent role in initiating chemotherapy-associated neuromuscular effects, these mediators can modulate downstream signaling molecules, which may represent suitable candidate targets for therapeutic intervention. Additionally, elucidation of the molecular pathways altered by chemotherapy in peripheral tissues will contribute to a better understanding of the mechanisms responsible for these side effects, which currently remain unclear. For the purpose of the following discussion, the focus will be on key molecular candidates in paclitaxel-induced neuromuscular effects.

4.1. Upstream Inflammatory Signaling Pathways

There is a compelling evidence for a role of toll-like receptor 4 (TLR4) in paclitaxel-induced peripheral neuropathy [33, 77 - 79]. TLR4 is activated by ROS in the DRG of paclitaxel-treated rats, and TLR4 antagonists can reduce mechanical hypersensitivity and block pain in rodent models [33, 79]. Another study involving TLR4 knockout mice found that animals without receptor expression were resistant to stress-induced neuroinflammation [80]. Interestingly, TLR4 activation may be closely associated with cytokine production, potentially leading to signaling events that engage other important downstream pathways involved in CIPN and muscle atrophy. In fact, there may even be some overlap with regards to the molecular changes occurring in response to chemotherapy in skeletal muscle and PNS tissues. Although the role of IL-6 is still unclear, upregulation of the Janus Kinase/Signal Transducer and Activator of Transcription 3 (JAK/STAT3) pathway, a major downstream mediator of IL-6 signaling, could be involved in taxane-induced neuromuscular symptoms. The STAT3 pathway, which signals from the cell surface to the nucleus in response to cytokines, is activated in spinal cord glial cells after nerve injury, and contributes to neuropathic pain, which can be attenuated by blockade with Suppressor of

Cytokine Signaling 3 (SOCS3) [81, 82]. Although inflammatory responses to paclitaxel have not been properly characterised in peripheral tissues, paclitaxel does induce IL-6 gene expression in ovarian cancer cell lines [83]. Furthermore, docetaxel, a taxane agent with a similar mechanism of action to paclitaxel, induced muscle atrophy and upregulated IL-6 protein expression in the gastrocnemius muscles of healthy mice [13]. This finding is particularly noteworthy, as muscle atrophy due to cancer cachexia is mediated by IL-6/JAK/STAT3 signaling, suggesting that there may be some parallels between cancer and chemotherapy-induced molecular alterations [17, 18, 51].

4.2. Endoplasmic Reticulum Stress

Endoplasmic reticulum (ER) stress, also known as the unfolded protein response (UPR), is a conserved eukaryotic process activated in the presence of unfolded and defective proteins [84]. When protein homeostasis cannot be restored, the UPR activates pro-apoptotic pathways and downregulates protein translation [85]. The ER stress response is of recent interest in relation to CIPN, with animal models demonstrating a connection between inflammation, oxidative stress and the UPR in the PNS [84, 86 - 88]. Since the induction of ER stress may be closely related to inflammatory responses, this could represent a viable downstream mechanism through which neuropathy is sustained after chemotherapy use. Importantly, paclitaxel can disrupt calcium signaling within the ER and mitochondria of cells [89]. Another study demonstrated that paclitaxel treatment elevates a number of ER stress markers *in vitro*, including C/EBP homologous protein (CHOP) and phosphorylated eIF2α, leading to caspase 3 and 4 activation [86]. However, despite this preliminary evidence, ER stress mechanisms need to be further explored *in vivo* and also in the context of skeletal muscle effects.

4.3. Paclitaxel-Specific Molecular Alterations

Aside from well-characterised inflammation-associated molecular alterations, and novel candidate molecular responses such as ER stress, which could potentially represent common targets across a variety of chemotherapy classes, drug-specific mechanisms can simultaneously contribute to functional effects, and should therefore be considered. Taxane compounds including paclitaxel and docetaxel primarily target microtubules, leading to microtubule stabilisation, polymerisation and disruption of cytoskeletal dynamics [2]. Based on this mechanism, one clinical study investigated the potential association between neuropathy incidence and gene variants in cancer patients by focusing on two relevant molecules: Microtubule-Associated Protein Tau (MAPT) and glycogen synthase kinase 3-beta (GSK3β) [90]. The MAPT protein is a cytoskeletal protein involved in microtubule assembly, and actually occupies the same binding site on beta-tubulin as paclitaxel [91]. Meanwhile, GSK3β is a protein kinase involved in MAPT phosphorylation [92]. Interestingly, polymorphisms in *GSK3B* but not *MAPT* were found to be associated with paclitaxel-induced peripheral neuropathy incidence in this patient cohort [90]. Furthermore, in both mice and rat models, inhibition of GSK3β protein activity by lithium attenuated paclitaxel-induced neuropathic pain [92, 93]. Therefore, although GSK3β is also closely associated with pathways involved in inflammation, it is clear that drug-associated molecular changes are another important consideration when targeting chemotherapy-induced neuromuscular effects. However, since few studies have actually examined the molecular alterations instigated by chemotherapy, instead focusing on morphological and physiological alterations, further investigation into candidate pathways of interest is required.

5. GENETIC SUSCEPTIBILITY TO CHEMOTHERAPY-INDUCED NEUROMUSCULAR EFFECTS

The significant inter-individual variability in CIPN incidence, severity, onset and progression suggests that host genetic factors may also play a role in the development of chemotherapy-induced neuromuscular effects [3, 4]. Of recent interest is the potential association between gene polymorphisms and neuropathy incidence as way of identifying individuals who might be at risk of developing CIPN. This is particularly important, as no definitive biomarkers have been identified to detect high-risk patients [3]. Predictive biomarkers for neuropathy associated with the use of certain chemotherapy drugs could potentially lead to the avoidance of serious, long-term neurotoxicity through pre-treatment modification in high-risk individuals.

Single Nucleotide Polymorphisms (SNPs) are the most common type of genetic variation among humans, and can be functionally important when they impact upon gene regulation and protein expression [94]. Consequently, both Genome-Wide Association Studies (GWAS) and focused candidate gene approaches have attempted to identify SNPs that may be associated with, or potentially play a role in, CIPN development. Notably, a bioinformatics study performing gene pathway analysis of numerous previous clinical investigations indicated that polymorphisms in inflammation-associated genes including *IL6, TNF, IL1B, STAT1, STAT3* and *IFNG* were most strongly associated with platinum-induced neuropathy [95]. Meanwhile, *TNF, P38 MAPK, PARP1* and *MYC* were the top genes associated with combined taxane-platinum-induced neuropathy. Along with genes related to cell growth, differentiation and inflammation, genes involved in DNA repair and oxidative stress were also associated with taxane and platinum-induced neuropathy [95]. These findings correlate with studies of pain in cancer patients, where SNPs in immune-response genes were shown to influence pain severity, and also support evidence in the literature, which implicates inflammation as a crucial process in chemotherapy-associated pathologies [96]. Furthermore, SNPs related to the specific mechanism of action of chemotherapy drugs have also been investigated. As mentioned, polymorphisms in *GSK3B* have previously been associated with paclitaxel-induced neuropathy [90]. Additionally, SNPs in the drug transporter genes *ABCC1* and *ABCC2* as well as voltage-gated sodium channels were associated with severe neurotoxicity in colorectal cancer patients receiving Folfox chemotherapy [97, 98]. Similarly, several SNPs in the *ABCB1* transporter and the cytochrome p450 enzymes *CYP3A4* and *CYP2C8*, which metabolise paclitaxel, have been associated with paclitaxel-induced sensory neuropathy [99 - 103].

Despite the growing use of GWAS in order to screen for genetic loci associated with CIPN, such studies are often statistically underpowered due to small sample sizes and the need to adjust for multiple testing [99, 104, 105]. Furthermore, these studies typically identify risk-alleles with only very small effect sizes, and generally no casual relationships can be determined. Since it is unclear whether isolated genetic variants can have a significant impact on CIPN risk, candidate gene pathway approaches may still therefore be useful in order to more comprehensively investigate gene variants and study rare SNPs. Finally, future studies using methodologies such as Next Generation Sequencing (NGS) in conjunction with candidate gene approaches may better inform an understanding of the complex pathophysiological mechanisms related to the development of CIPN and other treatment-associated effects such as muscle wasting.

6. CANCER-INDUCED AND CHEMOTHERAPY-INDUCED EFFECTS

The relationship between cancer-induced and chemotherapy-induced peripheral tissue effects is complex and not well understood. Fig. (**1**) summarizes the proposed common mechanisms of cancer and chemotherapy in peripheral tissues, involving the effects of inflammation on both skeletal muscle and the PNS. Unfortunately, the current understanding of the molecular and cellular alterations that occur in response to chemotherapy in the treatment setting is relatively limited, as studies have predominantly investigated peripheral effects in models using non-tumour-bearing rodents treated with chemotherapy. Therefore, the contribution of tumour-derived inflammation needs to be properly investigated by assessing functional and molecular changes in experimental models featuring chemotherapy administration in tumour-bearing rodents. In support of this, a recent study revealed that chemotherapy and cancer can induce similar molecular changes in skeletal muscle, indicating that future investigations are required to determine whether synergistic alterations in cellular signaling pathways might occur in response to the combination of cancer and treatment factors [10].

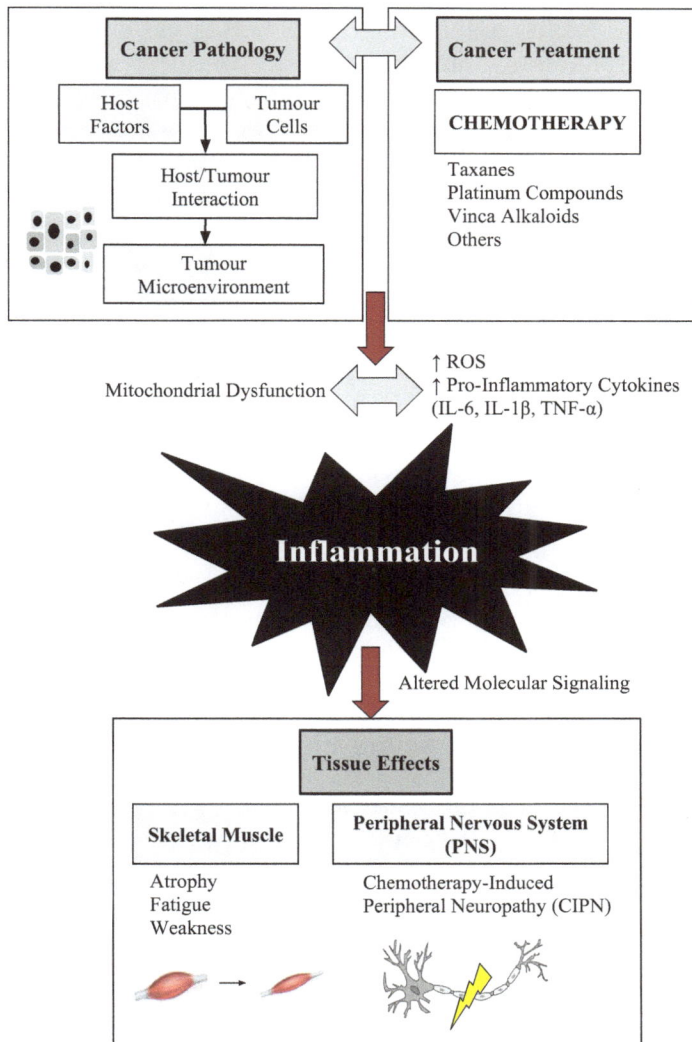

Fig. (1). Proposed contribution of cancer and chemotherapy to systemic inflammation and skeletal muscle and peripheral nervous system effects. Both cancer-related factors and chemotherapy treatment contribute to inflammation. Inflammation may involve the reciprocal interplay between mitochondrial dysfunction and the production of pro-inflammatory cytokines and Reactive Oxygen Species (ROS). Altered cellular molecular signaling downstream of these inflammatory mediators contributes to skeletal muscle and Peripheral Nervous System (PNS) effects, including muscle atrophy and Chemotherapy-Induced Peripheral Neuropathy (CIPN).

7.   RECENT   DEVELOPMENTS   IN   THE   TARGETING   OF CHEMOTHERAPY-INDUCED NEUROMUSCULAR EFFECTS

Extensive clinical and experimental investigation is being undertaken in order to discover successful strategies for the prevention and treatment of CIPN. As mentioned previously, despite numerous studies with a variety of drugs including antioxidants, growth factors, anticonvulsants, antidepressants and dietary supplements, there are currently no effective treatment options available that significantly reduce the severity of symptoms in patients with CIPN [3, 23]. Likewise, numerous candidate preventative treatments have been tested in either preclinical rodent models or patient cohort studies, including calcium, magnesium, vitamin E, glutamine, glutathione, *N*-acetylcysteine and lithium [93, 106 - 110]. However, despite these investigations, there is still a lack of sufficient evidence to recommend the use of any of these agents in the clinical setting. Instead, CIPN is generally managed through treatment modification, including dose reduction, increased intravenous dose infusion time and increased time between doses [111]. Unfortunately, in severe cases, cessation of treatment is sometimes required, which may compromise the anti-cancer effects of the treatment, reducing the overall success of potentially curative chemotherapy regimes. Some symptomatic treatments can be administered to manage pain and related symptoms, including non-steroidal anti-inflammatory drugs (NSAIDs), opioids, antidepressant agents such as duloxetine and antiepileptic drugs such as pregabalin [112]. The most promising intervention to date is the use of duloxetine, a neuronal serotonin and norepinephrine reuptake inhibitor [113]. In a Phase 3 randomized, double-blind, placebo-controlled trial, 30 mg of duloxetine daily taken over 5 weeks contributed to a significant reduction in pain in cancer patients with chemotherapy-induced sensory neuropathy [113].

Since there is still a clear unmet medical need for novel treatment options, numerous drug-related discoveries for the targeting of neuropathic pain and other sensory symptoms associated with CIPN have been patented in the past few years (Table 2) [114 - 127]. However, since the association between chemotherapy use and skeletal muscle atrophy is still relatively novel, very few patents have been developed specific to chemotherapy-induced muscle wasting. Together, these patents cover a wide range of drug types, including novel cyclic compounds, receptor antagonists, natural herbal derivatives, dietary supplements and mixed compositions. Although some of these patents are based upon the targeting of specific candidate mechanisms implicated in CIPN development, as derived from experimental studies, many are patents for drug-screening studies of newly designed compounds, which are being tested not only for CIPN, but also across a range of other conditions (Table 2).

Interestingly, over the past decade, a number of patents related to the targeting of inflammation-associated mediators and signaling pathways have been published. Most recently, targeting of the chemokine receptor CXCR2, a receptor for interleukin-8 (IL-8), by using selective receptor antagonists, has been patented as a prospective strategy for the treatment and prevention of CIPN, based on the putative role of pro-inflammatory mediators such as chemokines and cytokines in the induction of pain and sensory dysfunction [114]. Similarly, an older patent also grounded upon the role of pro-inflammatory signalling in CIPN pathogenesis involved the administration of a soluble IL-6 Receptor (sIL-6R)/IL-6 chimeric complex for the treatment of CIPN [128]. Since IL-6 can have pro-inflammatory and anti-inflammatory effects depending on the *in vivo* environmental conditions, this patent proposed that the biological activity of IL-6 when interacting with the sIL-6R may contribute to the survival and regeneration of neuronal cells, thereby representing a potential therapy for patients with neuropathy [128].

Table 2. Recent Patents Related to the Treatment and Prevention of Chemotherapy-Induced Peripheral Neuropathy and Skeletal Muscle Effects.

Patent Description	Patent Number	Patent Title	References
CIPN			
Using chemokine receptor CXCR2 antagonists for the treatment and/or prevention of CIPN	WO2016016178	Use of CXCR2 antagonists for the prevention and/or treatment of chemotherapy induced peripheral neuropathy (CIPN)	[114]
Inhibiting TLR4 signaling as a preventative or therapeutic option for inflammatory diseases, CIPN and other diseases	US20160326133	Cyclic compounds	[115]
Composition containing jaguen (lithospermi radix) to treat peripheral neuropathy, especially CIPN	WO2016182139	Composition, containing lithospermi radix extract as active ingredient, for preventing, alleviating, or treating peripheral neuropathy	[116]
Administering EPAC inhibitors for the treatment of chronic or neuropathic pain	US20160263088	Methods and compositions for treating chronic pain	[117]
Administering agents that increase NAD+ levels in patients to treat side effects of chemotherapy, including neuropathy	WO2016176437	Targeting NAD+ to treat chemotherapy and radiotherapy induced cognitive impairment, neuropathies and inactivity	[118]
Administering thiosemicarbazone compounds for the treatment of CIPN	US20160151339	Treatment for chemotherapy-induced peripheral neuropathy	[119]
Development of PARP inhibitors for the treatment of CIPN	US20120258180	Parp inhibitors for the treatment of CIPN	[120]
Novel methods and compositions for managing the negative side effects of cancer treatment, including neuropathy	US20160279094	Dietary and natural product management of negative side effects of cancer treatment	[121]

(Table 2) cont.....

Patent Description	Patent Number	Patent Title	References
Use of isothiocyanate derivatives to modulate peripheral pain, including diabetic neuropathy and chemotherapy-induced neuropathy	WO2016162246	Use of isothiocyanate derivatives as modulators of peripheral and neuropathic pain	[122]
Agents containing cysteine and theanine for reducing side effects of chemotherapy, including neuropathy	US20160143871	Agent for alleviating side effects in cancer chemotherapy	[123]
Chemotherapy-Induced Skeletal Muscle Effects			
Administration of flavonoids for the management of chemotherapy-induced muscle loss and alopecia	US20140187624	Method of managing chemotherapy induced alopecia or cachexia or both	[124]
Composition for the treatment and prevention of muscle atrophy related to age/drug treatment/immobilisation and/or cachexia	WO2016166480	Derivatives used in the treatment of muscle atrophy	[125]
Treatment of individuals with cancer or dose-limiting chemotherapy-associated cachexia with GDF 15 modulators combined with an anti-cancer agent	WO2016049470	Methods of reversing cachexia and prolonging survival comprising administering a gdf15 modulator and an anti-cancer agent	[126]
The use of myostatin antagonists such as bimagrumab for the treatment of cancer cachexia and cachexia due to chemotherapy treatment	WO2017081624	Uses of myostatin antagonists, combinations containing them and uses thereof	[127]

As previously mentioned, recent studies implicate TLR4 as a promising molecular candidate in paclitaxel-induced neuropathy. Accordingly, Kobayashi *et al.* [115] have patented an invention for novel cyclic compounds which inhibit TLR4 signaling in order to thoroughly investigate their potential use in the prevention and treatment of CIPN and other inflammatory conditions including ischemia-reperfusion injury. Importantly, the authors of this patent proposed the use of these newly designed TLR4 inhibitors not only for paclitaxel-induced neuropathy, but neuropathy caused by oxaliplatin, and preliminary data shows some promising analgesic properties of some of these compounds [115]. Another interesting recent patent claimed the benefit of using agents that increase nicotinamide adenine dinucleotide (NAD+) levels for the treatment of chemotherapy-induced neuropathy, as well as other cancer treatment-associated effects such as cognitive impairment, inactivity and fatigue [118]. It was proposed that the decline in NAD+ after chemotherapy treatment was related to altered gene expression, mitochondrial dysfunction and reduced metabolic capacity, and could be ameliorated through treatment with NAD+ modifying compounds [118]. This is supported by the previous discussion, which highlights a role of mitochondrial dysfunction and inflammation in chemotherapy-associated effects.

Although few patents have been developed specifically with the interest of targeting chemotherapy-induced muscle atrophy, one invention did involve the administration of procyanidin flavonoid compositions for the treatment of cachexia and alopecia in cancer patients undergoing chemotherapy treatment [124]. Furthermore, another patent for the management of muscle atrophy due to a range of conditions demonstrates the current interest in drug screening for the treatment of various forms of muscle wasting [125]. Finally, despite the lack of targeted designs for chemotherapy-associated cachexia, another patent for the use of biomarkers that are predictive for muscle atrophy across various settings indicates that other methods aside from drug screening are also being investigated in order to improve the current identification and management of treatment-associated side effects [129].

CONCLUSION

In summary, chemotherapy-induced peripheral neuropathy and muscle atrophy represent common side effects of cancer treatment that can significantly affect the quality of life of patients, contributing to impaired mobility and reduced long-term survival. Some potential overarching mechanisms including inflammation and mitochondrial dysfunction have been discussed, and may be relevant to both neuropathic and skeletal muscle effects. However, further elucidation of the mechanisms underlying these neuromuscular effects through experimental models is crucial so that targeted treatment options can be developed for future clinical use.

CURRENT & FUTURE DEVELOPMENTS

Since inflammation is strongly implicated in chemotherapy-induced neuromuscular effects, molecular alterations in peripheral tissues that occur downstream of inflammatory signaling should be investigated in future studies. It is likely that there are both common and drug-specific molecular changes that occur depending on the class of chemotherapy drug and whether it is administered in isolation or in combination. Furthermore, since host genetic factors are also important, future studies will need to more comprehensively investigate candidate gene pathways in order to elucidate the complex mechanisms involved in the development of drug-related toxicities, and to identify biomarkers of patient susceptibility. However, most crucially, to properly understand the pathophysiological basis of these effects, studies need to consider the contribution of both tumour and treatment factors, by using *in vivo* animal models that more closely represent the clinical setting. A number of recent patents in drug development demonstrate the extensive global interest in finding suitable treatments for CIPN, and based on the widespread investigation into the incidence, pathogenesis, prevention and treatment of chemotherapy-induced neuropathic and skeletal muscle effects, effective therapeutic options are readily anticipated in the future.

CONFLICT OF INTEREST

The authors declare no conflict of interest, financial or otherwise.

ACKNOWLEDGEMENTS

This study was supported by the Cancer Institute NSW Translational Program Grant – "Chemotherapy-induced Peripheral Neuropathy: Assessment strategies, Treatment and Risk Factors" (ID # 14/TPG/1-05).

REFERENCES

[1]   Stewart BW, Wild CP. World Cancer Report 2014. Lyon, France: International Agency for Research on Cancer 2014.

[2]   Park SB, Goldstein D, Krishnan AV, *et al.* Chemotherapy-induced peripheral neurotoxicity: A critical analysis. CA Cancer J Clin 2013; 63(6): 419-37.
[http://dx.doi.org/10.3322/caac.21204] [PMID: 24590861]

[3]   Seretny M, Currie GL, Sena ES, *et al.* Incidence, prevalence, and predictors of chemotherapy-induced peripheral neuropathy: A systematic review and meta-analysis. Pain 2014; 155(12): 2461-70.
[http://dx.doi.org/10.1016/j.pain.2014.09.020] [PMID: 25261162]

[4]   Miltenburg NC, Boogerd W. Chemotherapy-induced neuropathy: A comprehensive survey. Cancer Treat Rev 2014; 40(7): 872-82.
[http://dx.doi.org/10.1016/j.ctrv.2014.04.004] [PMID: 24830939]

[5]   Lees JG, Duffy SS, Moalem-Taylor G. Immunotherapy targeting cytokines in neuropathic pain. Front Pharmacol 2013; 4: 142.
[http://dx.doi.org/10.3389/fphar.2013.00142] [PMID: 24319429]

[6]   Bao T, Basal C, Seluzicki C, Li SQ, Seidman AD, Mao JJ. Long-term chemotherapy-induced peripheral neuropathy among breast cancer survivors: Prevalence, risk factors, and fall risk. Breast Cancer Res Treat 2016; 159(2): 327-33.
[http://dx.doi.org/10.1007/s10549-016-3939-0] [PMID: 27510185]

[7]   Hershman DL, Weimer LH, Wang A, *et al.* Association between patient reported outcomes and quantitative sensory tests for measuring long-term neurotoxicity in breast cancer survivors treated with adjuvant paclitaxel chemotherapy. Breast Cancer Res Treat 2011; 125(3): 767-74.
[http://dx.doi.org/10.1007/s10549-010-1278-0] [PMID: 21128110]

[8]   Kidwell KM, Yothers G, Ganz PA, *et al.* Long-term neurotoxicity effects of oxaliplatin added to fluorouracil and leucovorin as adjuvant therapy for colon cancer: Results from National Surgical Adjuvant Breast and Bowel Project trials C-07 and LTS-01. Cancer 2012; 118(22): 5614-22.
[http://dx.doi.org/10.1002/cncr.27593] [PMID: 22569841]

[9]   Argyriou AA, Cavaletti G, Briani C, *et al.* Clinical pattern and associations of oxaliplatin acute neurotoxicity: a prospective study in 170 patients with colorectal cancer. Cancer 2013; 119(2): 438-44.
[http://dx.doi.org/10.1002/cncr.27732] [PMID: 22786764]

[10]   Barreto R, Mandili G, Witzmann FA, Novelli F, Zimmers TA, Bonetto A. Cancer and chemotherapy contribute to muscle loss by activating common signaling pathways. Front Physiol 2016; 7(7): 472.

[PMID: 27807421]

[11]   Barreto R, Waning DL, Gao H, Liu Y, Zimmers TA, Bonetto A. Chemotherapy-related cachexia is associated with mitochondrial depletion and the activation of ERK1/2 and p38 MAPKs. Oncotarget 2016; 7(28): 43442-60.
[http://dx.doi.org/10.18632/oncotarget.9779] [PMID: 27259276]

[12]   Damrauer JS, Stadler ME, Acharryya S, Baldwin AS, Couch ME, Guttridge DC. Chemotherapy-induced muscle wasting: Association with NF-κB and cancer cachexia. Basic Appl Myol 2008; 18: 139-48.

[13]   Wang H, Li TL, Hsia S, Su IL, Chan YL, Wu CJ. Skeletal muscle atrophy is attenuated in tumor-bearing mice under chemotherapy by treatment with fish oil and selenium. Oncotarget 2015; 6(10): 7758-73.
[http://dx.doi.org/10.18632/oncotarget.3483] [PMID: 25797259]

[14]   Braun TP, Szumowski M, Levasseur PR, *et al.* Muscle atrophy in response to cytotoxic chemotherapy is dependent on intact glucocorticoid signaling in skeletal muscle. PLoS One 2014; 9(9): e106489.
[http://dx.doi.org/10.1371/journal.pone.0106489] [PMID: 25254959]

[15]   Sakai H, Sagara A, Arakawa K, *et al.* Mechanisms of cisplatin-induced muscle atrophy. Toxicol Appl Pharmacol 2014; 278(2): 190-9.
[http://dx.doi.org/10.1016/j.taap.2014.05.001] [PMID: 24823295]

[16]   Chen JA, Splenser A, Guillory B, *et al.* Ghrelin prevents tumour- and cisplatin-induced muscle wasting: Characterization of multiple mechanisms involved. J Cachexia Sarcopenia Muscle 2015; 6(2): 132-43.
[http://dx.doi.org/10.1002/jcsm.12023] [PMID: 26136189]

[17]   Bonetto A, Aydogdu T, Kunzevitzky N, *et al.* STAT3 activation in skeletal muscle links muscle wasting and the acute phase response in cancer cachexia. PLoS One 2011; 6(7): e22538.
[http://dx.doi.org/10.1371/journal.pone.0022538] [PMID: 21799891]

[18]   Bonetto A, Aydogdu T, Jin X, *et al.* JAK/STAT3 pathway inhibition blocks skeletal muscle wasting downstream of IL-6 and in experimental cancer cachexia. Am J Physiol Endocrinol Metab 2012; 303(3): E410-21.
[http://dx.doi.org/10.1152/ajpendo.00039.2012] [PMID: 22669242]

[19]   Prado CM, Baracos VE, McCargar LJ, *et al.* Sarcopenia as a determinant of chemotherapy toxicity and time to tumor progression in metastatic breast cancer patients receiving capecitabine treatment. Clin Cancer Res 2009; 15(8): 2920-6.
[http://dx.doi.org/10.1158/1078-0432.CCR-08-2242] [PMID: 19351764]

[20]   Jung HW, Kim JW, Kim JY, *et al.* Effect of muscle mass on toxicity and survival in patients with colon cancer undergoing adjuvant chemotherapy. Support Care Cancer 2015; 23(3): 687-94.
[http://dx.doi.org/10.1007/s00520-014-2418-6] [PMID: 25163434]

[21]   Antoun S, Borget I, Lanoy E. Impact of sarcopenia on the prognosis and treatment toxicities in patients diagnosed with cancer. Curr Opin Support Palliat Care 2013; 7(4): 383-9.
[http://dx.doi.org/10.1097/SPC.0000000000000011] [PMID: 24189893]

[22]   Bhatnagar B, Gilmore S, Goloubeva O, *et al.* Chemotherapy dose reduction due to chemotherapy induced peripheral neuropathy in breast cancer patients receiving chemotherapy in the neoadjuvant or adjuvant settings: a single-center experience. Springerplus 2014; 3: 366.
[http://dx.doi.org/10.1186/2193-1801-3-366] [PMID: 25089251]

[23]   Wolf S, Barton D, Kottschade L, Grothey A, Loprinzi C. Chemotherapy-induced peripheral neuropathy: Prevention and treatment strategies. Eur J Cancer 2008; 44(11): 1507-15.
[http://dx.doi.org/10.1016/j.ejca.2008.04.018] [PMID: 18571399]

[24]   Xiao WH, Zheng H, Bennett GJ. Characterization of oxaliplatin-induced chronic painful peripheral neuropathy in the rat and comparison with the neuropathy induced by paclitaxel. Neuroscience 2012;

203: 194-206.
[http://dx.doi.org/10.1016/j.neuroscience.2011.12.023] [PMID: 22200546]

[25] Xiao WH, Zheng H, Zheng FY, Nuydens R, Meert TF, Bennett GJ. Mitochondrial abnormality in sensory, but not motor, axons in paclitaxel-evoked painful peripheral neuropathy in the rat. Neuroscience 2011; 199: 461-9.
[http://dx.doi.org/10.1016/j.neuroscience.2011.10.010] [PMID: 22037390]

[26] Gouspillou G, Scheede-Bergdahl C, Spendiff S, *et al.* Anthracycline-containing chemotherapy causes long-term impairment of mitochondrial respiration and increased reactive oxygen species release in skeletal muscle. Sci Rep 2015; 5: 8717.
[http://dx.doi.org/10.1038/srep08717] [PMID: 25732599]

[27] Wang XM, Lehky TJ, Brell JM, Dorsey SG. Discovering cytokines as targets for chemotherapy-induced painful peripheral neuropathy. Cytokine 2012; 59(1): 3-9.
[http://dx.doi.org/10.1016/j.cyto.2012.03.027] [PMID: 22537849]

[28] Gornstein E, Schwarz TL. The paradox of paclitaxel neurotoxicity: Mechanisms and unanswered questions. Neuropharmacology 2014; 76(Pt A): 175-83.

[29] Callizot N, Andriambeloson E, Glass J, *et al.* Interleukin-6 protects against paclitaxel, cisplatin and vincristine-induced neuropathies without impairing chemotherapeutic activity. Cancer Chemother Pharmacol 2008; 62(6): 995-1007.
[http://dx.doi.org/10.1007/s00280-008-0689-7] [PMID: 18270703]

[30] Cata JP, Weng HR, Burton AW, Villareal H, Giralt S, Dougherty PM. Quantitative sensory findings in patients with bortezomib-induced pain. J Pain 2007; 8(4): 296-306.
[http://dx.doi.org/10.1016/j.jpain.2006.09.014] [PMID: 17175202]

[31] Cavaletti G, Cavalletti E, Oggioni N, *et al.* Distribution of paclitaxel within the nervous system of the rat after repeated intravenous administration. Neurotoxicology 2000; 21(3): 389-93.
[PMID: 10894128]

[32] Ledeboer A, Jekich BM, Sloane EM, *et al.* Intrathecal interleukin-10 gene therapy attenuates paclitaxel-induced mechanical allodynia and proinflammatory cytokine expression in dorsal root ganglia in rats. Brain Behav Immun 2007; 21(5): 686-98.
[http://dx.doi.org/10.1016/j.bbi.2006.10.012] [PMID: 17174526]

[33] Zhang H, Li Y, de Carvalho-Barbosa M, *et al.* Dorsal root ganglion infiltration by macrophages contributes to paclitaxel chemotherapy-induced peripheral neuropathy. J Pain 2016; 17(7): 775-86.
[http://dx.doi.org/10.1016/j.jpain.2016.02.011] [PMID: 26979998]

[34] Carozzi VA, Canta A, Chiorazzi A. Chemotherapy-induced peripheral neuropathy: What do we know about mechanisms? Neurosci Lett 2015; 596: 90-107.
[http://dx.doi.org/10.1016/j.neulet.2014.10.014] [PMID: 25459280]

[35] Aromolaran KA, Goldstein PA. [EXPRESS] Ion channels and neuronal hyperexcitability in chemotherapy-induced peripheral neuropathy; cause and effect? Mol Pain 2017; 13: 1744806917714693.
[http://dx.doi.org/10.1177/1744806917714693] [PMID: 28580836]

[36] Boehmerle W, Huehnchen P, Peruzzaro S, Balkaya M, Endres M. Electrophysiological, behavioral and histological characterization of paclitaxel, cisplatin, vincristine and bortezomib-induced neuropathy in C57Bl/6 mice. Sci Rep 2014; 4: 6370.
[http://dx.doi.org/10.1038/srep06370] [PMID: 25231679]

[37] Dougherty PM, Cata JP, Cordella JV, Burton A, Weng HR. Taxol-induced sensory disturbance is characterized by preferential impairment of myelinated fiber function in cancer patients. Pain 2004; 109(1-2): 132-42.
[http://dx.doi.org/10.1016/j.pain.2004.01.021] [PMID: 15082135]

[38] Boyette-Davis J, Xin W, Zhang H, Dougherty PM. Intraepidermal nerve fiber loss corresponds to the

development of taxol-induced hyperalgesia and can be prevented by treatment with minocycline. Pain 2011; 152(2): 308-13.
[http://dx.doi.org/10.1016/j.pain.2010.10.030] [PMID: 21145656]

[39]   Persohn E, Canta A, Schoepfer S, *et al.* Morphological and morphometric analysis of paclitaxel and docetaxel-induced peripheral neuropathy in rats. Eur J Cancer 2005; 41(10): 1460-6.
[http://dx.doi.org/10.1016/j.ejca.2005.04.006] [PMID: 15913989]

[40]   LaPointe NE, Morfini G, Brady ST, Feinstein SC, Wilson L, Jordan MA. Effects of eribulin, vincristine, paclitaxel and ixabepilone on fast axonal transport and kinesin-1 driven microtubule gliding: implications for chemotherapy-induced peripheral neuropathy. Neurotoxicology 2013; 37: 231-9.
[http://dx.doi.org/10.1016/j.neuro.2013.05.008] [PMID: 23711742]

[41]   Chen X, Green PG, Levine JD. Abnormal muscle afferent function in a model of Taxol chemotherapy-induced painful neuropathy. J Neurophysiol 2011; 106(1): 274-9.
[http://dx.doi.org/10.1152/jn.00141.2011] [PMID: 21562188]

[42]   Flatters SJ, Bennett GJ. Studies of peripheral sensory nerves in paclitaxel-induced painful peripheral neuropathy: Evidence for mitochondrial dysfunction. Pain 2006; 122(3): 245-57.
[http://dx.doi.org/10.1016/j.pain.2006.01.037] [PMID: 16530964]

[43]   Di Cesare Mannelli L, Zanardelli M, Failli P, Ghelardini C. Oxaliplatin-induced neuropathy: Oxidative stress as pathological mechanism. Protective effect of silibinin. J Pain 2012; 13(3): 276-84.
[http://dx.doi.org/10.1016/j.jpain.2011.11.009] [PMID: 22325298]

[44]   Barret M, Antoun S, Dalban C, *et al.* Sarcopenia is linked to treatment toxicity in patients with metastatic colorectal cancer. Nutr Cancer 2014; 66(4): 583-9.
[http://dx.doi.org/10.1080/01635581.2014.894103] [PMID: 24707897]

[45]   Zhang G, Li X, Sui C, *et al.* Incidence and risk factor analysis for sarcopenia in patients with cancer. Oncol Lett 2016; 11(2): 1230-4.
[http://dx.doi.org/10.3892/ol.2015.4019] [PMID: 26893724]

[46]   Garcia JM, Scherer T, Chen JA, *et al.* Inhibition of cisplatin-induced lipid catabolism and weight loss by ghrelin in male mice. Endocrinology 2013; 154(9): 3118-29.
[http://dx.doi.org/10.1210/en.2013-1179] [PMID: 23832960]

[47]   Mustian KM, Peoples AR, Peppone LJ, Lin P-J, Janelsins MC, Kleckner I. Effect of exercise on novel biomarkers of muscle damage and cancer-related fatigue: A nationwide URCC NCORP RCT in 350 patients with cancer. J Clin Oncol 2017; 35 (Suppl. 15): 10020.

[48]   Peoples AR, Peppone LJ, Lin P-J, Cole C, Heckler CE, Kleckner I. Effect of exercise on muscle immune response and mitochondrial damage and their relationship with cancer-related fatigue: A URCC NCORP study. J Clin Oncol 2017; 35 (Suppl. 15): 10119-9.

[49]   Gilliam LA, Ferreira LF, Bruton JD, Moylan JS, Westerblad H, St. Clair DK, *et al.* Doxorubicin acts through tumor necrosis factor receptor subtype 1 to cause dysfunction of murine skeletal muscle. J Appl Physiol (1985) 2009; 107(6): 1935-42.

[50]   Le Bricon T, Gugins S, Cynober L, Baracos VE. Negative impact of cancer chemotherapy on protein metabolism in healthy and tumor-bearing rats. Metabolism 1995; 44(10): 1340-8.
[http://dx.doi.org/10.1016/0026-0495(95)90040-3] [PMID: 7476295]

[51]   Shum AM, Mahendradatta T, Taylor RJ, *et al.* Disruption of MEF2C signaling and loss of sarcomeric and mitochondrial integrity in cancer-induced skeletal muscle wasting. Aging (Albany NY) 2012; 4(2): 133-43.
[http://dx.doi.org/10.18632/aging.100436] [PMID: 22361433]

[52]   Sorensen JC, Cheregi BD, Timpani CA, Nurgali K, Hayes A, Rybalka E. Mitochondria: Inadvertent targets in chemotherapy-induced skeletal muscle toxicity and wasting? Cancer Chemother Pharmacol 2016; 78(4): 673-83.

[http://dx.doi.org/10.1007/s00280-016-3045-3] [PMID: 27167634]

[53] Hussain G, Rizvi SA, Singhal S, Zubair M, Ahmad J. Serum levels of TNF-α in peripheral neuropathy patients and its correlation with nerve conduction velocity in type 2 diabetes mellitus. Diabetes Metab Syndr 2013; 7(4): 238-42.
[http://dx.doi.org/10.1016/j.dsx.2013.02.005] [PMID: 24290092]

[54] Wang XM, Hamza M, Wu TX, Dionne RA. Upregulation of IL-6, IL-8 and CCL2 gene expression after acute inflammation: Correlation to clinical pain. Pain 2009; 142(3): 275-83.
[http://dx.doi.org/10.1016/j.pain.2009.02.001] [PMID: 19233564]

[55] Beppu M, Sawai S, Misawa S, *et al.* Serum cytokine and chemokine profiles in patients with chronic inflammatory demyelinating polyneuropathy. J Neuroimmunol 2015; 279: 7-10.
[http://dx.doi.org/10.1016/j.jneuroim.2014.12.017] [PMID: 25669993]

[56] Fidanboylu M, Griffiths LA, Flatters SJ. Global inhibition of reactive oxygen species (ROS) inhibits paclitaxel-induced painful peripheral neuropathy. PLoS One 2011; 6(9): e25212.
[http://dx.doi.org/10.1371/journal.pone.0025212] [PMID: 21966458]

[57] Janelsins MC, Mustian KM, Palesh OG, *et al.* Differential expression of cytokines in breast cancer patients receiving different chemotherapies: Implications for cognitive impairment research. Support Care Cancer 2012; 20(4): 831-9.
[http://dx.doi.org/10.1007/s00520-011-1158-0] [PMID: 21533812]

[58] Cheung YT, Ng T, Shwe M, *et al.* Association of proinflammatory cytokines and chemotherapy-associated cognitive impairment in breast cancer patients: A multi-centered, prospective, cohort study. Ann Oncol 2015; 26(7): 1446-51.
[http://dx.doi.org/10.1093/annonc/mdv206] [PMID: 25922060]

[59] Groves TR, Farris R, Anderson JE, *et al.* 5-Fluorouracil chemotherapy upregulates cytokines and alters hippocampal dendritic complexity in aged mice. Behav Brain Res 2017; 316: 215-24.
[http://dx.doi.org/10.1016/j.bbr.2016.08.039] [PMID: 27599618]

[60] Pusztai L, Mendoza TR, Reuben JM, *et al.* Changes in plasma levels of inflammatory cytokines in response to paclitaxel chemotherapy. Cytokine 2004; 25(3): 94-102.
[http://dx.doi.org/10.1016/j.cyto.2003.10.004] [PMID: 14698135]

[61] Smith LB, Leo MC, Anderson C, Wright TJ, Weymann KB, Wood LJ. The role of IL-1β and TNF-α signaling in the genesis of cancer treatment related symptoms (CTRS): A study using cytokine receptor-deficient mice. Brain Behav Immun 2014; 38: 66-76.
[http://dx.doi.org/10.1016/j.bbi.2013.12.022] [PMID: 24412646]

[62] Krzystek-Korpacka M, Matusiewicz M, Diakowska D, *et al.* Impact of weight loss on circulating IL-1, IL-6, IL-8, TNF-alpha, VEGF-A, VEGF-C and midkine in gastroesophageal cancer patients. Clin Biochem 2007; 40(18): 1353-60.
[http://dx.doi.org/10.1016/j.clinbiochem.2007.07.013] [PMID: 17931612]

[63] Bossola M, Muscaritoli M, Bellantone R, *et al.* Serum tumour necrosis factor-alpha levels in cancer patients are discontinuous and correlate with weight loss. Eur J Clin Invest 2000; 30(12): 1107-12.
[http://dx.doi.org/10.1046/j.1365-2362.2000.00751.x] [PMID: 11122326]

[64] Cunha TM, Verri WA Jr, Silva JS, Poole S, Cunha FQ, Ferreira SH. A cascade of cytokines mediates mechanical inflammatory hypernociception in mice. Proc Natl Acad Sci USA 2005; 102(5): 1755-60.
[http://dx.doi.org/10.1073/pnas.0409225102] [PMID: 15665080]

[65] Ferreira SH, Lorenzetti BB, Bristow AF, Poole S. Interleukin-1 beta as a potent hyperalgesic agent antagonized by a tripeptide analogue. Nature 1988; 334(6184): 698-700.
[http://dx.doi.org/10.1038/334698a0] [PMID: 3137474]

[66] Peters CM, Jimenez-Andrade JM, Kuskowski MA, Ghilardi JR, Mantyh PW. An evolving cellular pathology occurs in dorsal root ganglia, peripheral nerve and spinal cord following intravenous administration of paclitaxel in the rat. Brain Res 2007; 1168: 46-59.

[http://dx.doi.org/10.1016/j.brainres.2007.06.066] [PMID: 17698044]

[67]   Peters CM, Jimenez-Andrade JM, Jonas BM, *et al*. Intravenous paclitaxel administration in the rat induces a peripheral sensory neuropathy characterized by macrophage infiltration and injury to sensory neurons and their supporting cells. Exp Neurol 2007; 203(1): 42-54.
[http://dx.doi.org/10.1016/j.expneurol.2006.07.022] [PMID: 17005179]

[68]   Alé A, Bruna J, Morell M, *et al*. Treatment with anti-TNF alpha protects against the neuropathy induced by the proteasome inhibitor bortezomib in a mouse model. Exp Neurol 2014; 253: 165-73.
[http://dx.doi.org/10.1016/j.expneurol.2013.12.020] [PMID: 24406455]

[69]   Kiguchi N, Maeda T, Kobayashi Y, Kondo T, Ozaki M, Kishioka S. The critical role of invading peripheral macrophage-derived interleukin-6 in vincristine-induced mechanical allodynia in mice. Eur J Pharmacol 2008; 592(1-3): 87-92.
[http://dx.doi.org/10.1016/j.ejphar.2008.07.008] [PMID: 18652822]

[70]   Shum AM, Polly P. Cancer cachexia: Molecular targets and pathways for diagnosis and drug intervention. Endocr Metab Immune Disord Drug Targets 2012; 12(3): 247-59.
[http://dx.doi.org/10.2174/187153012802002910] [PMID: 22385113]

[71]   Jiang Y, Guo C, Vasko MR, Kelley MR. Implications of apurinic/apyrimidinic endonuclease in reactive oxygen signaling response after cisplatin treatment of dorsal root ganglion neurons. Cancer Res 2008; 68(15): 6425-34.
[http://dx.doi.org/10.1158/0008-5472.CAN-08-1173] [PMID: 18676868]

[72]   Kelley MR, Jiang Y, Guo C, Reed A, Meng H, Vasko MR. Role of the DNA base excision repair protein, APE1 in cisplatin, oxaliplatin, or carboplatin induced sensory neuropathy. PLoS One 2014; 9(9): e106485.
[http://dx.doi.org/10.1371/journal.pone.0106485] [PMID: 25188410]

[73]   Areti A, Yerra VG, Naidu V, Kumar A. Oxidative stress and nerve damage: Role in chemotherapy induced peripheral neuropathy. Redox Biol 2014; 2: 289-95.
[http://dx.doi.org/10.1016/j.redox.2014.01.006] [PMID: 24494204]

[74]   Keeney JT, Miriyala S, Noel T, Moscow JA, St Clair DK, Butterfield DA. Superoxide induces protein oxidation in plasma and TNF-α elevation in macrophage culture: Insights into mechanisms of neurotoxicity following doxorubicin chemotherapy. Cancer Lett 2015; 367(2): 157-61.
[http://dx.doi.org/10.1016/j.canlet.2015.07.023] [PMID: 26225838]

[75]   van Norren K, van Helvoort A, Argilés JM, *et al*. Direct effects of doxorubicin on skeletal muscle contribute to fatigue. Br J Cancer 2009; 100(2): 311-4.
[http://dx.doi.org/10.1038/sj.bjc.6604858] [PMID: 19165199]

[76]   Cheregi B, Timpani C, Nurgali K, Rybalka E. Chemotherapy-induced mitochondrial respiratory dysfunction, oxidant production and death in healthy skeletal muscle C2C12 myoblast and myotube models. Neuromuscul Disord 2015; 25: S202.
[http://dx.doi.org/10.1016/j.nmd.2015.06.069]

[77]   Li Y, Adamek P, Zhang H, *et al*. The cancer chemotherapeutic paclitaxel increases human and rodent sensory neuron responses to TRPV1 by activation of TLR4. J Neurosci 2015; 35(39): 13487-500.
[http://dx.doi.org/10.1523/JNEUROSCI.1956-15.2015] [PMID: 26424893]

[78]   Li Y, Zhang H, Kosturakis AK, *et al*. MAPK signaling downstream to TLR4 contributes to paclitaxel-induced peripheral neuropathy. Brain Behav Immun 2015; 49: 255-66.
[http://dx.doi.org/10.1016/j.bbi.2015.06.003] [PMID: 26065826]

[79]   Yan X, Maixner DW, Yadav R, *et al*. Paclitaxel induces acute pain via directly activating toll like receptor 4. Mol Pain 2015; 11: 10.
[http://dx.doi.org/10.1186/s12990-015-0005-6] [PMID: 25868824]

[80]   Cheng Y, Pardo M, Armini RS, *et al*. Stress-induced neuroinflammation is mediated by GSK3-dependent TLR4 signaling that promotes susceptibility to depression-like behavior. Brain Behav

Immun 2016; 53: 207-22.
[http://dx.doi.org/10.1016/j.bbi.2015.12.012] [PMID: 26772151]

[81]   Dominguez E, Mauborgne A, Mallet J, Desclaux M, Pohl M. SOCS3-mediated blockade of JAK/STAT3 signaling pathway reveals its major contribution to spinal cord neuroinflammation and mechanical allodynia after peripheral nerve injury. J Neurosci 2010; 30(16): 5754-66.
[http://dx.doi.org/10.1523/JNEUROSCI.5007-09.2010] [PMID: 20410127]

[82]   Dominguez E, Rivat C, Pommier B, Mauborgne A, Pohl M. JAK/STAT3 pathway is activated in spinal cord microglia after peripheral nerve injury and contributes to neuropathic pain development in rat. J Neurochem 2008; 107(1): 50-60.
[http://dx.doi.org/10.1111/j.1471-4159.2008.05566.x] [PMID: 18636982]

[83]   Wang TH, Chan YH, Chen CW, *et al.* Paclitaxel (Taxol) upregulates expression of functional interleukin-6 in human ovarian cancer cells through multiple signaling pathways. Oncogene 2006; 25(35): 4857-66.
[http://dx.doi.org/10.1038/sj.onc.1209498] [PMID: 16547493]

[84]   Shin YK, Jang SY, Lee HK, *et al.* Pathological adaptive responses of Schwann cells to endoplasmic reticulum stress in bortezomib-induced peripheral neuropathy. Glia 2010; 58(16): 1961-76.
[http://dx.doi.org/10.1002/glia.21065] [PMID: 20830808]

[85]   Kim S, Joe Y, Kim HJ, *et al.* Endoplasmic reticulum stress-induced IRE1α activation mediates cross-talk of GSK-3β and XBP-1 to regulate inflammatory cytokine production. J Immunol 2015; 194(9): 4498-506.
[http://dx.doi.org/10.4049/jimmunol.1401399] [PMID: 25821218]

[86]   Tanimukai H, Kanayama D, Omi T, Takeda M, Kudo T. Paclitaxel induces neurotoxicity through endoplasmic reticulum stress. Biochem Biophys Res Commun 2013; 437(1): 151-5.
[http://dx.doi.org/10.1016/j.bbrc.2013.06.057] [PMID: 23806691]

[87]   Inceoglu B, Bettaieb A, Trindade da Silva CA, Lee KS, Haj FG, Hammock BD. Endoplasmic reticulum stress in the peripheral nervous system is a significant driver of neuropathic pain. Proc Natl Acad Sci USA 2015; 112(29): 9082-7.
[http://dx.doi.org/10.1073/pnas.1510137112] [PMID: 26150506]

[88]   Zhang E, Yi MH, Shin N, *et al.* Endoplasmic reticulum stress impairment in the spinal dorsal horn of a neuropathic pain model. Sci Rep 2015; 5: 11555.
[http://dx.doi.org/10.1038/srep11555] [PMID: 26109318]

[89]   Boehmerle W, Zhang K, Sivula M, *et al.* Chronic exposure to paclitaxel diminishes phosphoinositide signaling by calpain-mediated neuronal calcium sensor-1 degradation. Proc Natl Acad Sci USA 2007; 104(26): 11103-8.
[http://dx.doi.org/10.1073/pnas.0701546104] [PMID: 17581879]

[90]   Park SB, Kwok JB, Loy CT, *et al.* Paclitaxel-induced neuropathy: Potential association of MAPT and GSK3B genotypes. BMC Cancer 2014; 14: 993.
[http://dx.doi.org/10.1186/1471-2407-14-993] [PMID: 25535399]

[91]   Kar S, Fan J, Smith MJ, Goedert M, Amos LA. Repeat motifs of tau bind to the insides of microtubules in the absence of taxol. EMBO J 2003; 22(1): 70-7.
[http://dx.doi.org/10.1093/emboj/cdg001] [PMID: 12505985]

[92]   Gao M, Yan X, Weng HR. Inhibition of glycogen synthase kinase 3β activity with lithium prevents and attenuates paclitaxel-induced neuropathic pain. Neuroscience 2013; 254: 301-11.
[http://dx.doi.org/10.1016/j.neuroscience.2013.09.033] [PMID: 24070631]

[93]   Mo M, Erdelyi I, Szigeti-Buck K, Benbow JH, Ehrlich BE. Prevention of paclitaxel-induced peripheral neuropathy by lithium pretreatment. FASEB J 2012; 26(11): 4696-709.
[http://dx.doi.org/10.1096/fj.12-214643] [PMID: 22889832]

[94]   Bosó V, Herrero MJ, Santaballa A, *et al.* SNPs and taxane toxicity in breast cancer patients.

Pharmacogenomics 2014; 15(15): 1845-58.
[http://dx.doi.org/10.2217/pgs.14.127] [PMID: 25495407]

[95]   Reyes-Gibby CC, Wang J, Yeung SJ, Shete S. Informative gene network for chemotherapy-induced peripheral neuropathy. BioData Min 2015; 8: 24.
[http://dx.doi.org/10.1186/s13040-015-0058-0] [PMID: 26269716]

[96]   Reyes-Gibby CC, Spitz MR, Yennurajalingam S, *et al.* Role of inflammation gene polymorphisms on pain severity in lung cancer patients. Cancer Epidemiol Biomarkers Prev 2009; 18(10): 2636-42.
[http://dx.doi.org/10.1158/1055-9965.EPI-09-0426] [PMID: 19773451]

[97]   Cecchin E, D'Andrea M, Lonardi S, *et al.* A prospective validation pharmacogenomic study in the adjuvant setting of colorectal cancer patients treated with the 5-fluorouracil/leucovorin/oxaliplatin (FOLFOX4) regimen. Pharmacogenomics J 2013; 13(5): 403-9.
[http://dx.doi.org/10.1038/tpj.2012.31] [PMID: 22868256]

[98]   Argyriou AA, Cavaletti G, Antonacopoulou A, *et al.* Voltage-gated sodium channel polymorphisms play a pivotal role in the development of oxaliplatin-induced peripheral neurotoxicity: Results from a prospective multicenter study. Cancer 2013; 119(19): 3570-7.
[http://dx.doi.org/10.1002/cncr.28234] [PMID: 23821303]

[99]   Abraham JE, Guo Q, Dorling L, *et al.* Replication of genetic polymorphisms reported to be associated with taxane-related sensory neuropathy in patients with early breast cancer treated with Paclitaxel. Clin Cancer Res 2014; 20(9): 2466-75.
[http://dx.doi.org/10.1158/1078-0432.CCR-13-3232] [PMID: 24599932]

[100] Sissung TM, Mross K, Steinberg SM, *et al.* Association of ABCB1 genotypes with paclitaxel-mediated peripheral neuropathy and neutropenia. Eur J Cancer 2006; 42(17): 2893-6.
[http://dx.doi.org/10.1016/j.ejca.2006.06.017] [PMID: 16950614]

[101] de Graan AJ, Elens L, Sprowl JA, *et al.* CYP3A4*22 genotype and systemic exposure affect paclitaxel-induced neurotoxicity. Clin Cancer Res 2013; 19(12): 3316-24.
[http://dx.doi.org/10.1158/1078-0432.CCR-12-3786] [PMID: 23640974]

[102] Kus T, Aktas G, Kalender ME, *et al.* Polymorphism of CYP3A4 and ABCB1 genes increase the risk of neuropathy in breast cancer patients treated with paclitaxel and docetaxel. Onco Targets Ther 2016; 9: 5073-80.
[http://dx.doi.org/10.2147/OTT.S106574] [PMID: 27574448]

[103] Lam SW, Frederiks CN, van der Straaten T, Honkoop AH, Guchelaar HJ, Boven E. Genotypes of CYP2C8 and FGD4 and their association with peripheral neuropathy or early dose reduction in paclitaxel-treated breast cancer patients. Br J Cancer 2016; 115(11): 1335-42.
[http://dx.doi.org/10.1038/bjc.2016.326] [PMID: 27736846]

[104] Schneider BP, Li L, Radovich M, *et al.* Genome-wide association studies for taxane-induced peripheral neuropathy in ECOG-5103 and ECOG-1199. Clin Cancer Res 2015; 21(22): 5082-91.
[http://dx.doi.org/10.1158/1078-0432.CCR-15-0586] [PMID: 26138065]

[105] Leandro-García LJ, Inglada-Pérez L, Pita G, *et al.* Genome-wide association study identifies ephrin type A receptors implicated in paclitaxel induced peripheral sensory neuropathy. J Med Genet 2013; 50(9): 599-605.
[http://dx.doi.org/10.1136/jmedgenet-2012-101466] [PMID: 23776197]

[106] Hochster HS, Grothey A, Childs BH. Use of calcium and magnesium salts to reduce oxaliplatin-related neurotoxicity. J Clin Oncol 2007; 25(25): 4028-9.
[http://dx.doi.org/10.1200/JCO.2007.13.5251] [PMID: 17664456]

[107] Kottschade LA, Sloan JA, Mazurczak MA, *et al.* The use of vitamin E for the prevention of chemotherapy-induced peripheral neuropathy: Results of a randomized phase III clinical trial. Support Care Cancer 2011; 19(11): 1769-77.
[http://dx.doi.org/10.1007/s00520-010-1018-3] [PMID: 20936417]

[108] Vahdat L, Papadopoulos K, Lange D, *et al.* Reduction of paclitaxel-induced peripheral neuropathy with glutamine. Clin Cancer Res 2001; 7(5): 1192-7.
[PMID: 11350883]

[109] Cascinu S, Catalano V, Cordella L, *et al.* Neuroprotective effect of reduced glutathione on oxaliplatin-based chemotherapy in advanced colorectal cancer: A randomized, double-blind, placebo-controlled trial. J Clin Oncol 2002; 20(16): 3478-83.
[http://dx.doi.org/10.1200/JCO.2002.07.061] [PMID: 12177109]

[110] Lin PC, Lee MY, Wang WS, *et al.* N-acetylcysteine has neuroprotective effects against oxaliplatin-based adjuvant chemotherapy in colon cancer patients: Preliminary data. Support Care Cancer 2006; 14(5): 484-7.
[http://dx.doi.org/10.1007/s00520-006-0018-9] [PMID: 16450089]

[111] Cavaletti G, Marmiroli P. Chemotherapy-induced peripheral neurotoxicity. Curr Opin Neurol 2015; 28(5): 500-7.
[http://dx.doi.org/10.1097/WCO.0000000000000234] [PMID: 26197027]

[112] Kaley TJ, Deangelis LM. Therapy of chemotherapy-induced peripheral neuropathy. Br J Haematol 2009; 145(1): 3-14.
[http://dx.doi.org/10.1111/j.1365-2141.2008.07558.x] [PMID: 19170681]

[113] Smith EM, Pang H, Cirrincione C, *et al.* Effect of duloxetine on pain, function, and quality of life among patients with chemotherapy-induced painful peripheral neuropathy: A randomized clinical trial. JAMA 2013; 309(13): 1359-67.
[http://dx.doi.org/10.1001/jama.2013.2813] [PMID: 23549581]

[114] Igboko E, Wren PB. Use of CXCR2 antagonists for the prevention and/or treatment of chemotherapy induced peripheral neuropathy (CIPN). WO2016016178, 2016.

[115] Kobayashi T, Saitoh M, Wada Y, *et al.* Cyclic compounds. US20160326133, 2016.

[116] Kim NS, Park J-S, Lee J-M, *et al.* Composition, containing lithospermi radix extract as active ingredient, for preventing, alleviating, or treating peripheral neuropathy. WO2016182139, 2016.

[117] Cheng X, Mei F, Kavelaars A, *et al.* Methods and compositions for treating chronic pain. US20160263088, 2016.

[118] Sinclair DA, Wu L. Targeting NAD$^+$ to treat chemotherapy and radiotherapy induced cognitive impairment, neuropathies and inactivity. WO2016176437, 2016.

[119] Ghanbari HA, Jiang Z. Treatment for chemotherapy-induced peripheral neuropathy. US20160151339, 2016.

[120] Giranda VL, Shoemaker AR, Browman KE, *et al.* Parp inhibitors for the treatment of CIPN. US20120258180, 2012.

[121] Deleyrolle LP, Reynolds BA. Dietary and natural product management of negative side effects of cancer treatment. US20160279094, 2016.

[122] Morazzoni P, Iori R. Use of isothiocyanate derivatives as modulators of peripheral and neuropathic pain. WO2016162246, 2016.

[123] Kurihara S, Tsuchiya T. Agent for alleviating side effects in cancer chemotherapy. US20160143871, 2016.

[124] Bhaskaran S, Vishwaraman M. Method of managing chemotherapy induced alopecia or cachexia or both. US20140187624, 2014.

[125] Raynal SN, Kergoat MR, Autier V, *et al.* Derivatives used in the treatment of muscle atrophy. WO2016166480, 2016.

[126] Gyuris J, Lerner L, Lin J. Methods of reversing cachexia and prolonging survival comprising administering a gdf15 modulator and an anti-cancer agent. WO2016049470, 2016.

[127] Klickstein LB, Roubenoff R, Feige J, *et al.* Uses of myostatin antagonists, combinations containing them and uses thereof. WO2017081624, 2017.

[128] Revel M, Chebath J, Krug H. IL6R/IL6 chimera for therapy of chemotherapy-induced peripheral neuropathy. US20110274647, 2011.

[129] Reinker S, Roubenoff R, Wang YK, *et al.* Biomarkers predictive of muscle atrophy, method and use. WO2015111008, 2015.

CHAPTER 7

Recent Advances in Nutrigenomics: Patent Applications

Elvan Y. Akyuz[a]**, Ozlem Aytekin**[a]**, Banu Bayram**[a] **and Yusuf Tutar**[a,b,*]

[a] *Nutrition and Dietetics Department, Health Sciences Faculty, University of Health Sciences, Istanbul, Turkey*

[b] *Department of Basic Pharmaceutical Sciences, Division of Biochemistry, Faculty of Pharmacy, Istanbul, Turkey*

Abstract: Nutrition and dietary habits are investigated as environmental factors in cancer development and a strong relationship has been found between diet and cancer. Nutrients affect gene expression, gene regulation and eventually individuals' genome. Genes related to carcinogen metabolism, steroid hormone metabolism and DNA repair are involved in cancer progress. Therefore, it is crucial to understand the factors affecting the change in cancer-related genes. Nutrigenomics is a new multidisciplinary field, investigating the effect of nutrients on genome and its expression through molecular techniques. Nutrigenomics enables to unveil how nutrients regulate cellular metabolism via gene and protein expressions and provide information on the functions of genome. The resulting differences or similarities in gene expressions as response to diets, will enable to understand diet-gene interactions at personalized levels that will implement the concept of personalized nutrition. The genetic variations among individuals will explain the health and disease status of human to be used to determine the cancer risk of individuals. In this chapter, it is aimed to review nutrient-cancer interaction, nutrigenomics approaches and patents related to the implications of nutrigenomics in cancer treatments.

Keywords: Bioenergetic capacity, cancer, cancer prevention, diagnostics, diet, epigenetics, food components, genome stability, metabolic syndrome, metabolism, nutraceuticals, nutrients, nutrigenomics, nutrition, patent, personalized nutrition, predictive markers, single nucleotide polymorphism, well-being.

1. INTRODUCTION

Cancer is a complicated disease with a high prevalence that threatens human health and decreases the quality of life. There are several therapies for the

** Corresponding author Yusuf Tutar:** Nutrition and Dietetics Department, Health Sciences Faculty, University of Health Sciences, Department of Basic Pharmaceutical Sciences, Division of Biochemistry, Faculty of Pharmacy, Mekteb-i Tibbiye-i Sahane Kulliyesi, Selimiye Mah. Tibbiye Cad. No: 38, 34668 Uskudar, Istanbul, Turkey; Tel: +90 216 418 96 16; Fax: +90 216 418 96 20; E-mail: ytutar@outlook.com

Atta-ur-Rahman and Khurshid Zaman (Eds.)

treatment and prevention of cancer. As the most common method, chemotherapy has many drawbacks such as serious side effects, low response, low efficacy, and poor specificity in cancer treatment. Therefore, alternative techniques have been investigated.

Dietary habits influence cancer risk and tumor behavior. The genome is affected by bioactive food compounds and nutrition. The molecules affect receptors and transcription factors and depending on the nature of the food compound, the interaction alters gene expression. It is estimated that diet influences at least one-third of the cancer cases however, specific components of diet and nutrient-nutrient interaction may provide solid data. Therefore, the interaction of food components with human genome is one of the essential determinants of cancer and current research in this field has provided limited knowledge so far. Technological advancements in omics technologies now enable researchers to detect key molecules at biochemical mechanisms.

Nutrigenomics reveals genomic principles in nutritional researcher and elucidates associations between specific food component and genetic factors. Food components influence gene expression and nutrigenomics identifies molecular mechanism that underlies these genetic predispositions. Eventually, it will be possible to understand the pathogenesis and mechanism of chronic diseases including cancer. The interaction between nutrition, gene expression and metabolism is crucial for the maintenance of health status. Highlighting the "nutrition-genome black box" will be possible through "omics" technologies for the analysis of genome, transcriptome, proteome, and metabolome in dietary intervention studies. The resulting differences or similarities in gene expressions as a response to different diets, will enable to understand the diet-gene interactions at personalized levels. The genetic variations among individuals will explain the health and disease status of human. Further, inherited genetic makeup of individual may lead to different responses to various nutrients and nutrigenomics may reveal this coordination. Databases are common in the field of cancer-drug omics technologies, however, information deposition to databases is new at nutrigenomics research [1].

Personal evaluation of hereditary genetic background as well as individual's transcriptome provide insights into cancer prevention, onset, progression, and therapy. Omics technologies help in understanding molecular mechanism; however, nutrient-nutrient interactions as well as differences in individual's response over food components make nutrigenomic studies complicated. The accumulation of data will be helpful for the clinicians and dietetic practitioners for cancer therapy and will be useful for scientists to understand the molecular mechanisms in detail for dietary interventions. Recent advances in nutrigenomics

- cancer relevant patents were reported in this work.

1.1. Nutrigenomics and its Relation to Cancer

Nutrigenomics focuses on the relationship between a person's diet and genes. Absorption of bioactive food components and their molecular targets can be enhanced by this relationship. Therefore, nutrigenomics benefits from genetics, epigenetics, transcriptomics, proteomics, and metabolomics [2].

The effects of food components on genes have been implicated in cancer risk with different results on individuals. Further, similar dietary habits of individuals may account for different results. Therefore, these suggest that not all individuals respond to diet identically.

Personalized diet may provide dietary change for those individuals at risk and nutrigenomics may provide molecular insights into individual's well-being. Eating behaviors across individuals and its health consequences are investigated in nutrigenomics. Food components may act on individual's health divergently depending on individual's genetic context such as Single-Nucleotide Polymorphisms (SNPs), transcriptome, copy number variation, and epigenetic events by modulating biochemical pathways of human metabolism and increasing the risk of systemic diseases [3].

Food choices and availability differ greatly by cultural and economic factors. Taste perception i.e sugar and fat uptake also determines the food components. Lifestyle and eating habits may also contribute to the composition of food ingredients. Vegan's diet may deficient for some vitamins and minerals and overeating may cause excess triacylglycerol and cholesterol levels in the blood. The deficiency-excess food components may affect gene expression and genome stability through mutations and genomic instability. Furthermore, inherited genome diversity and single nucleotide polymorphisms of ethnic groups are other factors to be considered for nutrigenomics research. Diet and genetic factors may lead to phenotypic changes throughout life. Understanding these mechanisms is crucial to elucidate systematic disease as well as cancer mechanisms. To identify molecular targets of nutrigenomic research, omics technologies underpin solid data. Omics technologies are essential for personalized nutrition since transcriptomic, proteomic, and metabolomic data allow to screen individual's response (failure in response) to dietary intervention strategies. Omics data help to determine an individual's genetic properties and allow defining instead of determining nutritional requirements since all these factors may alter by age, diet preferences, and physical activity. Gathering all omics data will determine an individual's nutritional phenotype and healthy diet plan. Cancer is a disease where biochemical pathways are not working properly. Inherited (mutations, SNPs) or acquired (epigenetic changes) genetic background of an individual is difficult to correct but it is possible to compensate deficiencies by diet intervention strategies [4, 5].

Food components' effect on human metabolism and diseases have been studied and results indicate that the components modify cancer risk and tumor behavior. These diverse food components originate from animal and plant sources. Food industry also introduces modified and packaged food for consumption. Genetically modified plant or animal foods as well as fast foods are part of modern life food consumption. The effect of modified, processed, and animal-plant food on human genome has not been fully studied yet. However, the increase in cancer rates has a good correlation with packed food consumption.

To establish nutritional needs and therapeutic strategies to reduce chronic diseases, genetic susceptibility has been determined for different types of cancers. Array technologies enable the detection of gene expression alteration upon perturbation and food component's effect on individuals can be determined. In cancer, all biochemical pathways are deregulated and molecular targets can be determined by investigating cell proliferation, apoptosis, differentiation, and angiogenesis. Key targets at these pathways are modified by food components but one major disadvantage in determining the molecular mechanism is to determine nutrient-nutrient interaction [6]. Bioactive components may affect multiple pathways as well. One bioactive compound may promote whereas the other may inhibit apoptosis. This may lead to counter effects in dietary therapy and the overall effect results in alteration of gene expression [7, 8].

Cancer finds alternative mechanisms for cell survival using multiple signaling pathways and therefore, diet therapy must evaluate multiple cancer pathways simultaneously. Thus food bioactive compound interaction with genes must be properly evaluated in order to promote better health and reduce the risk of cancer [9].

1.2. Nutrition, Epigenetics, and Genome Stability

All cells have identical genomes in an individual's body, however; each cell has its own unique epigenome. Epigenetic modification mechanisms such as DNA methylation and histone acetylation modulate gene expression through changes in the chromosomes' structure.

In nutrigenomics, epigenetics is an essential mechanism since food bioactive compounds can modify epigenetic mechanism and alter gene expression. Therefore, nutrients may reverse or alter epigenetic mechanisms. It should be noted that tumor suppressor genes are silenced in cancer cells compared to that of the healthy cells [10].

Genome is actively involved in cellular processes during replication and recombination and at this stage, it is susceptible to different damages. Cell maintains DNA stability/fidelity by repair mechanisms and prevents tumor development. Inappropriate nutrient supply can cause genome mutation and alter the expression of genes responsible for genome maintenance. Therefore, deficiencies of micronutrients may cause DNA damage and cancer [11, 12].

1.3. Diet and Cancer Prevention

Only a small percent of human cancers originate from inherited genome but most of the cases originate from mutations and these sporadic events occur because of environmental contaminants and dietary compounds [13]. Researches indicated that certain genes can be regulated by bioactive compounds from the diet and these molecular differences can be used in an individual's diet therapy for cancer prevention. Food components modulate cancer onset and progression which are targets for anticancer treatments [14 - 16]. Anticancer treatment by nutrigenomics strategy can be applied for prevention of cancer. Epigenetic events mediate gene expression and age-increased susceptibility to cancer may develop from an accumulation of these events. These changes are also targets of bioactive compounds. Bioactive compounds mediate nuclear receptors and transcription factors, thus transcriptome of an individual depends on diet and eating habits [17].

To sum up, genetic variations, epigenetic modulations, and interactions among dietary bioactive compounds modulate cancer onset and progress. Therefore, identification of gene targets specific for cell and tissue pathways can help nutrigenomics researchers to develop diagnostic and preventive strategies.

Diet and cancer correlation studies suggest that vegetarian food is usually associated with food but animal based food is usually associated with cancer risk [18, 19]. However, these judgments-correlations must be proved at the molecular level to understand the interaction between biochemical molecules and dietary bioactive compounds. Magnitude and response to bioactive food components are affected by genetic context including SNPs, indels (insertions-deletions), copy number variations, and translocations. Therefore, molecular-level understanding of optimized health benefits by nutrigenomics depends on an individual's genetic background and its interaction with food components.

Interventions based on nutrigenomics have been growing continuously during this last decade. Current efforts on patents over these interventions are reported here. The first three patents covered here based on personalized formulations-nutraceuticals and relationship to genetic properties of an individual. These nutraceuticals improve health and well-being; i. Composition and method to optimize and customize nutritional supplement formulations by measuring genetic and metabolomic contributing factors to disease diagnosis, stratification, prognosis, metabolism, and therapeutic outcomes- US20060062859 [20]; ii: Nutraceutical compositions and methods with biologically active ingredients- US20080317734 [21], iii: Diagnostic system for selecting nutrition and pharmacological products for animals-US7873482 [22].

The genome has not been well characterized and studies are underway to understand it. Nutrition and gene interactions are covered in two consecutive patents. The patents also cover food sensitivity and provide a highlight for the future personalized nutraceuticals: iv. System and method for evaluating and providing nutrigenomic data, information and advice-US7877273 [23], v: Method for determining personalized nutrition and diet using nutrigenomics and physiological data US20100113892 [24], vi: Multi-stage nutrigenomic diagnostic food sensitivity testing in animals US8450072 [25].

Nutrigenomics also elucidates potential markers for cancer and searches for natural products for health improvement. Two patents that cover these topics here are: vii: Predictive markers for cancer and metabolic syndrome US2013045535 [26] and viii: Novel compositions from *Nigella sativa* - US20150004266 [27].

Finally not only genetics but also epigenetic factors are covered and to understand dietary treatment and bioenergetic capacity, important information about metabolic diseases is also provided. Two patents covering these topics are the following: ix: Method of dietary treatment for genetic and epigenetic diseases and disorders- US20170056357 [28] and x: Bioenergetics profiling of circulating blood cells and systems, devices, and methods relating thereto- US2015024795 [29].

1.4. Composition and Method to Optimize and Customize Nutritional Supplement Formulations by Measuring Genetic and Metabolomic Contributing Factors to Disease Diagnosis, Stratification, Prognosis, Metabolism, and Therapeutic Outcomes - US20060062859

To customize individual nutritional supplements to optimize health outcomes, genetic and metabolic factors which affect disease diagnosis, prognosis, and metabolism have been monitored. The aim of the patent is to understand genome response to drugs and nutrients. Completion of human genome remains unrevealed in terms of functionality among health professionals since metabolomics duress may cause critical disease as the condition modify gene expression. Further, epigenetic events and several molecules may also alter gene expression. Specific genes are also expressed differently at the tissue level. Even though two individuals differs only 0.1%, DNA sequences vary at millions of bases. The variants are called SNPs. Certain SNPs have a direct influence on health. And it is known that individuals respond differently to nutraceuticals and medications. Individual's age and health status (liver, kidney function and metabolic competence) mediate the response. Thus, genetic variants, SNPs, and inherited differences in the metabolism as well as disposition of nutrients and drugs, determine clinical variables.

Therefore, nutritional environment formed by dietary compounds influence health by altering an individual's gene expression. Common dietary substances acting on the genome may create a risk for certain genetic diseases on onset, incidence, and progression of the disease. In other terms, diet affects an individual based on his/her genetic makeup. Thus, dietary intervention may be useful for prevention, mitigation, or curing diseases.

This patent provides a novel approach for body recomposition termed as neurogenobolics and healthy body mass management technology by custom nutraceutical formulations based on individual's genes. The patent uses a natural factor to induce recomposition. It has been introduced as unique as it requires sufficient nutrition. The technology provides healthy metabolism for energy management. The ingredients also provide better stress inflammation management along with pleasure/food craving management.

To sum up, the invention replenishes nutritional needs to regulate energy management of biochemical mechanisms, attenuate the effects of chronic stress and inflammation, block food cravings, promote and support immune system, and support neuroendocrine system for healthy weight management. The patent employed nutrigenomics for controlling body weight which is essential for the prevention of systemic diseases such as cancer [20].

1.5. Nutraceutical Compositions and Methods with Biologically Active Ingredients -US20080317734

Another invention tests an individual's blood and nutrient deficiency to formulate necessary vitamins, minerals, antioxidants, growth factors, metabolites, protease, natural extract, and biomolecules. Then, these are encapsulated in nanosome for oral intake. The personalized nutraceutical formulations are based on nutrient deficiencies and improve health function.

SNPs or other mutations may lead to breakdown or inefficient flow of a biological pathway. The result may cause a deficiency in growth factor production or uptake of nutrients. This invention helps in maintaining health and well-being and/or prevents systemic diseases [21].

1.6. Diagnostic System for Selecting Nutrition and Pharmacological Products for Animals - US7873482

An important part of this patent reveals molecular dietary signature based on the genetic profile of animals to reveal nutrition and related genetic makeup. Thus, nutrition-related disorder background can be elucidated to reduce morbidity and mortality and improve the lifespan of the animal. The innovative part of this work is based on nutrition assessment and genetic data but current tests do not provide data for nutrition based disorder predictions. The study selected genes, proteins, and metabolites from animals by array, serial analysis of gene expression, gene sequencing, proteomic and metabolomic assays [22].

1.7. System and Method for Evaluating and Providing Nutrigenomic Data, Information and Advice - US7877273

Development of systems, methods and applications for personalized nutrition/diets, to pursue well-being and implement health in individuals using artificial intelligence methods has gained interest in recent years in order to improve human health.

Nutritional imbalance is associated with a variety of chronic diseases and it is possible to prevent or delay the onset of particular diseases with dietary adjustments. The lifestyle, medical history, and genetic profile of the individuals play important roles in predisposition to diseases. Furthermore, the diet, amounts of micronutrients, macronutrients, and food constituents affect the development of many diseases including heart diseases, diabetes, obesity, osteoporosis as well as cancer. The Patent US7877273 aims to provide nutritional information and recommendations depending on the individual's genetic background, medical history, susceptibility to diseases, behavior, lifestyle, and diet using methods and systems. A system composed of a wireless communication device, remote system and a database was invented to develop a personalized lifestyle database using artificial intelligence and data mining processes. The database includes four main domains including scientific knowledge, genetics, lifestyle, and transactional.

The invention provides food planning, personalized advice for eating and supplementing the individual's diet using information in an individual's database. Through artificial intelligence methods, it is possible to introduce the code of the product to the remote system and provide nutritional information about the product, whether it is advisable for the individuals considering their predisposition to diseases and lifestyle factors. The invention intends to decrease an individual's predisposition for developing a disease. The application program operational on a system, provides information to individuals about the benefits of the food item via its barcode whenever and wherever they need information. Additionally, it is possible to forward this information to the call center where the individual's personal lifestyle database is located. By means of health professionals from the call center or automated systems, recommendations or advice on purchase of the products are provided in terms of side effects, problems or benefits. The methods and systems in this invention also timely remind individuals the intake of medications or supplements that they need and allow the tracking of these supplements.

Knowing the genetic background of the individual provides controlling genes that are linked to specific diseases by specific combinations of various nutrients, bioactive foods, and dietary supplements, also it is probable to manufacture personalized nutraceuticals specific to individuals' unique problems through this invention [23].

Similarly, the patent US20100113892 entitled *"Method for Determining Personalized Nutrition and Diet Using Nutrigenomics and Physiological Data"* has been developed as an e-health intervention based on reducing the likelihood of chronic diseases, where nutrient-gene interactions are involved, by means of personalized nutrition [24]. A nutrigenomic research supermarket with collected nutritional, genetic, clinical, physiological, metabolic and lifestyle information from individuals including health or disease outcomes has been established to be used in personalized nutrition. The purchased food products by individuals can be tracked through barcode or RFID tag systems and the amount of consumed nutrients and their components are recorded to be used in databases. The data carried by barcodes also include nutrigenomic data describing gene-nutrient interactions of the particular products for research purposes. This model may also be used as an evaluation tool of ingredients, food products for food ingredient manufacturers in order to determine their effect on health maintenance and disease management [24].

1.8. Multi-Stage Nutrigenomic Diagnostic Food Sensitivity Testing in Animals - US8450072

The patent is related to food sensitivity testing in animals. Food sensitivity in people may lead to gastrointestinal, neurological, pulmonary, dermatologic, ear, nose and throat, musculoskeletal, genitourinary, cardiovascular and endocrine problems. Animals also have the same clinical problems with food sensitivity [25].

The studies have shown that specialized nutrition intake helps to remain healthy and enhances the life of animals as well. A rapid, commercially useful, practical testing and screening method was developed to determine the sensitivity and intolerance of foods in animals. In the test, firstly saliva and other bodily fluid samples were collected from animals to determine the presence of at least one of IgA or IgM, secondly the presence of at least one of IgA, IgM, IgG or immune complexes were determined from blood samples. The amount or the presence of the antibodies indicates a food sensitivity or intolerance against a specific food ingredient or composition. Finally, a biologically active nutrient from a molecular dietary signature was determined by using the responses of the test. Molecular dietary signature may change according to the animal genotype.

Because of using one ingredient removing technique, classical food sensitivity testing is time consuming. Moreover some of the tests cause to unsightly skin due to injection. Multi-stage nutrigenomic diagnostic food sensitivity testing in animals such as dogs, cats, rabbits, hamsters and horses, diagnoses food sensitivity or intolerance based on the presence of antibodies. The technique is more rapid and easier than classical testing.

In the test, it is possible to predict latent or pre-clinical gastrointestinal disease by detecting IgA and IgM antibodies from saliva to food ingredients. Therefore, 'leaky gut syndrome' or 'inflammatory bowel disease' may be diagnosed before gastrointestinal biopsy. The amounts of immunoglobulins may differ in blood, body fluids and tissues to each animal. Generally, salivary immunoglobulin amounts remain constant in cats. However, it varies daily in dogs. There is a good correlation between blood and saliva concentrations, but it is important to know this correlation for reliability of the test.

By using the diagnostic test system, common allergens and peptides from grains (wheat, corn and soy), meats (mostly beef, fish and other meats), dairy products, eggs, botanicals, seed oils, vegetables and fruits are screened in domestic animals, like dogs or cats, for sensitivity or intolerance to complete pet food or food supplements in dry, semi-dry or wet forms. Also, the diagnostic test system is used to determine the effects of biologically active nutrients on DNA polymorphisms and genomic responses in individual animals.

According to the disclosure, pre-packaged and pre-mixture foods (pet food meals, biscuits, snacks, treats, sprinkles, candies and other forms of foods) are tested to determine which ingredient(s) leads to food sensitivity or intolerance in animals. In the test, there are three test protocols; saliva-based test protocol, serum-based test protocol and DNA/RNA nutrigenomic test protocol. The very practical saliva test protocol can be performed even by the owner of animals easily. Blood serum is needed for serum test protocol and experience is necessary to take blood from the animal. DNA/RNA nutrigenomic test protocol is a very special protocol which is performed to a very limited number of animals in a laboratory.

The test samples of saliva, blood or other bodily fluid are collected by a swab, absorbent paper or straws about 1-5 ml or 1-15 g and portioned to 96-well plate. Common animal food antigens are added to the wells for Enzyme-Linked Immunosorbent Assay (ELISA). Quantitative or semi-quantitative analyses are conducted by Point-of-Service (POS) test kit system to detect IgA, IgM, IgG or immune complexes and the amount of IgA, IgM, IgG or immune complexes in serum, and the amount of IgA or IgM or IgG in saliva is determined against a food ingredient. These reactive immune responses create four different types of food sensitivity or intolerance reactions. Type I is called as immediate hypersensitivity, and IgE antibody is responsible for the reaction. An allergic reaction occurs in 2 hours, after the allergen exposure. Measuring IgE antibody amount is a very costly process to diagnose food sensitivity or intolerance. IgG or IgM antibodies responsible for type II reaction. It is called as delayed hypersensitivity, and an allergic reaction occurs in 2 days to several days. Type III is also called as delayed hypersensitivity. IgG antibody leads to the immune complex at the end of a few reactions. Immune complex in the blood causes blood vessel damages and increases inflammatory process. The allergic reactions occur in days to weeks in type IV, causing granulomatous tissue rejection.

According to the present disclosure, collected samples are screened by ELISA or other immunoassay methods. The amount of IgA or IgG or immune complex in serum samples and the amount of IgA or IgM in saliva, blood spot and other bodily fluid samples are compared with healthy animals' antibodies at the end of the method. The results are assessed as high, normal or lower than normal. Lower than normal levels and normal levels indicate healthy animals, and higher than normal levels indicate food sensitivity or intolerance against food composition containing wheat or other gluten foods, corn, soy, beef or but not limited to other meats, fish, dairy products, eggs, other grains, botanicals, seed oils or fish, botanicals, vegetables, nuts, or fruit, and macro-micro components such as vitamins, amino acids, plants, plant extracts having nutraceutical, therapeutic and functional properties. The amounts of antibodies for healthy and unhealthy animals are shown in Table **1**.

In DNA/RNA nutrigenomic test protocol, two groups of animals (healthy and unhealthy) are fed with a specific nutrient and placebo for a period. Gene variations are determined from blood samples of these two groups. In the test kit, the number of up and down regulated genes is classified according to stress, external stimuli, immune system process and cell communication [25].

1.9. Predictive Markers for Cancer and Metabolic Syndrome - US2013045535

The patent is about using a predictive biomarker for determination of type 2 diabetes, insulin resistance, and cardiovascular disease associated with obesity. It is based on determining the level of SNPs and resulting genetic metabolic syndrome. The first step is to measure the level of protein expressions of FASN, USP2A, GSTΩ1, SOD2, KCNE2 and BNP at the detectable levels *via* immunohistochemical applications. Moreover, determination of blood pressure, Body Mass Index (BMI), and analysis the levels of insulin, blood sugar, triglycerides, HDL, LDL and C-reactive protein were conducted. Variants and the levels of SNPs indicate the recurrence and cancer type. Similarly, the expression of one or more genes consisting of FTO (fat mass and obesity associated) gene, MC4R (melanocortin 4 receptor), TMEM18 (transmembrane protein 18), GNPDA2 (glucosamine6 phosphate deaminase 2), ETV5 (Ets variant 5), BDNF (brain derived neurotrophic factor), SH2B1 (SH2B adapter protein 1), and PCSK1 (proprotein convertase subtilisin/kexin type 1) indicates the recurrence and cancer type.

Table 1. Levels of Antibodies for Healthy and Unhealthy Dog and Cats.

Salivary IgA (U/mL)	Salivary IgM (U/mL)	Tested Animal	Health Condition	Allergy Intensity
10	-	Dog	Healthy	-
25	-	Cat	Healthy	-
-	25	Dog or cat	Healthy	-
15	-	Dog	Unhealthy	Moderate
30	-	Cat	Unhealthy	Moderate
-	35	Dog or cat	Unhealthy	Moderate
20	-	Dog	Unhealthy	Severe
35	-	Cat	Unhealthy	Severe
-	40	Dog or cat	Unhealthy	Severe

A kit was produced to predict the prognostic outcome or response to treatment that includes some of the gene-specific or gene-selective probes and/or primers for measuring the expression levels of related gen and/or genes (*e.g.*, one or more genes from the GPEPs or FASN).

In the test, firstly DNA was extracted from Caucasian subject's blood samples for the detection of SNPs. The obtained SNPs were compared by using HapMap database from NCBI and by the web-based tagger application from Broad Institute at Harvard University. SNPs, alone or in combination with mapping can show the certain damaged chromosome regions. These chromosomal regions may indicate metabolic syndrome or cancer [26].

The expression intensity of genes is evaluated by using signal to noise (S/N) scores. Insulin resistance biomarkers and insulin sensitivity are evaluated by measuring FASN, USP2A and FASN/USP2A combinations as biomarkers [26].

1.10. Novel Compositions from *Nigella Sativa* - US20150004266

This patent is about the production of four super critical fluid extracts containing high-level Thymoquinone (TQ) through supercritical CO_2 extraction from *Nigella sativa* seeds. It is believed that the biological effects of the *Nigella sativa* that are beneficial for health, stem from the TQ, which is the main fat component in fixed oil. However, in experiments conducted so far, it was determined that there were effects that stemmed from other components aside from the TQ. In addition, the fractions obtained have more antioxidant, thermogenic, anti-inflammatory effects than *Nigella sativa*; and for this reason, it has been reported that it may be used in the treatment of inflammation-related diseases as a supplement in diets.

The *N. sativa* seeds extract or its oil, which is used as nutritional supplement, is non-toxic even in high amounts, and therefore it is used safely. The novel product may be used orally in capsule, plastic bag, tablet, soft gel, lozenge, dust or granule form with a certain amount of active content. Aside from these, it may be applied safely through implantation or intramuscular injection.

In order to obtain the product, nearly 100 kg *N. sativa* seeds were crushed in the dust form, and extracted with supercritical CO_2. As a result TQ with 39% was obtained which is the highest intensity for the first time. Studies were conducted on the extracts that were produced, for example;

It was determined that the free radical eliminating capacity of *N. sativa* extract that contained 39% TQ (NS9) was higher than the TQ alone at a rate of nearly 3-fold.

With another study, the issue of whether the *N. sativa* extract affected the Prostate Specific Antigen (PSA) release in benign prostate cells was investigated. In the end, TQ decreased the PSA in only low dosage; and it was determined that the *N. sativa* extract which contained 39% TQ decreased the PSA more than the other extracts and more than the TQ alone.

The issue of whether the *N. sativa* dust seeds obtained with supercritical CO_2 extracts decreased directly the mitochondrial membrane potential in the adipocytes when compared with pure TQ or DNP was investigated, and it was determined that it decreased more in a relative manner.

In another trial, the issue of whether the supercritical fluid CO_2 extracts of

N. sativa formed lipolysis in adipocytes or myocytes was investigated. The forskolin was used as the positive control in this study, and it was determined that all the NS supercritical extracts led to the release of free fatty acids more than the TQ.

In a trial in which the effects of *N. sativa* extracts on the AMPK activation in C2C12 myocytes were compared with the AICAR, it was determined that while the fractions obtained in 140-bar, 50°C and after 30 minutes, and the fractions obtained under the same pressure and temperature but after 120 minutes activated the AMPK in myocytes, the fraction obtained under 300-bar, 60°C in 3 hours did not have any effects. When compared with the AICAR, which was used as the positive control, it was observed that the fraction that was obtained under 140-bar, 50°C and in 120 minutes, was more effective in activating the AMPK than the AICAR.

In a trial in which the effect of the extract that contained nearly 40% TQ (NS9) on adaptive thermogenesis was investigated, a male who was at the age of 61 and who did aerobic exercises at a medium level was given 2 capsules of NS9 3 times a day for 1 year, and the changes in the weight were observed. In the end, it was determined that there was a 3% decrease in the weight with only 40mg, *N. Sativa* supplement per kilogram. This shows that the product has an effect that facilitates weight-losing by increasing the adaptive thermogenesis.

As the last item, in a study in which the effects of the extracts on adiponectin release and IL6 release in adipocytes induced by t10CLA were investigated, it was demonstrated that all the supercritical CO_2 extracts of the *N. sativa* and the TQ inhibited the IL6 secretion in the adipocytes stimulated with t10CLA, and decreased the release of adiponectin. In addition to this, it was emphasized that the extracts might be positively influential on insulin resistance associated with t10CLA.

All the supercritical CO_2 extracts of *N. sativa* and the TQ inhibit the Trans-Epithelial Electrical Resistance (TEER) loss in $CaCO_2$ epithelium cells stimulated with trans10CLA isomer (t10CLA), and have an anti-inflammatory effect. In this way, the damage decreased in the single layer epithelium in the intestines and ensures the membrane integrity of the intestines.

In addition to these studies, it was also reported that the use of these extracts in combination with CLA mixed isomers that contain t10CLA might be beneficial in losing weight, metabolic syndrome or Type 2 diabetes in order to increase efficacy [27].

1.11. Method of Dietary Treatment for Genetic and Epigenetic Diseases and Disorders - US20170056357

This patent is related with nutrition supplements and the therapeutic use of nutraceutical foods that might have epigenetic effects. This invention is presented as a functional food or as a nutritional supplement in capsule form.

Although many epigenetic markers are inherent, this may change with the diet. The majority of genetic diseases appear as a result of the interaction and combination between genetic factors and alleles or their variants, which are normally not the cause for diseases alone, with the environmental factors. Quitting smoking and alcohol, living an active life, having healthy nutrition habits and similar changes in lifestyles are the recommendations for a healthy life; however, they are not easy to apply. It is not clear how a personalized diet should be due to lack of knowledge on nutrients.

Today, trinucleotide-repeat diseases like the Rett Syndrome (RTT) and Fragile X Syndrome, which are among genetic and epigenetic diseases, memory disorders, chronic inflammation, cancerous cells that exist despite the cancer treatment, may be treated with the nutrition supplements or nutraceutical foods in this invention, which is approved by FDA. The invention is focused to fix the disorder in the histone acetylation in these diseases. Acetate is a very good acetyl group resource for histone acetylation. Other resources of acetate may be used to treat various genetic and epigenetic diseases or disorders. The low toxicity of dietary acetate like calcium acetate, sodium acetate and potassium acetate, which are food additives approved by the FDA, provide wide therapeutic field for treatments. Similarly, the magnesium acetate, which is produced as 700 mg capsule containing 600 mg acetate used as the dietary supplement in this invention, is also a good acetate resource.

This invention uses dietary contents to modify the epigenetic patterns in some cells in the body; and therefore, they will be converted into genetic patterns that will reduce the diseases and disorders. Especially dietary contents that provide acetate with high bioavailability increase the acetylation of other biomolecules that have effects on gene expressions of the cells and proteins, and disrupt the dysfunctional epigenetic patterns. In this way, they ensure that more suitable patterns are selected for the treatment of diseases and disorders.

In order to increase the histone acetylation, various pharmacological treatment methods have been investigated; however, these treatments also have several side effects. Treatments must have very little or no toxicity. Epigenetic treatments are generally not toxic due to the epigenetic feedback mechanisms of the body. This invention includes the studies conducted on acetate whose toxic effects are very little in increasing the histone acetylation. The desired dosages for treatment were achieved by using the invention as a capsule or a drink.

Acetate intake may increase the protein acetylation to develop memory, learning, motor function; and synaptic formation, and Brain-Derived Neurotrophic Factor Protein (BDNF) expression. Based on this, it is recommended that acetate from 100 mg a day to 15.000 mg a day used as one single dose or magnesium acetate, calcium acetate, sodium acetate, potassium acetate or ethyl acetate are used for the treatment of Rett Syndrome. In addition, acetate intake inhibits the growth of tumors and the proliferation of cancer cells, reduces the size of the tumors, decreases the methylation of cancerous cells in CpG islets, and increases the expression of one or more tumor-suppressing genes. Because of these effects, the treatment for Non-Hodgkin's Lymphoma and trinucleotide repetition disorder includes the use of substances that will provide acetate to the patients, which is also the case in Rett Syndrome as 100mg and 15.000mg acetate a day.

In all these diseases or disorders, it is expected that 900 mg acetate provides positive responses for treatment; however, the use of 1500 mg acetate is recommended until the Phase I clinical trials are done [28].

1.12. Bioenergetics Profiling of Circulating Blood Cells and Systems, Devices, and Methods Relating Thereto - US2015024795

The patent US2015024795 is based on the invention for measuring the respiratory capacity: in other words, bioenergetic capacity of the cells isolated from a blood sample obtained from a subject. Bioenergetic capacity provides important information about metabolic diseases such as diabetes, obesity, heart diseases, and several disorders including inflammation and neurodegeneration. It has been stated that the loss of bioenergetic capacity is associated with these diseases. Therefore, it is a powerful parameter to determine the wellness of the elderly suffering from these diseases, whether they pursue a healthy ageing.

The metabolic profile of blood cells migrating through the circulatory system and tissues has been proposed as an important biomarker to examine the metabolism of tumor cells that they interact. It has been reported that the glycolysis rate in tumor cells is very high, which is followed by lactic acid fermentation in the cytosol. Especially glycolytic rates of rapidly growing tumor cells (malignant cells) are reported as 200 times higher than those of their normal tissues of origin. Additionally, inflammation and immune responses are involved in the development of numerous diseases. The change in circulating factors, such as inflammatory cytokines, affects bioenergetic capacity of tumors and mitochondrial function. For that reason, circulating blood cells are crucial biomarkers as they may reflect the metabolic conditions of tumor cells such as lung, pancreatic, breast, kidney, prostate, hepatic tumor cells. It is possible to apply the best treatment strategy for the individuals depending on their bioenergetics profile through the invention stated in patent US2015024795. If a subject has found to have the high respiratory capacity, an aggressive treatment (an aerobic exercise program, weight loss diet, dietary supplements or monitoring respiratory capacity of blood cells) is applied. On the other hand, an improvement therapy is applied as a non-aggressive treatment, if a subject has the low respiratory capacity. This invention is expressed as the first well-accepted blood biomarker that accurately predicts the overall wellness of the individual and recovery rate after various treatments for diseases [29].

CONCLUSION

Nutrigenomics allows screening genetic makeup and diet response of an individual for cancer prevention and progression. Genetic modifications and nutritional status of an individual can be integrated for personalized diet therapy. To understand the mechanism, omics technologies and bioinformatics offer valuable data however, nutrient-nutrient interactions complicate the molecular mechanism. Therefore, establishing databases may provide information to understand multifactorial effectors and facilitate elucidation of different mechanisms. Further, new technologies-patents may help highlighting molecular mechanisms.

CURRENT & FUTURE DEVELOPMENTS

Nutrigenomics is the interaction between nutrients in the foods and individual's genetic structure. Soon it will be possible to know what kind of diet a person needs to lower the risk of diseases including cancer. Omics technologies (proteomics, lipidomics, microbiomics and metabolomics) are powerful tools to identify new biomarkers which can be applied in metabolic interventions leading to better understanding of the metabolism of nutrients and thus customized diets can be determined. Leading research groups, food manufacturers, and medical companies are searching to discover innovative approaches through omics technologies both in nutrition and metabolism and develop personalized food products for well-being and disease free life, and finally combine drug discovery studies with nutrigenomic studies to elucidate new therapeutic outcomes. Food products including bioactive nutrients will be determined against specific DNAs to combat against diseases. Discovering new genes with new technologies, gene interactions, and their roles in specific biochemical pathways that play a role in nutritional metabolism will open a new route for personalized nutrition. Furthermore, nutrition-related epigenetics studies are required to identify new epigenetic markers for the risk, diagnosis, and prognosis of the diseases.

CONSENT FOR PUBLICATION

Declared none.

CONFLICT OF INTEREST

The authors confirm that this chapter content has no conflict of interest.

ACKNOWLEDGEMENTS

Declared none.

REFERENCES

[1]   Saito K, Arai S, Kato H. A nutrigenomics database-integrated repository for publications and associated microarray data in nutrigenomics research. Br J Nutr 2005; 94(4): 493-5.
[http://dx.doi.org/10.1079/BJN20051536] [PMID: 16197571]

[2]   Davis CD, Milner J. Frontiers in nutrigenomics, proteomics, metabolomics and cancer prevention. Mutat Res 2004; 551(1-2): 51-64.
[http://dx.doi.org/10.1016/j.mrfmmm.2004.01.012] [PMID: 15225581]

[3]   Carsten C, Stine MU, Ferdinand M. Adaption of the human genome to dietary changes. Nutrigenomics. Springer 2016; pp. 71-86.

[4]   Nicastro HL, Trujillo EB, Milner JA. Nutrigenomics and cancer prevention. Curr Nutr Rep 2012; 1(1): 37-43.
[http://dx.doi.org/10.1007/s13668-011-0007-6] [PMID: 24910810]

[5]   Thunders M, Mangai S, Cooper R. Nutrigenetics, nutrigenomics, and the future of dietary advice. Food Nutr Sci 2013; 4: 999-1003.
[http://dx.doi.org/10.4236/fns.2013.410129]

[6]   Milner JA, Romagnolo DF, *et al.* Bioactive Compounds and Cancer 2010; 469-96.

[7]   Martin KR. Using nutrigenomics to evaluate apoptosis as a preemptive target in cancer prevention. Curr Cancer Drug Targets 2007; 7(5): 438-46.
[http://dx.doi.org/10.2174/156800907781386650] [PMID: 17691903]

[8]   Davis CD, Emenaker NJ, Milner JA. Cellular proliferation, apoptosis and angiogenesis: Molecular targets for nutritional preemption of cancer. Semin Oncol 2010; 37(3): 243-57.
[http://dx.doi.org/10.1053/j.seminoncol.2010.05.001] [PMID: 20709208]

[9]   Nepomuceno JC. Nutrigenomics and cancer prevention. Cancer treatment-conventional and innovative approaches. InTech Open Science 2013; pp. 391-416.

[10]   Choi SW, Friso S. Epigenetics: A new bridge between nutritionand health. Adv Nutr 2010; 1(1): 8-16.
[http://dx.doi.org/10.3945/an.110.1004] [PMID: 22043447]

[11]   Dutta D, Shatalin K, Epshtein V, Gottesman ME, Nudler E. Linking RNA polymerase backtracking to genome instability in *E. coli*. Cell 2011; 146(4): 533-43.
[http://dx.doi.org/10.1016/j.cell.2011.07.034] [PMID: 21854980]

[12]   Ames BN, Wakimoto P. Are vitamin and mineral deficiencies a major cancer risk? Nat Rev Cancer 2002; 2(9): 694-704.
[http://dx.doi.org/10.1038/nrc886] [PMID: 12209158]

[13]   Sales NMR, Pelegrini PB, Goersch MC. Nutrigenomics: Definitions and advances of this new science. J Nutr Metab 2014; 2014: 202759.

[http://dx.doi.org/10.1155/2014/202759] [PMID: 24795820]

[14]   Cozzolino SMF, Cominetti C. Biochemical and Physiological Bases of Nutrition in Different Stages of Life in Health and Disease. 1ˢᵗ ed., Sao Paulo, Brazil: Monole 2013.

[15]   Cozzolino SMF. The Bioavailability of Nutrients. 4ᵗʰ ed., Sao Paulo, Brazil: Monole 2012.

[16]   Norheim F, Gjelstad IMF, Hjorth M, *et al.* Molecular nutrition research: The modern way of performing nutritional science. Nutrients 2012; 4(12): 1898-944.
        [http://dx.doi.org/10.3390/nu4121898] [PMID: 23208524]

[17]   Milner JA, Romagnolo DF. Cancer Biology and Nutrigenomics. Nutrition and health: Bioactive compounds and cancer. Totowa, NJ: Humana Press 2010; pp. 25-43.
        [http://dx.doi.org/10.1007/978-1-60761-627-6_2]

[18]   Berrino F, Krogh V, Riboli E. Epidemiology studies on diet and cancer. Tumori 2003; 89(6): 581-5.
        [http://dx.doi.org/10.1177/030089160308900601] [PMID: 14870822]

[19]   Riscuta G, Dumitrescu RG. Nutrigenomics: Implications for breast and colon cancer prevention. Cancer Epigenetics, Methods and Protocols. Totowa, NJ: Humana Press 2012; pp. 343-58.
        [http://dx.doi.org/10.1007/978-1-61779-612-8_22]

[20]   Blum K, Meshkin B, Downs B. Composition and method to optimize and customize nutritional supplement formulations by measuring genetic and metabolomic contributing factors to disease diagnosis, stratification, prognosis, metabolism, and therapeutic outcomes. US20060062859, 2006.

[21]   Azimi N, Kharazmi MS. Nutraceutical compositions and methods with biologically active ingredients. US20080317734, 2008.

[22]   Stefanon B, Dodds WJ. Diagnostic system for selecting nutrition and pharmacological products for animals. US7873482, 2011.

[23]   Abramson FD. System and method for evaluating and providing nutrigenomic data, information and advice. US7877273, 2011.

[24]   Kaput J. Method for determining personalized nutrition and diet using nutrigenomics and physiological data. US20100113892, 2010.

[25]   Dodds WJ. Multi stage nutrigenomic diagnostic food sensitivity testing in animals. US8450072, 2010.

[26]   Muraca PJ. Predictive markers for cancer and metabolic syndrome. US2013045535, 2013.

[27]   Babish JG. Novel compositions from *Nigella Sativa*. US20150004266, 2015.

[28]   Ott DM. Method of dietary treatment for genetic and epigenetic diseases and disorders. US20170056357, 2017.

[29]   Molina AJA, Williamson J, Kritchevsky S. Bioenergetics profiling of circulating blood cells and systems, devices, and methods relating thereto. US2015024795, 2015.

Author Index

Akyuz, Elvan Y.
Ayik, Erdem
Aytekin, Ozlem
Bayram, Banu
Chatterji, Biswa P.
Dash, Aiswarya
Elpek, Gulsum O.
Feather, Claire E.
Haeri, Azadeh
Kaku, Tanvi S.
Khan, Maria
Kwok, John B.

López-Martínez, Alfonso F.
Mehryab, Fatemeh
Moalem-Taylor, Gila
Moghimi, Hamid R.
Murcia, Laura
Navarro-Mendoza, María I.
Nicolás, Francisco E.
Pérez-Arques, Carlos
Polly, Patsie
Sultana, Shaheen
Tutar, Yusuf
Yusuf, Mohammad

SUBJECT INDEX

www.ingramcontent.com/pod-product-compliance
Lightning Source LLC
Chambersburg PA
CBHW050828220326
41598CB00006B/335

* 9 7 8 1 6 8 1 0 8 6 2 8 6 *